W9-BZG-552

Rating Scales in Mental Health

2nd Edition

Martha Sajatovic, MD
Luis F. Ramirez, MD

LEXI-COMP

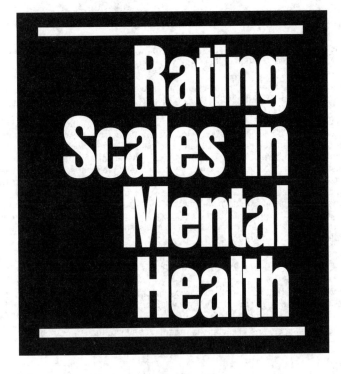

Rating Scales in Mental Health

2nd Edition

Martha Sajatovic, MD
Associate Professor of Psychiatry
Case Western Reserve University
Cleveland, Ohio

Luis F. Ramirez, MD
Adjunct Associate Professor of Psychiatry
Case Western Reserve University
Cleveland, Ohio

LEXI-COMP INC
Hudson (Cleveland)

NOTICE

This handbook is intended to serve the user as a handy quick reference and not as a complete rating scales information resource. It does not include information on every rating scale available.

While great care has been taken to ensure the accuracy of the information presented, the reader is advised that the authors, editors, reviewers, contributors, and publishers cannot be responsible for the continued currency of the information or for any errors, omissions, or the application of this information, or for any consequences arising therefrom. Therefore, the author(s) and/or the publisher shall have no liability to any person or entity with regard to claims, loss, or damage caused, or alleged to be caused, directly or indirectly, by the use of information contained herein. The editors are not responsible for any inaccuracy of quotation or for any false or misleading implication that may arise due to the text or formulas as used or due to the quotation of revisions no longer official. Actual dosing amounts for any specific drug should be based on an in-depth evaluation of the individual patient's therapy requirement and strong consideration given to such issues as contraindications, warnings, precautions, adverse reactions, along with the interaction of other drugs. The manufacturers most current product information or other standard recognized references should always be consulted for such detailed information prior to drug use.

The editors, authors, and contributors have written this book in their private capacities. No official support or endorsement by any federal agency or pharmaceutical company is intended or inferred.

The publishers have made every effort to trace the copyright holders for borrowed material. If they have inadvertently overlooked any, they will be pleased to make the necessary arrangements at the first opportunity.

If you have any suggestions or questions regarding any information presented in this handbook, please contact Lexi-Comp at 330-650-6506.

This manual was produced using the FormuLex™ Program — a complete publishing service of Lexi-Comp, Inc.

LEXI-COMP

1100 Terex Road
Hudson, Ohio 44236
(330) 650-6506

ISBN 1-59195-052-X

TABLE OF CONTENTS

TABLE OF CONTENTS *(Continued)*

3

TABLE OF CONTENTS *(Continued)*

ABOUT THE AUTHORS

Martha Sajatovic, MD

Dr. Sajatovic is Associate Professor of Psychiatry at Case Western Reserve University School of Medicine in Cleveland, Ohio. She has a strong interest in assessment instruments in psychiatry, and has served as a consultant to pharmaceutical companies for rating scales training, as well as publishing in this area.

Dr. Sajatovic received her BS in biology at Ohio State University and completed medical school at the Medical College of Ohio at Toledo. She completed her residency training in psychiatry at University Hospitals of Cleveland where she was Chief Resident in Research. Following completion of her residency, Dr. Sajatovic was Clinical Director of Inpatient Schizophrenia Research at University Hospitals of Cleveland, and later, was the Associate Chief of Psychiatry and Chief of the Mood Disorders Program at the Cleveland Veterans Affairs Medical Center in Cleveland, Ohio. Dr. Sajatovic has extensive experience with the management of serious mental illness through her work as a state hospital Chief Clinical Officer (Cleveland Campus Northcoast Behavioral Healthcare), in her own private practice, and in consulting with agencies providing community services to the seriously mentally ill.

Dr. Sajatovic has published a number of original papers on treatment of serious mental illness and treatment outcomes including work with special populations such as the elderly, women with psychosis, and individuals with developmental disorder. She has been a guest lecturer at numerous academic and community settings including speaking to consumer and family advocacy groups for individuals with psychiatric illness. Dr. Sajatovic has a long-standing commitment to education including supervision of medical students and residents in psychiatry, lecturing at Case Western Reserve University School of Medicine, psychiatric resident supervision, and seminar teaching for residents in psychiatry.

Luis F. Ramirez, MD

Dr. Ramirez is Adjunct Clinical Associate Professor of Psychiatry at Case Western Reserve University, President of Quality Outcomes Training, and a research psychiatrist with North Coast Clinical Trials in Cleveland, Ohio.

Dr. Ramirez completed his medical training in Cali, Colombia and his psychiatric training in Cleveland. During his professional career, he has worked with University Hospitals of Cleveland, the Cleveland Veterans Health Administration, West Side Community Mental Health Center, and pharmaceutical corporations.

Dr. Ramirez has conducted research in the areas of schizophrenia, depression, and pathological gambling and has been active in training professionals in the United States, Europe, Africa, Australia, and Latin America in the prevention and management of disturbed behavior, patient-doctor communication, professional presentations, and how to use and apply rating scales. Dr. Ramirez serves as a consultant for several pharmaceutical companies and other private institutions.

PREFACE

The measurement of health outcomes has undergone significant change in the last decade. Due to a number of factors, including technological advances and a greater emphasis on consumer satisfaction, it has become increasingly important to objectively define illness, and response to treatment. Unlike many other branches of medicine, the field of psychiatry has few biologic or laboratory measures to quantify illness severity in psychiatric disorders. This situation has given rise to a number of psychiatric rating scales that can be utilized to define, categorize, and evaluate a wide variety of psychiatric problems.

Our goal in writing this book is to provide mental health clinicians with information on assessment tools that may be used to evaluate clinical outcomes in a variety of domains. In addition to discussing conceptual issues around rating scales, we present many specific scales. There is a mix of self-rated and clinician-rated measures. We have attempted to primarily present scales that are brief and relatively simple to administer. Selection of specific rating scales for inclusion was one of the most difficult tasks in assembling this book, and we realize that many excellent scales have not been included in this volume. Additionally, many scales exist in multiple formats/versions. We have made an attempt to provide a copy of what we believe to be the most commonly used version in our rating scale monographs.

This second edition of *Rating Scales in Mental Health* contains a number of new scales. In response to suggestions and requests from readers of our first edition, we have added more scales for children/adolescents, scales for other domains of interpersonal functioning, scales for premenstrual dysphoric disorder, eating disorders, and additional self-rated scales. Readers of the first edition of this book have noted that our monographs, intended to provide a brief overview and review of "key points" for each scale, due to space limitations, frequently do not provide detailed scoring instructions. Readers who desire further details on scale administration/scoring are advised to utilize the references provided in each monograph to provide more information in each scale. In cases where scale manuals are available, contact information for these are provided in the monographs as well.

We hope that this volume will be practical and easy to use. Your comments are encouraged and appreciated, as we consider these suggestions for future editions. Comments and/or suggestions can be sent via the Lexi-Comp website - www.lexi.com - and will be forwarded to the authors.

— Martha Sajatovic, MD

COPYRIGHT ISSUES

Scales that were developed by or for government agencies are generally in the public domain and, thus, may be reproduced without requesting permission. However, many scales have been copyrighted by individuals or groups. These scales should only be reproduced in full or in part only with specific permission from the copyright holders.

ACKNOWLEDGMENTS

The *Rating Scales in Mental Health* handbook exists in its present form as the result of the concerted efforts of the following individuals: Robert D. Kerscher, publisher and president of Lexi-Comp Inc; Lynn D. Coppinger, managing editor; Ginger Stein, project manager; David C. Marcus, director of information systems; Libby Young, product manager; and Tracey J. Reinecke, cover design.

Special acknowledgment is given to everyone on the Lexi-Comp staff who helped in the production of this handbook.

In addition, the authors wish to thank their families, friends, and colleagues who supported them in their efforts to complete this handbook.

HOW THIS BOOK IS ORGANIZED

The *Rating Scales in Mental Health* handbook discusses and presents various rating scales in psychiatry.

The first section of this book discusses general concepts in the use of rating scales, history of rating scales, statistical evaluation of rating scales, and rating scale domains. Finally, there are two clinical vignettes which describe typical scenarios of how rating scales may be used to assess multidimensional mental health outcomes.

The second section of this book contains 113 psychiatric rating scales that can be applied in a variety of clinical and/or research settings. Scales are grouped in categories such as psychiatric diagnoses (eg, scales to assess depression), functional domains (eg, quality of life), and special populations (eg, psychiatric ratings used in children). Each scale is presented as a monograph which describes the scale and various aspects of the scale. If copyright permission has been obtained, the scale will be reproduced in full or in part at the end of the monograph. Publishers produce additional copies of the scale, often with accompanying training manuals, to explain the use of the scale. It is highly recommended that scale raters thoroughly read and understand how to administer a scale before using the scale in research or clinical settings. Some scales and training/scoring materials are also available in electronic format.

The third section of this book contains an appendix with charts and tables in a quick reference format. Using the appendix, clinicians may rapidly identify categories and characteristics of rating scales.

The last section of this book contains three indexes: 1) an acronyms listing, 2) an alphabetical listing of all rating scales found in this handbook, and 3) an author listing based on the included scales.

All scales will be described utilizing the following fields of information:

Overview	Brief description of the scale, which may include strengths and weaknesses of the scale, comments regarding differing versions of the scale, frequency of use/citation, and particular issues related to scale administration.
General Applications	Concisely states what is being measured and the populations/settings in which the scale is generally used.
Selected Psychometric Properties	Provides selected brief information on statistical properties of the scale.
References	Journals and/or books which discuss and/or display the scale.
Copyright	Cites individual / group / publisher having copyright.
Scale Generally Done By	Describes person/discipline who typically administers this scale.
Time to Complete Scale	Gives time in minutes generally required to administer and complete the scale.
Representative Study Utilizing Scale	Cites a publication which utilizes the scale as an assessment tool. This may provide an example of a typical use of this scale.
RATING SCALE	The scale will appear here if it is in the public domain or if permission has been granted to reproduce the scale. Scales that are copyrighted should be reproduced only with permission from the copyright holders. Some scales will be presented only in part as agreed upon with the copyright holder. Many scales have additional instructions which should be obtained from the references cited in the monograph.

PURPOSE AND HISTORY OF RATING SCALES IN PSYCHIATRY

For many years, the nations of the world have collected data on birth and death rates, education, crime, employment, and many other measures of social, economic, and political situations. These data have helped governments to plan and make decisions about how to deal with the problems of society. Among these measurements, those involving health have always been of great importance and have been used to set policies and allocate resources. An accurate accounting of health indexes has become more critical (and more complicated) due to the exponential growth of the cost of health care. The concept of health is an abstract concept that has been very difficult to measure, and like many other things of similar nature, generally cannot be measured directly. Because of this difficulty, indirect measures of health, such as symptom severity, disability level, change over time, and change with treatment, have been utilized to evaluate health outcomes.

According to the World Health Organization (WHO), health is defined as complete "physical, mental, and social well-being, and not merely the absence of disease and infirmity." This definition, written more than 50 years ago, is important because it emphasizes the importance of biopsychosocial factors in achieving that elusive goal of being "healthy." A corollary of this definition may be the recommendation that we need to consider multiple factors in the evaluation of health outcomes. With this in mind, we must measure symptoms, quality of life, work, interpersonal relations, intrapsychic foundations, disabilities, and responses to treatment in order to judge our ability to treat patients.

The development of health measurements has been very impressive during the last 50 years with important methodological advances made around the time of World War II. During the war, large numbers of recruits were evaluated for physical and mental fitness with a variety of screening tests which later formed the basis for the development of psychological well-being measurements.

Another development during this era was the application of numerical scaling techniques to health indices. This provided the ability to translate subjective statements about pain or anxiety into a numerical figure which could be used for statistical analysis. Around this time, the first randomized trial was conducted in England. In 1946, the British health authorities wanted to know if the use of streptomycin in the treatment of tuberculosis justified its cost. British medical experts worried that the evidence for the drug's effectiveness came from the observation of single cases without good controls. To prove or disprove this point, the Medical Research Council commissioned Austin Bradford Hill, a professor at the University of London, to do the necessary analysis. Hill was influenced by experiments done in the agricultural field to eliminate bias using the laws of chance. He set up a statistical series of random sampling numbers to determine which patients in the tuberculosis clinical trial would receive which therapy. At the same time he set up inclusion and exclusion criteria and tried to eliminate extraneous factors that might influence the outcome. After six months of treatment, Hill was able to demonstrate that the treatment with streptomycin saved lives, with only 7% of the streptomycin treated patients dying in comparison with 27% of the patients in the control group. After the publication of the results in the *British Medical Journal* in 1948, the randomized clinical trial became the state-of-the-art in determining efficacy of medications in the management of disease.

It is more than coincidental that the greatest advances in pharmacological treatments of disease have been accomplished in the last 50 years, with psychiatric treatments being no exception. The discovery of the antipsychotic effects of phenothiazines, the antidepressant effects of the tricyclics, the antianxiety effects of the benzodiazepines, and the development of randomized clinical trials created the need for instruments that could assign numerical values based upon observations of patient behaviors, affects, and feelings. Psychiatric rating scales such as the Hamilton Scales for Anxiety and Depression, and the Brief Psychiatric Rating Scale were created to serve this purpose and demonstrate the undisputed value of these medications in the treatment of mental disorders when compared to placebo. Since then hundreds of scales have been developed for different purposes providing many alternatives to investigators. At the same time, scales were also developed to assist in making psychiatric diagnoses, to measure side effects of medications, and to evaluate other areas of functioning such as physical capabilities, disabilities, or quality of life.

PURPOSE AND HISTORY OF RATING SCALES IN PSYCHIATRY
(Continued)

The exponential developments in health assessments have created various areas of interest including: Quality Assurance, Quality Improvement, Outcome Management, and Pharmacoeconomics. Growth in our understanding of these topics has produced a substantial amount of information and literature with many different evaluation instruments, some of which are presented in this book.

Quality was defined by Donabedian as "a property of, and a judgment upon, some definable unit of (health)care" which emphasizes the relationship between quality, outcomes, and measurements. In the case of patient care, these have to do with personal and technical issues. In the personal area, we have to consider issues such as patient satisfaction, access to care, and in general, the quality of the relationships between providers (at different levels) and the patient. In the technical area, the health measurements are related to diagnostic issues, prognostic measurements, descriptive systems, and evaluative processes.

In summary, scales are important clinical and research tools that allow us to measure psychiatric conditions at different points in time. This provides us with enough information to evaluate health outcomes, which may assist in determining the usefulness of different treatments and their cost-effectiveness value. This data may ultimately allow us to improve patient care, correct mistakes, and optimize health outcomes for patients receiving psychiatric services.

WHAT RATING SCALES MEASURE

Health assessments measure a variety of components of health. Some are functional measures which focus on the diagnosis, prognosis, and evaluation methods of different illnesses. For example, the measurement of the blood pressure is a health measure that has diagnostic value. Prognostic measures such as Apgar scores or IQ can give us information about expectation of an individual's future health, while some evaluative indices can help to look at the changes that happened with time.

Other health measurements have to do with the topic domains. For example, they are concerned with a particular organ, organ system, or with a disorder. They can be specific, generic, broad spectrum, or classified according to the method used, such as questionnaires or rating scales. In a rating scale, an interviewer, usually a clinician trained in how to use the scale, assesses different aspects of health utilizing an open clinical interview or an interview with different degrees of structure, but finally making the determination depending on his/her clinical experience.

Most of the scales used in psychiatric research are *ordinal* scales in which numbers are used as labels for different categories reflecting an increased order for the item being measured. For instance: 0 = normal, 1 = slight, 2 = mild, 3 = moderate, 4 = severe. This system has the shortcoming of lacking the accuracy of *interval* scales where the unit changes are constant and always represent the same value. In order to achieve consistency with the ordinal scales, it is important to have definitions and/or guidelines for the items/anchoring points in order to assign the proper numerical values and to minimize the personal bias of the rater. Bias in assigning a number could be due to a series of factors. The role of experience in the clinical evaluations is very important. This experience is something that cannot be learned, but is lived, and may be influenced by the professional orientation of the person doing the rating. The next chapter will outline some recommendations on how to execute scales properly, but in general the idea is to provide a number to an observation, statement, affect, symptom, behavior, etc that will permit the statistical manipulation of clinical data in order to assess change.

Other important issues with regard to rating scales and the quality of the measurements are the concepts of *reliability* and *validity*. Reliability is the ability of the scale to convey consistent and reproducible information. Some experts prefer the use of consistency rather than reliability, emphasizing the concept of stability of the measurements across time, patients, and raters.

Validity is the degree to which the scale measures what it is supposed to measure. Most validation studies about a scale start with an assessment of the *content validity*, referring to the clinical appropriateness of the measure and how adequately the questions reflect the aims that were specified in the scope of the measure. These attributes are more subjective than statistical with the clinical credibility of a measure inferred from the comments of experts and/or patients. The statistical attributes are referred to as *criterion validity* which looks at the correlation of the instrument in comparison to a "gold standard." Other concepts associated with the validity of a scale are the *construct validity* and the *factorial validity*. Construct validation begins with a conceptual definition of the topic to be measured and the factorial analysis has to do with the underlying conceptual structure of the instrument and how the items may or may not fall into groupings. See "Selected Psychometric Terms Used to Describe Rating Scales" in the Appendix *on page 448.*

THE PSYCHIATRIC INTERVIEW AND APPLICATION OF RATING SCALES

THE RATING SCALE INTERVIEW

Each scale has its own manual or guideline that explains how to use the scale, the rating system, and other specific information, including definitions of the items and the scale anchoring points. In general, most scales evaluate the patient/patient behavior over a defined period of time, that is usually 7 days prior to the administration of the scale. Most of the information needed to complete rater-administered scales is obtained with a clinical interview which can be structured, semistructured, or nonstructured depending on the preference of the rater and/or the condition of the scale. During the rating process, it is important to rate what is observed or what is reported without taking into consideration psychological, psychodynamic, or any other kinds of explanations. In the case of having difficulties in selecting a severity/ grading number (2 vs 3 or 3 vs 4, etc), the rater is advised to select the higher number. It is also advisable that the rater be familiar or have all the information available and necessary to make the appropriate ratings. Inexperienced raters must do ratings under supervision until their "competence" in using a particular scale has been corroborated but, in general, a rater can do a good job if s/he is capable of doing a good interview, is familiar with the scale, and follows the manual.

STEPS TO DOING A GOOD RATING

The following are important points to keep in mind for doing a good scale rating:

1. Have all the information available
2. Be familiar with the scale
3. Perform a good interview
4. Ask all the items
5. Make sure you have established the severity of the symptoms

In several studies, it has been shown that the interview is the main source of error. The reasons are multiple, but in general they have to do with the interviewer not asking about all the items or failing to clarify inconsistencies or completely missing components for the accurate assessment of symptoms severity.

It is important for the interviewer to prepare himself/herself, to prepare the environment, and to prepare the patient in order to eliminate all barriers of communication. It is necessary that the interviewer establish an atmosphere of trust and professionalism, where the patient feels safe and secure to answer all the questions appropriately and accurately.

The interviewer should prepare himself/herself by reviewing all the information available about the patient, and by becoming familiar with the interview and the different items. It is important that s/he be focused and calm. The environment has to be clean, accessible, warm, and conducive to good communication. The patient must be greeted properly and instructed regarding the purpose of the interview with an appropriate introduction to the questions that are going to be asked.

The art of interviewing is knowing which questions to ask and how to ask them. In the case of rating scales, the type of questions are determined by the items composing the scale. It is important to cover all the items and to determine the severity of the symptoms. In many cases, and with the proposed idea of increasing accuracy, the questions are preprepared making the interview semi or structured. In this case, the interviewer has to be careful not to relinquish the control of the interview to the structure of the questioning or to the "leading" quality of preprepared questions. It must be kept in mind that the structured interview is still a clinical activity designed to collect information about the illness of the patient.

The interviewer must ask questions about all items, and once the presence of the symptoms is established, then s/he must ask questions to ascertain the severity of the symptoms. During this process, the interviewer needs to become aware of inconsistencies presented by the patient and must clarify them using appropriate techniques. The repetitive asking of questions to clarify items often gives a mechanical quality to the interviews, which the interviewer should resist, making sure s/he does not interfere with the free associations of the patient and his/her presentation of the different symptoms. It is also important that the interviewer be fully aware of the utilization of time, as the longer the interview, the more difficult it is to keep the attention of the patient.

The interviewer must finish the interview by asking the patient's input at the end, and by summarizing the data obtained in order to make sure that all the questions have been asked, and there are no items being left out. At this time, arrangements for next visits can be made and an outline of what is going to happen next should be presented to the patient and/or family.

It is important to practice interviewing patients with different scales. As we have mentioned, practitioners cannot learn experience from books and/or watching others. They need to interview patients, record these experiences, and be able to discuss their interviews and ratings with colleagues who can give their opinions and comments about the techniques utilized. In addition, scoring can be discussed to reach some sort of consensus, which will help with interrater reliability and homogeneity of the scorings. In summary, if the interviewer is familiar with the scale, uses the manual, and does a good interview, the rating scale scoring will usually accurately reflect the condition of the patient.

SPECIFIC RATING SCALE TYPES

Rating scales may be used for a variety of purposes in differing clinical settings. Some scales are designed to be used as a one-time assessment, while others are meant to be repeated sequentially, so that change over time can be evaluated. Major categories include:

A. DIAGNOSTIC SCALES

Psychiatric diagnostic scales are assessment tools that identify specific mental disorders. Most of these are lengthy instruments, designed generally as a one-time assessment, often taking 45-90 minutes to administer. Diagnostic scales may be paired with other clinical assessments, or may be done independently. Research studies frequently utilize diagnostic scales to select a homogenous group of research subjects at study initiation. Diagnostic scales are more rarely used in clinical settings, primarily because of the time required for their administration. Diagnostic scales for adults include the Present State Examination (PSE) *on page 28*, a diagnostic assessment tool which was developed to standardize diagnostic procedures in international studies of mental illness. The PSE was used in the World Health Organization's (WHO) International Pilot Study of Schizophrenia. The PSE is not used a great deal currently, but has been replaced by other instruments, including the Composite International Diagnostic Interview (CIDI) *on page 24* and the Schedules for Clinical Assessment in Neuropsychiatry (SCAN) *on page 32*. Both of these scales were developed using items from the PSE. Both the CIDI and the SCAN were developed by the WHO. Additional information on these scales, including opportunities for training in these instruments, may be obtained on the WHO internet site at www.who.int.

Other commonly used diagnostic scales include the Structured Clinical Interview for Axis I DSM-IV Disorders (SCID) *on page 33*, the Schedule for Affective Disorders and Schizophrenia (SADS) *on page 31*, and the Diagnostic Interview Schedule (DIS) *on page 25*, developed by the National Institute of Mental Health (NIMH).

There are a number of popular instruments to identify and evaluate severity of psychiatric illness in children and adolescents. These include the Schedule for Affective Disorder and Schizophrenia for School-Age children (K-SADS), The National Institute of Mental Health Diagnostic Interview Schedule for Children (NIMH-DISC), and the Child Behavior Checklists (CBCL). Both the K-SADS and the DISC are structured or semistructured interviews which ultimately categorize subjects along DSM diagnostic lines. The CBCL does not furnish a diagnosis, but rather identifies broad groups of symptoms in evaluated subjects.

Because of the length and detail of most diagnostic measures, intensive training is usually required to properly administer these instruments. Clinicians and administrators contemplating the use of diagnostic scales in outcomes studies, must carefully consider the costs and time involved in adequate training versus the potential benefits of using these measures.

B. SYMPTOM-BASED SCALES

Many rating scales in psychiatry are based on the assessment of a particular symptom or set of symptoms, and are not targeted to a specific psychiatric diagnosis. An example of this is the Brief Psychiatric Rating Scale (see BPRS *on page 130*), which evaluates a variety of symptoms including depression, hostility, and uncooperativeness. The BPRS has been used to evaluate individuals with many different psychiatric disorders, including schizophrenia and bipolar disorder.

C. DIAGNOSIS-SPECIFIC SCALES

There are a smaller number of rating scales in psychiatry designed to be used for specific psychiatric diagnoses. These include the Positive and Negative Symptom Scale for Schizophrenia (PANSS *on page 158*) and the Calgary Scale for Depression in individuals with schizophrenia who have depressive symptoms. Diagnosis-specific scales exist for many diagnostic categories including depression, anxiety disorders, and cognitive disorders. Some scales, such as the Hamilton Rating Scale for Depression (HAM-D *on page 100*), were originally intended as diagnosis-specific scales, but over the years have been used in clinical/research settings as symptom-based scales.

D. SELF-RATED VS RATER-ADMINISTERED SCALES

Some rating scales in psychiatry are designed to be self-rated. Advantages to self-rated scales are primarily the ease of administration, with no clinician or professional staff time required for scale administration. Self-rated scales may be useful in evaluating subtle, subjective states. Additionally, self-rated scales can be used in psycho-educational interventions to raise awareness in patient self-identification of illness target symptoms and monitoring of clinical progress. An example is use of the Beck Depression Inventory (see BDI *on page 80*), a self-rated depression scale used to identify and monitor mood symptoms in a patient being treated for a major depressive episode.

Disadvantages of self-rated scales primarily center around reliability. This may be more of a problem in disorders where lack of insight is often a key feature of illness, such as may be the case with schizophrenia. Often, to optimize reliability of outcome determinations, a self-rated scale will be paired with a clinician-rated measure (eg, the Beck Depression Inventory and the Hamilton Rating Scale for Depression being used together).

E. OTHER DIMENSIONS OF OUTCOME

Other scales in psychiatry are neither symptom- nor disorder-based. This includes the important domain of quality of life. As healthcare has become more consumer-oriented, and as medical technology has advanced, there has been increasing emphasis on the expectation that treatment should lead to not only a reduction in psychopathology, but should also lead to an improved quality of life. There are many instruments that have been developed to evaluate quality of life (QOL). These include the Quality of Life Interview (QOLI *on page 256*) by Lehman, the Quality of Well Being Scale (QWB *on page 281*), and the Sickness Impact Profile (SIP *on page 284*), among others. A disadvantage of many of the currently utilized instruments to evaluate quality of life is their length and complexity. It must be remembered that QOL scales are usually accompanied by at least one measure of illness severity. When designing outcome study plans, the study organizer must take into account the total amount of time which will be required at each assessment interval. The "time to complete scale" portion of the monographs in this book may be helpful in providing this information. However, when clinical data is obtained via a standard clinical interview, it is often possible to rate multiple scales from a single interview.

Another domain of outcome that may be evaluated by rating scales is functional level. Frequently, a functional level scale paired with a symptom severity scale will provide important outcome information. For example, it is not enough to know that the atypical antipsychotic clozapine reduces Brief Psychiatric Rating Scale (BPRS) scores in treatment-refractory schizophrenia. It is also important to identify that the clozapine-related BPRS score reduction is associated with an improvement in patient functional level.

Another increasingly recognized critical factor in clinical outcomes is patient satisfaction and patient perception of care. Many new scales are being developed in this area. Patient perception of care measures include the Client Satisfaction Questionnaire (CSQ *on page 249*) and the Patient Satisfaction Questionnaire, (PSQ *on page 247*), among others. Patient satisfaction may be helpful in determining how desirable or acceptable treatment or care systems are from the point of view of the patient/consumer. As with all scales, care must be taken in selecting an appropriate sample of individuals to assess using patient satisfaction scales. The sample surveyed should be representative of all patients who use the care system unless it is determine *a priori* that a more select sample is being evaluated. Finally, it must be remembered that patient satisfaction does not necessarily correlate with reduction in symptoms severity.

SPECIFIC RATING SCALE TYPES *(Continued)*

There are many other domains of clinical outcome including general health status, adverse events, and resource utilization. The best outcome analysis will often evaluate multiple domains of outcome, rather than relying on single dimension, such as symptoms severity. Other important factors of outcome evaluation include sample selection, sample size, and timing of assessment. These will be further discussed in the section entitled "Statistical Evaluation of Outcome Data" *on page 17.*

STATISTICAL EVALUATION OF OUTCOME DATA

It must be remembered that in order for clinical outcomes to be most accurately assessed, the investigator/clinician must develop a plan which addresses the following points: What outcomes will be measured? Which patients will be included? When will the outcomes be measured? Who is going to use the information provided by the outcomes data? Answering these basic questions will allow for optimal scale selection, subject assignment, study design, and methodology. Collecting extensive amounts of data on all patients is expensive and time-intensive, as well as impractical for the most part. When the investigator clearly defines the study question and determines the study population, it is likely that data collection and interpretation will be more successful. Additional factors which must be considered in study set-up include data on the use of a scale in a given population, validity and reliability of the scale, availability of staff resources for scale administration (including both training and scale administration time), scale standardization, and ease of subject participation.

Scales should be selected which have demonstrated validity and reliability with the clinical population in question. Staffing resources are also important in determining feasibility of using any particular scale. In today's healthcare environments, staff time for outcomes data collection is often minimal or nonexistent. For this reason, self-rated scales may be an attractive option, although their reliability is generally less good than rater-administered scales. Finally, the desire to collect data must be balanced with what is comfortable and acceptable for patients. Many patients, particularly those with more severe mental illness, are unable to tolerate prolonged interview sessions. A maximum "one-sitting" session might be 45-60 minutes for such individuals.

The data or information produced by rating scales can be used to evaluate change in single, individual patients over time or to compare groups of patients. The data can be assessed using statistical or nonstatistical methods. To better illustrate the various ways of assessing outcomes with the use of rating scales, the following four situations are discussed:

- A. A single patient
- B. Two or more patients
- C. Two or more groups of patients
- D. The prediction of outcomes

A. A SINGLE PATIENT

Rating scales are often utilized to assess treatment response in an individual patient. In one approach, the patient is rated before and after treatment. This provides a time-limited, quantified assessment of the amount of change in the patient's clinical status during the time that treatment was administered. A second approach involves evaluating a patient repeatedly at some established intervals during the time that treatment is administered. Ideally, this should begin before treatment is initiated, and end with a final rating sometime after the treatment is completed. Such an extended course of repeated measure provides quantified treatment outcomes or a psychiatric functional history. In either the first or the second approach, the patient's progress in response to treatment could be evaluated by comparing the scores on the repeated rating scales. In this manner, the scores derived from rating scales administered to the patient could be used to monitor the individual's clinical status during the time that treatment was provided.

While both of these approaches provide useful and quantifiable information, the comparison upon which final status is based is the patient's own baseline score. An assumption is made that the change from baseline to final score results from the effects of treatment, and not from other characteristics of either the patients' or of their surroundings. The investigator/clinician must be cautious in interpreting data from comparisons based upon a single patient. Although comparing a patient's response to their own baseline is a useful clinical exercise, the information provided can only be generalized to the patient being rated.

Rating scales may also be used for other comparisons. This includes comparisons that assess treatment response between different types of patients, or those that evaluate the effects of

STATISTICAL EVALUATION OF OUTCOME DATA *(Continued)*

specific differences between patients such as gender or pre-treatment history. These are comparisons that involve two or more patients.

B. TWO OR MORE PATIENTS

Rating scales are easily used with data from two or more patients. Between-patient comparisons are used to assess the effectiveness of different treatments provided to similar patients (eg, a comparison of psychotherapy vs medication treatment in individuals with major depression). Between-patient comparisons are also used to assess the effectiveness of the same treatment when it is provided to two different kinds of patients (eg, a comparison of treatment response in individuals with depression with psychotic features, and those with depression without psychotic features). A representative scenario of a between-patient comparison is as follows: A new type of group psychotherapy has been developed for individuals with schizophrenia that supposedly provides greater improvement compared to the current psychotherapy generally provided to individuals with schizophrenia. The investigator/clinician wishes to see if this improvement is true for his/her clinic. To answer this question, the clinician identifies two individuals with schizophrenia who have generally the same type of illness in terms of severity, duration of illness, etc, and who also have similar demographic characteristics such as age, gender, educational level, etc. Both patients are rated on well-accepted, well-validated rating scales such as the Brief Psychiatric Rating Scale (BPRS *on page 130*) or the Positive and Negative Symptom Scale for Schizophrenia (PANSS *on page 158*) before and after treatment. One individual is given the new treatment, while the other individual is given the established, older treatment (standard of care). When treatment is completed, a comparison of the two patient's scores gives some idea as to whether the new treatment may be associated with more positive outcomes. Although the result of this comparison is useful in assisting with clinic-based treatment planning, it must be cautioned that this is still a relatively uncontrolled comparison. As with the individual patient data, results cannot fairly be generalized beyond the patients originally assessed. For this reason, larger numbers of patients are generally included in most clinical trials in order to more accurately make decisions regarding optimum clinical outcomes.

C. TWO OR MORE GROUPS OF PATIENTS

Comparisons involving two or more groups of patients are generally utilized when specific questions regarding clinical outcomes are researched. Usually, the groups of patients differ from each other in specific ways. An example is individuals with major depression, with and without comorbid substance abuse. As with the comparison involving two individual patients, it is preferable that all or most other characteristics of the patients are similar. Another way of evaluating group comparisons is comparing outcomes between two different types of treatment in two similar groups of patients. An example is administration of a new antidepressant medication compared to an older antidepressant medication. Ideally, the groups of patients are selected at random, and asked to participate in the study. The patients are then assigned, in random fashion, to receive either one of the new treatments. Patients might be rated on such rating scales as the Hamilton Rating Scale for Depression *on page 100* or the Montgomery-Asberg Depression Rating Scale *on page 106*.

Rating scales are administered in both groups prior to treatment and again at the end of treatment or at some predetermined time after treatment is initiated. The use of random sampling and the random assignment of patients to treatment groups is critical, as it reduces the chance that the groups will differ prior to treatment. An example of how this could give biased results is if patients are allowed to select which of two treatments they receive. It is possible that individuals who select the new treatments may be more treatment-refractory to older treatments (and thus more ill), or conversely, these individuals may be more motivated to improve.

When groups of patients are compared, it is often necessary to use statistical tools and rules. These provide a standard means of determining whether or not the two groups truly differ from each other. They also give some indication regarding how likely it is that other groups from the same general population of patients would show similar differences if it were possible to include them in the analysis. Overall, the use of statistical tools allows the investigator to have more confidence in his/her conclusions. The statistical tools also provide information that enable an assessment regarding the degree of certainty with which conclusions are drawn. Finally, statistical tools provide a statistical means of controlling for pre-existing group differences that could not be taken into account by random selections and/or random assignment.

Two common statistical tools for comparing groups of patients are t-tests and analysis of variance (also abbreviated as ANOVA). Both of the tools provide a standardized, mathematical-, and probability-based means of ascertaining if observed differences between groups of patients are large and consistent enough to conclude that they truly differ from one another. In other words, that the observed difference is not due merely to chance variation between the groups. When only two groups of patients are compared, t-tests and analysis of variance are identical. When more than two groups of patients are being compared, analysis of variance is a better choice. For example, comparing depression outcomes in three groups of patients, with each group having received treatment with a different antidepressant medication, can be done using analysis of variance. Analysis of variance also can be used to compare groups across time, or when the participants are being compared on more than one characteristic (eg, depressed patients with or without comorbid substance abuse and treatment with two different antidepressant medications). Analysis of variance can also be used to control baseline group differences. There are a number of good statistical computer-based packages available. While many of these packages are relatively easy to use and provide high quality statistical tests, it is important that the investigator understand the statistical techniques to ensure their correct application. Consultation with a statistician or researcher well-versed in statistical techniques is recommended in order to provide the most accurate results and use of statistical software.

D. PREDICTION OF OUTCOMES

Data obtained from the use of rating scales can be used in prediction models to identify those factors that contribute to treatment outcomes. For example, outcome data may be used to identify which clinical characteristics of patients with schizophrenia are associated with the best response to a novel antipsychotic therapy. Outcome information can be used to identify groups of patients using logistic regression (eg, recovery vs continued illness), to target an event using survival analysis (the eventual occurrence of an event, or to predict the time to an event, such as illness relapse), or to predict a continuous indicator of outcome using ordinary least squares regression analysis (to predict the level of an outcome variable that ranges continuously from most severe to least severe). Using these three types of outcome data, statistical models can be developed to predict outcome level, outcome groups, or outcome events. "Common Statistical Techniques Used in Rating Scale Analysis" found in the Appendix *on page 449*, summarizes some common statistical tools. As with the use of t-tests and analysis of variance, consultation with an individual well-versed in statistical techniques is recommended prior to study design/implementation.

VIGNETTES DEMONSTRATING THE USE OF RATING SCALES

VIGNETTE I

CLINICAL VIGNETTE WITH DEPRESSED PATIENT

Mr A is a 42-year-old married man with a history of recurrent depression. He has a history of alcohol abuse but has maintained sobriety for the last 16 years. He has experienced moderate depressive symptoms for the last month, and at the urging of his wife, makes an appointment to see a psychiatrist.

When dealing with a depressed patient, it is important to keep in mind several things besides the evaluation of his/her depressive symptoms. These include:

1. Comorbid conditions

2. Quality of life or functional impairments associated with the illness

3. Risk of suicide

4. Patient satisfaction with health care or treatment

A diagnostic scale may be utilized to assist in verifying a psychiatric diagnosis, according to DSM-IV or some other standardized criteria. Comorbid conditions, such as substance abuse, might be evaluated with a specialized screen rating scale (eg, the CAGE questionnaire or the MAST). Once the diagnosis is established and it is clear that the patient is suffering a major depressive disorder without any comorbid conditions, at least two scales are recommended for the assessment and follow-up of depressive symptoms: A self-reported scale such as the Beck Depression Inventory (BDI *on page 80*) and a clinician-administered scale. The two most frequently utilized clinician-administered scales are the Hamilton Rating Scale for Depression (HAM-D *on page 100*) and the Montgomery-Asberg Depression Rating Scale (MADRS *on page 106*). The MADRS may be a more functional scale, shorter and easier to administer. At the same time, a scale for the estimation of suicidal risk can be utilized. Any of the scales in this book are acceptable. The California Risk Estimator for Suicide *on page 326* is brief, but less well validated than the Beck scales. It is very important to emphasize here that these scales are only guides and cannot replace, under any circumstances, the clinical evaluation of the patient. In terms of the Quality of Life and/or disability caused by the illness, the Dartmouth COOP Functional Assessments Charts (see The COOP Charts for Adult Primary Care Practice *on page 194*) are simple, elegant, and easy to score. Quality of life may be assessed with either a clinician-administered or a self-rated scale. Functional level can be assessed with a simple scale such as the GAS *on page 176* or GAF. All scales should be done at least once at baseline (before treatment) and should be repeated sequentially. An example of frequency of administration in depressed patients is baseline, end of week 1, end of week 2, week 4, week 8, and quarterly thereafter. Finally, consumer satisfaction with healthcare services is critical in today's healthcare environment. Scales such as the CSQ or the SSS-30 may be utilized to evaluate consumer satisfaction with provider services.

Not all scales must be done at each of the follow-up points. In general, symptom assessments require more frequent administration compared to variables that may change/develop more slowly, such as quality of life or client satisfaction.

VIGNETTE II

EVALUATION OF A NEW ANTIDEPRESSANT BY A DRUG COMPANY

A drug company has a new antidepressant, that in phase II studies, has shown to have antidepressant properties in a sample of 300 patients. The phase II study showed the possibility that the medication has a short onset of action.

Determine the clinical goals of the phase III studies:

1. Antidepressant efficacy
2. Side effects
3. Patient satisfaction/tolerability
4. Quality of life issues/utilities
5. Onset of action
6. Potential indications different than depression

1. **Antidepressant activities:** An excellent scale for the evaluation of the antidepressant effect of a medication, at the present time, is the Montgomery-Asberg Depression Rating Scale (MADRS) due to the fact that it is short, easy to administer, with little influence from changes in somatic symptoms as the commonly used Hamilton-D (HAM-D) scale.

   The studies evaluating the antidepressant effects of medication will benefit from the addition of self-reported scales such as the Beck Inventory for Depression (BDI).

2. **Side effects:** In these days of many antidepressants with very similar clinical profiles, it is important to evaluate the side effect profile of novel medications carefully. Therefore, scales such as the UKU are effective and comprehensive. It is also important to evaluate the sexual side effects considering that many of the currently-used antidepressants may be associated with this problem. If the new medication being tested were an antipsychotic, a scale like the Barnes Akathisia Scale could be used as part of an assessment for medication-induced involuntary movements.

3. **Patient satisfaction/treatment tolerability:** This area can be analyzed using the side effect profile determined by the UKU or other side effect scales/questionnaires. It is important here to look at the patient's beliefs about the medication, if s/he likes to take it and if s/he believes the medication is helping or not. If the new medication being tested were an antipsychotic, a scale like the Drug Attitude Inventory (DAI) could be used.

4. **Quality of life:** There are several scales that can be utilized to look at quality of life. For studies with patients suffering depression, general scales like the Quality of Life Inventory (QOLI) or the SF-36 Health Survey can be utilized. To obtain information about utilities, it is necessary to get some data utilizing a Standard Gamble situation or a Trade-off technique. These techniques take into account multiple aspects of quality of life.

5. **Onset of action:** In order to have some idea about the onset of action of a medication, it is important to have frequent observations and ratings. These observations should be done every 3 days at the beginning of the study. Generally, in longer-term studies, ratings become more infrequent once medication dosage/response is stabilized.

6. **Other potential indications:** Scales such as the HAM-D or the HAM-A can be utilized to see the effect the medication has over symptoms of anxiety or sleep dysfunction.

DIAGNOSTIC SCALES

IN PSYCHIATRY

TABLE OF CONTENTS

Due to the length of these scales, descriptions only are provided here. Copies of the scales themselves, as well as detailed instructions or information on obtaining training in scale administration, should be obtained from listed copyright holders or literature references.

A. COMPOSITE INTERNATIONAL DIAGNOSTIC INTERVIEW (CIDI)

OVERVIEW

This diagnostic scale is an epidemiological instrument like the DIS *on page 25*, sharing a significant number of questions with the DIS. It also has items from the PSE *on page 28* and has modified DIS questions to improve the interpretations from other cultures. The CIDI was developed by Kessler, et al, for the World Health Organization (WHO) to provide a diagnostic tool for international and cross-cultural epidemiological studies. The CIDI collects information to diagnose patients using DSM or the ICD. The CIDI and related information, including how to obtain training in the use of CIDI, may be viewed on the internet website of the WHO.

GENERAL APPLICATIONS

The CIDI is used to diagnose psychiatric illness.

SELECTED PSYCHOMETRIC PROPERTIES

The CIDI, as the DIS, was developed to be administered by a nonclinical skilled interviewer. It has good reliability and good validity.

REFERENCES

Kessler RC, Andrews G, Mroczek D, et al, "The World Health Organization Composite International Diagnostic Interview-Short Form (CIDI-SF)," *International Journal of Methods in Psychiatric Research*, 1998, 7:171-85.

Robins LN, Wing J, Wittchen HU, et al, "The Composite International Diagnostic Interview: An Epidemiological Instrument Suitable for Use in Conjunction With Different Diagnostic Systems and in Different Cultures," *Arch Gen Psychiat*, 1988, 45(12):1069-77.

World Health Organization, Composite International Diagnostic Interview (CIDI), Geneva, World Health Organization, 1990.

COPYRIGHT/PUBLISHER

World Health Organization (WHO)
Headquarter Office
Avenue Appia 20
1211 Geneva 27, Switzerland
Tel: (+ 00 41 22) 791 21 11; Fax: (+ 00 41 22) 791 31 11
e-mail: publications@who.int
Website: www.who.int

SCALE GENERALLY DONE BY

Trained interviewer

TIME TO COMPLETE SCALE

60-90 minutes

REPRESENTATIVE STUDY UTILIZING SCALE

Kessler RC, DuPont RL, Berglund P, et al, "Impairment in Pure and Comorbid Generalized Anxiety Disorder and Major Depression at 12 Months in Two National Surveys," *Am J Psychiatry*, 1999, 156(12):1915-23.

B. DIAGNOSTIC INTERVIEW SCHEDULE (DIS)

OVERVIEW

This scale, developed by LN Robins and colleagues, is an epidemiological instrument to be utilized by nonclinicians in large-scale epidemiological studies. The scale is designed to obtain information that can be used for the diagnosis of most of the major psychiatric disorders according to different diagnostic criteria (eg, DSM, Feighner criteria, and RDC). The information for the DIS is collected utilizing a structured interview performed by a trained rater.

GENERAL APPLICATIONS

The DIS is utilized to diagnose major psychiatric illness in adults.

SELECTED PSYCHOMETRIC PROPERTIES

Interrater reliability of the DIS is good. Validity of the DIS has been demonstrated in several studies in which the diagnosis made by a nonclinical interviewer was compared with the diagnosis made by a psychiatrist using the DIS or another traditional assessment.

REFERENCES

Robins LN, Helzer JE, and Croughan J (eds), National Institute of Mental Health Diagnostic Interview Schedule, Version III, PHS Publication ADM-T-42-3, Rockville, MD: NIMH, 1981.

Robins LN, Helzer JE, Croughan J, et al, "National Institute of Mental Health Diagnostic Interview Schedule. Its History, Characteristics, and Validity," *Arch Gen Psychiatry*, 1981, 38(4):381-9.

COPYRIGHT

Dr Lee Robins
Washington University School of Medicine
Department of Psychiatry
4940 Children's Place
St Louis, MO 63110-1093

SCALE GENERALLY DONE BY

Trained interviewer

TIME TO COMPLETE SCALE

90-120 minutes

REPRESENTATIVE STUDY UTILIZING SCALE

Appelbaum PS, Robbins PC, and Monahan J, "Violence and Delusions: Data From the MacArthur Violence Risk Assessment Study," *Am J Psychiatry*, 2000, 157(4):566-72.

C. MINI INTERNATIONAL NEUROPSYCHIATRIC INVENTORY (MINI)

OVERVIEW

The Mini-International Neuropsychiatric Interview (MINI) is a short, structured diagnostic interview developed by an International group of psychiatrists and clinicians. The MINI is designed to diagnose DSM-IV and ICD-10 psychiatric disorders for multicenter clinical trials and epidemiology studies as well as a first step in outcome tracking in nonresearch clinical settings. The MINI is a relatively brief instrument that is divided into modules corresponding to diagnostic categories such as major depressive episode, dysthymia, mania/hypomania, panic disorder, social phobia, post-traumatic stress disorder, nonalcohol psychoactive substance use disorders, psychotic disorders, anorexia nervosa, and generalized anxiety disorder. The MINI can be administered by raters after a relatively brief training and has been translated into multiple different languages.

GENERAL APPLICATIONS

The MINI is used to diagnose major Axis I psychiatric disorders in DSM-IV and ICD-10.

SELECTED PSYCHOMETRIC PROPERTIES

The MINI has good validity and reliability and compares well as a diagnostic instrument with the CIDI and the SCID.

REFERENCES

Sheehan DV, Lecrubier Y, Sheehan KH, et al, "The Mini-International Neuropsychiatric Interview (MINI): The Development and Validation of a Structured Diagnostic Psychiatric Interview for DSM-IV and ICD-10," *J Clin Psychiatry*, 1998, 59(Suppl 20):22-33.

COPYRIGHT

David Sheehan, MD, MBA
University of South Florida
Institute for Research in Psychiatry
3515 East Fletcher Avenue
Tampa, FL 33613-4788
Tel: 813-974-4544
e-mail: dsheehan@com1.med.usf.edu

Yves Lecrubier, MD/Thierry Hergueta, MD
Hopital de la Salpetriere
47, Boulevard de l'Hopital
F. 75651 Paris, France
Tel: 33(0) 1 42 16 16 59
e-mail: hergueta@ext.jussieu.fr

SCALE GENERALLY DONE BY

Trained rater

TIME TO COMPLETE SCALE

15-20 minutes

REPRESENTATIVE STUDY UTILIZING SCALE

Houeto JL, Mesnage V, Mallet L, et al, "Behavioural Disorders, Parkinson's Disease and Subthalamic Stimulation," *J Neurol Neurosurg Psychiatry*, 2002, 72(6):701-7.

D. PRESENT STATE EXAMINATION
Ninth Edition (PSE-9)

OVERVIEW

This scale was developed by JK Wing and collaborators for the World Health Organization (WHO). Its purpose was to provide a diagnostic instrument for international studies. It was used for the first time in projects looking at the diagnosis of patients in the USA and England, and later in the World Health Organization's International Pilot Study of Schizophrenia. The scale is administered by a trained person using a semistructured interview concentrated on the signs and symptoms at the time of the interview, and symptoms during the month prior to the interview. Only information obtained from the subject is acceptable; information from other parties can be used as a guide for questioning but are not utilized for scoring. Use of the PSE has declined in favor of more recently developed diagnostic scales, such as the SCAN *on page 32* and the CIDI *on page 24.*

There are 140 items to be rated on the PSE, which include information about psychopathology collected during the interview. The main areas rated are health worry, tension, autonomic anxiety, thinking, depressed mood, sociality, appetite, libido, sleep, retardation, irritability, expansive mood, speech, obsessions, depersonalization, perceptual disorders, thought reading, hallucinations, delusions, sensorium, memory, insight, drug abuse, affect, and mood.

The PSE is available in many languages and has been validated in most of them including Spanish, Russian, and Japanese.

There is also an "American version" called the Psychiatric Assessment Interview (PAI) developed by Carpenter and collaborators, which is based on the PSE and utilizes the same interviewing technique.

GENERAL APPLICATIONS

The PSE is used to diagnose major psychiatric illness in adults.

SELECTED PSYCHOMETRIC PROPERTIES

The scale has excellent interrater reliability with trained interviewers. Validity is good. A strength of the scale is the tremendous amount of psychopathological information that can be obtained and then organized by a computer program called CATEGO.

REFERENCES

Wing JK, Cooper JE, and Sartorious N, *Measurement and Classification of Psychiatric Symptoms. An Instruction Manual for the PSE and Catego Program*, London, New York: Cambridge University Press, 1974.

World Health Organization, The International Pilot Study of Schizophrenia, WHO, Geneva, 1973, Vol 1.

COPYRIGHT/PUBLISHER

Cambridge University Press
Edinburgh Building
Shaftesbury Rd
Cambridge CB2 2RU
e-mail: information@cup.cam.ac.uk

SCALE GENERALLY DONE BY

Trained interviewer

TIME TO COMPLETE SCALE

90-120 minutes

REPRESENTATIVE STUDY UTILIZING SCALE

Harris T, Brown GW, and Robinson R, "Befriending as an Intervention for Chronic Depression Among Women in an Inner City. 1: Randomized Controlled Trial," *Br J Psychiatry*, 1999, 174:219-24.

E. PRIMARY CARE EVALUATION OF MENTAL DISORDERS (PRIME-MD)

OVERVIEW

The Primary Care Evaluation of Mental Disorders (PRIME-MD) is a relatively brief, rater-administered scale designed to assist primary care physicians in diagnosing individuals with mental disorders most commonly encountered in primary care settings. The PRIME-MD has two sections: A one-page patient questionnaire (PQ) which screens for mental disorders, and a longer clinician evaluation guide (CEG) which is used to follow up on positive items from the PQ. The PQ consists of 25 items answered "yes" or "no" where a "yes" answer would be further evaluated on the CEG. The CEG includes five diagnostic modules in DSM-IV: Mood disorders, anxiety disorders, alcohol use, eating disorders, and somatoform disorders. Each question in the CEQ evaluates a simplified version of a DSM-IV criterion for mental disorders. Final diagnoses are checked off on a diagnostic summary sheet.

GENERAL APPLICATIONS

The PRIME-MD is used to diagnose commonly seen mental disorders in a primary care setting.

SELECTED PSYCHOMETRIC PROPERTIES

The reliability of the PRIME-MD varies by diagnosis with a kappa value of 0.73 for eating disorder to 0.15 for minor depressive disorder. Kappa values for major depressive disorder has been reported as 0.61 and for panic disorder as 0.60.

REFERENCES

Spitzer RL, Williams JB, Kroenke K, et al, "Utility of a New Procedure for Diagnosing Mental Disorders in Primary Care. The PRIME-MD 1000 Study," *JAMA*, 1994, 272(22):1749-56.

COPYRIGHT

Pfizer, Inc

Copies of the PRIME-MD may be obtained from:
Robert L Spitzer, MD
Biometrics Research Department, Unit 60
New York State Psychiatric Institute
1051 Riverside Dr
New York, NY 10032

SCALE GENERALLY DONE BY

Patient Questionnaire: Self-rated
Clinician Guide: Primary care physician

TIME TO COMPLETE SCALE

10-20 minutes

REPRESENTATIVE STUDY UTILIZING SCALE

Goodwin RD, Hoven CW, and Spitzer RL, "Diabetes and Eating Disorders in Primary Care," *Int J Eat Disord*, 2003, 33(1):85-91.

F. SCHEDULE FOR AFFECTIVE DISORDERS AND SCHIZOPHRENIA (SADS)

OVERVIEW

This scale, developed by J Endicott and RL Spitzer, attempts to resolve the diagnostic dilemma between schizophrenic and mood disorders that has existed in psychiatry for many years. The SADS uses a semistructured interview, in some ways similar to the PSE (see PSE *on page 28*), with open-ended questions designed to obtain information to make a diagnosis utilizing the Research Diagnostic Criteria (RDC). The interviewer can alter the order of the questioning and is permitted to use all the information available. The SADS has two parts. In Part I the symptoms are rated in two periods, the week before the interview and the one week period during the past year when the symptoms were the worst the patient experienced. Part II deals with the past history and treatment history. A variety of versions of the SADS are available from the publisher. A children's version of the SADS (K-SADS) has also been developed.

GENERAL APPLICATIONS

The SADS is used to diagnose major psychiatric disorders.

SELECTED PSYCHOMETRIC PROPERTIES

Interrater reliability for this scale has been found to be high. The SADS has also been reported to have a high degree of concordance with the National Institute of Mental Health Diagnostic Interview Schedule (NIMH-DIS).

REFERENCES

Endicott J and Spitzer RL, "A Diagnostic Interview: The Schedule for Affective Disorders and Schizophrenia," *Arch Gen Psychiatry*, 1978, 35(7):837-44.

Hasselbrock V, Stabenau J, Hasselbrock M, et al, "A Comparison of Two Interview Schedules. The Schedule for Affective Disorders and Schizophrenia-Lifetime and the National Institute of Mental Health Diagnostic Interview Schedule," *Arch Gen Psychiatry*, 1982, 39(6):674-7.

COPYRIGHT

Jean Endicott, PhD
Chief, Department of Research, Assessment and Training
New York State Psychiatric Institute
1051 Riverside Drive
123 New York, NY 10032

SCALE GENERALLY DONE BY

Trained interviewer

TIME TO COMPLETE SCALE

60 minutes

REPRESENTATIVE STUDY UTILIZING SCALE

Perlick DA, Rosenheck RA, Clarkin JF, et al, "Symptoms Predicting Inpatient Service Use Among Patients With Bipolar Affective Disorder," *Psychiatr Serv*, 1999, 50(6):806-12.

G. SCHEDULES FOR CLINICAL ASSESSMENT IN NEUROPSYCHIATRY (SCAN)

OVERVIEW

The SCAN is a diagnostic scale which was developed within the framework of the World Health Organization (WHO) and the National Institute of Mental Health (NIMH) Joint Project on Diagnoses and Classification of Mental Disorders, Alcohol, and Related Problems. The SCAN is a variation on the PSE (see PSE *on page 28*), with a more comprehensive assessment. The SCAN allows the rater to evaluate the patient's present state, the present episode, or the "lifetime ever". The SCAN includes an Item Group Checklist which collects information from other sources, such as medical records or information by family members. It also has a Clinical Information Schedule which contains summary items about areas such as social disability and/ or clinical diagnosis. Like the PSE, the data collected from all the assessments is analyzed by a computer program called CATEGO-5. CATEGO can make the diagnosis according to ICD or DSM criteria plus providing the axial diagnosis.

GENERAL APPLICATIONS

The SCAN is used to diagnose psychiatric illness in adults.

SELECTED PSYCHOMETRIC PROPERTIES

The overall intraclass correlation coefficient is 0.67, with overall reliability of lifetime diagnoses 0.60.

REFERENCES

Wing JK, Babor T, Brugha T, et al, "SCAN. Schedules for Clinical Assessment in Neuropsychiatry," *Arch Gen Psychiatry*, 1990, 47(6):589-93.

COPYRIGHT

World Health Organization (WHO)
Headquarter Office
Avenue Appia 20
1211 Geneva 27
Switzerland
Tel: (+ 00 41 22) 791 2111
Fax: (+ 00 41 22) 791 3111
e-mail: publications@who.int

The SCAN is distributed in the U.S. by:
American Psychiatric Press
1400 K Street NW
Washington, DC 20005
e-mail: www.appi.org

SCALE GENERALLY DONE BY

Psychiatrist or psychologist

TIME TO COMPLETE SCALE

90-120 minutes

REPRESENTATIVE STUDY UTILIZING SCALE

Eaton WW, Anthony JC, Romanoski A, et al, "Onset and Recovery From Panic Disorder in the Baltimore Epidemiologic Catchment Area Follow-up," *Br J Psychiatry*, 1998, 173:501-7.

H. STRUCTURED CLINICAL INTERVIEW FOR AXIS I DSM-IV DISORDERS (SCID)

OVERVIEW

This multimodular scale was developed to obtain information, using a structured interview, for making the major Axis I diagnosis according to the fourth edition of DSM (DSM-IV). Before covering the different modules (mania, psychosis, depression, substance abuse disorders, anxiety disorders, post-traumatic stress disorders, somatization disorders, eating disorders, and adjustment disorders), the clinician focuses on the main problem affecting the patient in order to get enough information to decide which module to use.

This instrument is one of the most widely utilized diagnostic instruments in psychiatric research. The format of the instrument is useful for clinicians as it allows for a comprehensive review of criteria utilized to make the major DSM-IV psychiatric diagnoses.

GENERAL APPLICATIONS

The SCID is used to diagnose major psychiatric illness in adults.

SELECTED PSYCHOMETRIC PROPERTIES

The SCID has been extensively utilized in many studies, with a variety of patient populations, clinical and nonclinical settings, and in different countries. Interrater reliability has been good and the test-retest reliabilities are above 0.6.

REFERENCES

First MB, Spitzer RL, Gibbon M, et al, *Structured Clinical Interview for DSM-IV Axis I Disorders*, New York, NY: State Psychiatric Institute, Biometrics Research, 1995.

Spitzer RL, Williams JWB, and Gibbon M, *Instruction Manual for the Structured Clinical Interview for DSM-III-R* (SCID, 4/1/87 Revision).

COPYRIGHT

MB First
RL Spitzer
M Gibbon
JWB Williams
American Psychiatric Press
1400 K Street NW, Suite 1101
Washington, DC 20005

SCALE GENERALLY DONE BY

Trained interviewer

TIME TO COMPLETE SCALE

60-90 minutes

REPRESENTATIVE STUDY UTILIZING SCALE

Olfson M, Guardino M, Struening E, et al, "Barriers to the Treatment of Social Anxiety," *Am J Psychiatry*, 2000, 157(4):521-7.

ANXIETY

RATING SCALES

TABLE OF CONTENTS

I. GENERAL ANXIETY

A. COVI ANXIETY SCALE (COVI)

OVERVIEW

The Covi Anxiety Scale, developed by L Covi et al, is a simple three-item scale used to measure the severity of anxiety symptoms. The Covi scale measures anxiety along three separate dimensions - verbal report, behavior, and somatic symptoms of anxiety. Each dimension is rated on a 1 to 5 spectrum (1 = not at all, 5 = very much). The scale is very simple to administer; however, as it only as has three general ratings, it is usually paired with another more comprehensive scale (such as the HAM-A *on page 38*).

GENERAL APPLICATIONS

The Covi Anxiety Scale is used to measure severity of anxiety symptoms.

SELECTED PSYCHOMETRIC PROPERTIES

Although there is limited psychometric data on this scale, the Covi Anxiety Scale has been reported to accurately distinguish groups of anxious patients from patients with depressive symptoms.

REFERENCES

Lipman RS, "Differentiating Anxiety and Depression in Anxiety Disorders: Use of Rating Scale," *Psychopharmacol Bull*, 1982, 18(4):69-77.

Lipman RS, Covi L, Downing RW, et al, "Pharmacotherapy of Anxiety and Depression," *Psychopharmacol Bull*, 1981, 17(3):91-103.

COPYRIGHT

Not applicable

SCALE GENERALLY DONE BY

Clinician or trained rater

TIME TO COMPLETE SCALE

5-10 minutes

REPRESENTATIVE STUDY UTILIZING SCALE

Chouinard G, Saxena B, Belanger MC, et al, "A Canadian, Multicenter, Double-Blind Study of Paroxetine and Fluoxetine in Major Depressive Disorder," *J Affect Disord*, 1999, 54(1-2):39-48.

COVI ANXIETY SCALE

Rate each of the following according to the degrees of severity below:

1 = not at all; 2 = somewhat; 3 = moderately; 4 = considerably; 5 = very much

I. _____ Verbal report: Feels nervous, shaky, jittery, suddenly fearful or scared for no reason, tense, has to avoid certain situations, places, or things because of getting frightened, difficulty in concentrating

II. _____ Behavior: Looks scared, shaking, apprehensive, restless, jittery

III. _____ Somatic symptoms of anxiety: Trembling, sweating, rapid heartbeat, breathlessness, hot or cold spells, restless sleep, discomfort in stomach, lump in throat, having to go to the bathroom frequently

B. HAMILTON RATING SCALE FOR ANXIETY (HAM-A)

OVERVIEW

The HAM-A, developed by M Hamilton, is the most widely utilized assessment scale for anxiety symptoms, and was originally intended to be used to evaluate individuals who are already diagnosed with anxiety disorders. The HAM-A may be less useful in evaluating anxiety symptoms in those with other psychiatric disorders. The HAM-A consists of 14 items and, like the HAM-D, is heavily focused on somatic symptoms, with a great reliance on the patient's subjective report. Each item is rated on a 0 to 4 scale (0 = not present, 4 = severe) with a final item which rates behavior at interview. The scale is designed to evaluate change in symptoms over time. Strengths of the scale include its brevity and widely accepted use. Limitations include its lack of generalizability to anxiety symptoms in other psychiatric disorders and the predominant focus on somatic, self-reported symptoms. When the HAM-A is used in patients with major depression, it should be paired with a scale that measures severity of depressive symptoms, such as the HAM-D (see HAM-D *on page 100* or the MADRS *on page 106*).

GENERAL APPLICATIONS

The HAM-A is a very widely used scale to evaluate anxiety symptoms at baseline and in response to treatment.

SELECTED PSYCHOMETRIC PROPERTIES

The HAM-A has very good internal consistency with Cronbach's alphas of 0.79-0.86. One week test-retest reliability value of 0.64 has been demonstrated.

REFERENCES

Hamilton M, "Diagnosis and Rating of Anxiety," *Studies of Anxiety*, Lader MH, ed, *Brit J Psychiatr* Spec Publication, 1969, 3:76-9.

Hamilton M, "Hamilton Anxiety Scale," *ECDEU Assessment Manual for Psychopharmacology*, Guy W, ed, Rockville, MD: U.S. Department of Health, Education, and Welfare, 1976, 193-8.

Danish University Antidepressant Group, "Citalopram: Clinical Effect Profile in Comparison With Clomipramine. A Controlled Multicenter Study. Danish University Antidepressant Group," *Psychopharmacology*, 1986, 90(1):131-8.

Hamilton M, "The Assessment of Anxiety States by Rating," *Br J Med Psychol*, 1959, 32:50-5.

COPYRIGHT

ECDEU version - not applicable

SCALE GENERALLY DONE BY

Clinician or trained rater

TIME TO COMPLETE SCALE

20 minutes

REPRESENTATIVE STUDY UTILIZING SCALE

Bakker A, van Dyck R, Spinhoven P, et al, "Paroxetine, Clomipramine, and Cognitive Therapy in the Treatment of Panic Disorder," *J Clin Psychiatry*, 1999, 60(12):831-8.

HAMILTON ANXIETY SCALE

(ECDEU Version)

Mark and score as follows:

0 = Not present; 1 = Mild; 2 = Moderate; 3 = Severe; 4 = Very severe

ANXIOUS MOOD

_____ Worries, anticipation of the worst, fearful anticipation, irritability

TENSION

_____ Feelings of tension, fatigability, startle response, moved to tears easily, trembling, feelings of restlessness, inability to relax

FEARS

_____ Of dark, of strangers, of being left alone, of animals, of traffic, of crowds

INSOMNIA

_____ Difficulty in falling asleep, broken sleep, unsatisfying sleep and fatigue on waking, dreams, nightmares, night terrors

INTELLECTUAL

_____ Difficulty in concentration, poor memory

DEPRESSED MOOD

_____ Loss of interest, lack of pleasure in hobbies, depression, early waking, diurnal swing

SOMATIC (Muscular)

_____ Pains and aches, twitchings, stiffness, myoclonic jerks, grinding of teeth, unsteady voice, increased muscular tone

SOMATIC (Sensory)

_____ Tinnitus, blurring of vision, hot and cold flushes, feelings of weakness, pricking sensation

B. HAMILTON RATING SCALE FOR ANXIETY (HAM-A) *(Continued)*

CARDIOVASCULAR SYMPTOMS

_____ Tachycardia, palpitations, pain in chest, throbbing of vessels, fainting feelings, sighing, dyspnea

RESPIRATORY SYMPTOMS

_____ Pressure or constriction in chest, choking feelings, sighing, dyspnea

GASTROINTESTINAL SYMPTOMS

_____ Difficulty in swallowing, wind, abdominal pain, burning sensations, abdominal fullness, nausea, vomiting, borborygmi, looseness of bowels, loss of weight, constipation

GENITOURINARY SYMPTOMS

_____ Frequency of micturition, urgency of micturition, amenorrhea, menorrhagia, development of frigidity, premature ejaculation, loss of libido, impotence

AUTONOMIC SYMPTOMS

_____ Dry mouth, flushing, pallor, tendency to sweat, giddiness, tension headache, raising of hair

BEHAVIOR AT INTERVIEW

_____ Fidgeting, restlessness or pacing, tremor of hands, furrowed brow, strained face, sighing or rapid respiration, facial pallor, swallowing, etc

C. SHEEHAN DISABILITY SCALE

OVERVIEW

The Sheehan Disability Scale, developed by D Sheehan, is a simple and commonly used rating scale used to evaluate impairments in the domains of work, social life/leisure, and family life/home responsibility as a result of an anxiety disorder. Each domain is rated on an 11-point continuum from 0 = no impairment to 10 = most severe. There are ranges within each continuum of mild (1-3), moderate (4-6), and marked (5-9). The use of the Sheehan disability scale is usually paired with another scale that measures symptom severity, such as the SPRAS *on page 64*, or a clinician-rated severity of illness scale.

GENERAL APPLICATIONS

The Sheehan Disability Scale is used to evaluate disability related to having an anxiety disorder.

SELECTED PSYCHOMETRIC PROPERTIES

Internal consistency of the Sheehan Disability Scale is high, with alphas of 0.89 for the 3-item scale.

REFERENCES

Sheehan DV, *The Anxiety Disease*, New York, NY: Scribner, 1983, 144-3.

Sheehan DV, Harnett-Sheehan K, and Raj BA, "The Measurement of Disability," *Int Clin Psychopharmacol*, 1996, 11(Suppl 3):89-95.

COPYRIGHT

David V Sheehan, MD, MBA
University of South Florida
Institute for Research in Psychiatry
3515 East Fletcher Avenue
Tampa, FL 33613-4788
Tel: 813-974-4544
Fax: 813-974-4575

SCALE GENERALLY DONE BY

Clinician or trained rater

TIME TO COMPLETE SCALE

5 minutes or less

REPRESENTATIVE STUDY UTILIZING SCALE

Bakker A, van Dyck R, Spinhoven P, et al, "Paroxetine, Clomipramine, and Cognitive Therapy in the Treatment of Panic Disorder," *J Clin Psychiatry*, 1999, 60(12):831-8.

C. SHEEHAN DISABILITY SCALE *(Continued)*

SHEEHAN DISABILITY SCALE

Please mark one box for each scale

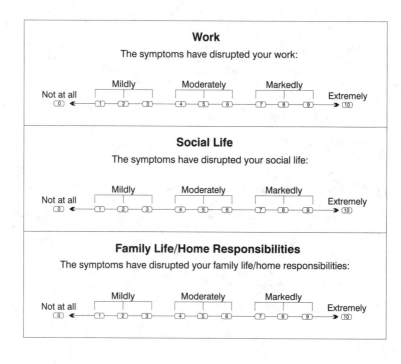

D. STATE-TRAIT ANXIETY INVENTORY (STAI)

OVERVIEW

The STAI, developed by C Spielberger, is a 40-item self-report assessment that differentiates between state anxiety, a temporary condition experienced in specific situations, and trait anxiety, the general chronic anxiety experienced by some individuals. The STAI has two 20-item scales, the first of which evaluates how likely an individual is to feel anxiety (trait), while the second evaluates how the individual feels at that moment (state). A computer version of the STAI is available.

GENERAL APPLICATIONS

The STAI may be used to differentiate between state (temporary/situational) and trait (long-term) anxiety.

SELECTED PSYCHOMETRIC PROPERTIES

The STAI has good correlation with other widely-used anxiety scales, such as the Beck Anxiety Inventory and the Fear Questionnaire.

REFERENCES

Spielberger CD, *State-Trait Anxiety Inventory: A Comprehensive Bibliography*, Consultant Psychologists Press: Palo Alto, CA, 1984.

COPYRIGHT

Charles D Spielberger, PhD
Mind Garden, Inc
1690 Woodside Road #202
Redwood City, CA 94061
Tel: (650) 261-3500

SCALE GENERALLY DONE BY

Clinician or trained rater

TIME TO COMPLETE SCALE

10 minutes

REPRESENTATIVE STUDY UTILIZING SCALE

Chouinard G, Saxena B, Belanger MC, et al, "A Canadian, Multicenter, Double-Blind Study of Paroxetine and Fluoxetine in Major Depressive Disorder," *J Affect Disord*, 1999, 54(1-2):39-48.

D. STATE-TRAIT ANXIETY INVENTORY (STAI) *(Continued)*

SAMPLE ENTRIES OF THE

STATE TRAIT ANXIETY INVENTORY (STAI)

➔ The **S-Anxiety scale** consists of twenty statements that evaluate how respondents feel *"right now*, at this moment"

1 = NOT AT ALL   **2** = SOMEWHAT   **3** = MODERATELY SO   **4** = VERY MUCH SO

A. I feel at ease 1   2   3   4

B. I feel upset... 1   2   3   4

➔ The **T-Anxiety scale** consists of twenty statements that assess how respondents feel "generally"

1 = ALMOST NEVER   **2** = SOMETIMES   **3** = OFTEN   **4** = ALMOST ALWAYS

A. I am a steady person.. 1   2   3   4

B. I lack self-confidence... 1   2   3   4

II. PHOBIAS/SOCIAL ANXIETY

E. BRIEF FEAR OF NEGATIVE EVALUATION
SCALE (Brief-FNE)

OVERVIEW

The Brief-FNE, developed by M Leary, is based upon the FNE, a widely utilized, 30-item questionnaire to assess social phobia, specifically, the fear of receiving negative evaluations from others. The 30 items of the FNE have true/false answers and yield a total phobia score that may be compared to established norms for individuals with and without social phobia. Scores on the FNE indicate a fear of the loss of social approval. The Brief-FNE appears to preserve the excellent properties of the FNE while reducing the scale length to 12 items. The Brief-FNE items are rated on a 5-point continuum ranging from "not at all" to "extremely." Items 2, 4, 7, and 10 are reverse scored. The Brief-FNE has good correlation with the Social Phobia and Anxiety Inventory (see SPAI *on page 51*).

GENERAL APPLICATIONS

The Brief-FNE is a scale to evaluate severity of social phobia.

SELECTED PSYCHOMETRIC PROPERTIES

The inter-item reliability of the Brief-FNE is quite high, with Cronbach's alpha = 0.90. This compares favorably with the reliability coefficient of 0.92 for the full-length FNE.

REFERENCES

Leary MR, "A Brief Version of the Fear of Negative Evaluation Scale," *Personality and Social Psychology*, 1983, 9:371-5.

COPYRIGHT

Mark R Leary
Wake Forest University
PO Box 7778
Winston Salem, NC 27109-7778

SCALE GENERALLY DONE BY

Self-rated

TIME TO COMPLETE SCALE

5-10 minutes

REPRESENTATIVE STUDY UTILIZING SCALE

Van Ameringen M, Mancini C, and Oakman JM, "Nefazodone in Social Phobia," *J Clin Psychiatry*, 1999, 60(2):96-100.

II. PHOBIAS/SOCIAL ANXIETY *(Continued)*

BRIEF FEAR OF NEGATIVE
EVALUATION SCALE (Brief-FNE)

INSTRUCTIONS: Read each of the following statements carefully and indicate how characteristic it is of you according to the following scale:

1 = Not at all characteristic of me
2 = Slightly characteristic of me
3 = Moderately characteristic of me
4 = Very characteristic of me
5 = Extremely characteristic of me

Reverse score items were marked (R) before summing.

	Item-Total Corr.
(1) I worry about what other people will think of me even when I know it doesn't make any difference.	.54
(2) I am unconcerned even if I know people are forming an unfavorable impression of me. (R)	.53
(3) I am frequently afraid of other people noticing my shortcomings.	.64
(4) I rarely worry about what kind of impression I am making on someone. (R)	.57
(5) I am afraid that others will not approve of me.	.67
(6) I am afraid that people will find fault with me.	.66
(7) Other people's opinions of me do not bother me. (R)	.43
(8) When I am talking to someone, I worry about what they may be thinking about me.	.60
(9) I am usually worried about what kind of impression I make.	.68
(10) If I know someone is judging me, it has little effect on me. (R)	.56
(11) Sometimes I think I am too concerned with what other people think of me.	.75
(12) I often worry that I will say or do the wrong things.	.73

F. FEAR QUESTIONNAIRE (FQ)

OVERVIEW

The Fear Questionnaire, developed by IM Marks and AM Matthews, is a 24-item, self-rated scale that is used mainly for the assessment of phobias. One component of the fear questionnaire evaluates phobic behaviors associated with a series of phobic situations, while another component of the questionnaire evaluates symptoms of anxiety, depression, and general distress caused by a phobia. The questionnaire evaluates five social situations, five body-injury phobic situations, and five agoraphobic situations, which separately, can be used as subscales. Each item is rated on a 0 to 8 scale (0 = no phobia, 8 = most severe). The scale arrives at a total phobia score as well as subscale scores for agoraphobia, body-injury, and social phobia.

GENERAL APPLICATIONS

The fear questionnaire assesses phobic symptoms and other psychiatric symptoms resulting from phobias such as depression, anxiety, and general distress.

SELECTED PSYCHOMETRIC PROPERTIES

Good test-retest reliability has been reported. The correlation for the three subscales combined was 0.82. Test-retest correlation was 0.93 for main target phobia, 0.79 for global phobia rating, and 0.82 for the anxiety-depression subscale.

REFERENCES

Marks IM and Mathews AM, "Brief Standard Self-Rating for Phobic Patients," *Behav Res Ther*, 1979, 17(3):263-7.

COPYRIGHT

Isaac Marks, MD
Maudsley Hospital
Institute for Psychiatry
DeCrespigny Park
London SE4 8AF, UK

SCALE GENERALLY DONE BY

Self-rated by patient

TIME TO COMPLETE SCALE

10 minutes

REPRESENTATIVE STUDY UTILIZING SCALE

Van Ameringen M, Mancini C, and Oakman JM, "Nefazodone in Social Phobia," *J Clin Psychiatry*, 1999, 60(2):96-100.

F. FEAR QUESTIONNAIRE (FQ) *(Continued)*

FEAR QUESTIONNAIRE

Name _____ Age ____ Sex ____ Date _____

Choose a number from the scale below to show how much you would avoid each of the situations listed below because of fear or other unpleasant feelings. Then write the number you chose in the box opposite each situation.

0	1	2	3	4	5	6	7	8
Would not avoid it		Slightly avoid it		Definitely avoid it		Markedly avoid it		Always avoid it

1. Main phobia you want treated (describe in your own words) ☐
   _____

2. Injections or minor surgery ☐
3. Eating or drinking with other people ☐
4. Hospitals ☐
5. Travelling alone by bus or coach ☐
6. Walking alone in busy streets ☐
7. Being watched or stared at ☐
8. Going into crowded shops ☐
9. Talking to people in authority ☐
10. Sight of blood ☐
11. Being critcized ☐
12. Going alone far from home ☐
13. Thought of injury or illness ☐
14. Speaking or acting to an audience ☐
15. Large open spaces ☐
16. Going to the dentist ☐
17. Other situations (describe) ☐

Leave blank → ☐☐☐ ☐

Ag + Bl + Soc = Total
2-16

Now choose a number from the scale below to show how much you are troubled by each problem listed, and write the number in the box opposite.

0	1	2	3	4	5	6	7	8
Hardly at all		Slightly troublesome		Definitely troublesome		Markedly troublesome		Very severely troublesome

18. Feeling miserable or depressed ☐
19. Feeling irritable or angry ☐
20. Feeling tense or panicky ☐
21. Upsetting thoughts coming into your mind ☐
22. Feeling you or your surroundings are strange or unreal ☐
23. Other feelings (describe) ☐ ☐

Total ☐

How would you rate the present state of your phobic symptoms on the scale below?

0	1	2	3	4	5	6	7	8
No phobias present		Slightly disturbing/ not really disabling		Definitely disturbing/ disabling		Markedly disturbing/ disabling		Very severely disturbing/ disabling

Please circle one number between 0 and 8

G. LIEBOWITZ SOCIAL ANXIETY SCALE (LSAS)

OVERVIEW

The Liebowitz Social Anxiety Scale (LSAS), also called the Liebowitz Social Phobia Scale, developed by M Liebowitz, rates fear/anxiety and avoidance on 24 commonly feared "perform-ance" or "social situations". Each phobic situation, such as talking to people in authority or being the center of attention, is rated on a 0 to 3 spectrum (0 = none/never, 3 = severe or usually). There are 13 performance-related items and 11 social-related items. Each situation is also rated in terms of fear/anxiety and in degree of avoidance.

GENERAL APPLICATIONS

The LSAS is used to evaluate degree of fear and avoidance in common social situations.

SELECTED PSYCHOMETRIC PROPERTIES

The LSAS has good internal consistency, with Cronbach's alphas of 0.82 to 0.92 across its subscales.

REFERENCES

Liebowitz MR, "Social Phobia," *Mod Probl Pharmacopsychiatry*, 1987, 22:141-73.

Heimberg RG, Horner KJ, Juster HR, et al, "Psychometric Properties of the Liebowitz Social Anxiety Scale," *Psychol Med*, 1999, 29(1):199-212.

COPYRIGHT

Dr Michael Liebowitz
New York State Psychiatric Institute
722 W 168th St
New York, NY 10032

SCALE GENERALLY DONE BY

Clinician or trained rater

TIME TO COMPLETE SCALE

15 minutes

REPRESENTATIVE STUDY UTILIZING SCALE

Pallanti S, Quercioli L, Rossi A, et al, "The Emergence of Social Phobia During Clozapine Treatment and Its Response to Fluoxetine Augmentation," *J Clin Psychiatry*, 1999, 60(12):819-23.

G. LIEBOWITZ SOCIAL ANXIETY SCALE (LSAS) *(Continued)*

LIEBOWITZ SOCIAL ANXIETY SCALE (LSAS)

	Fear or Anxiety	Avoidance
	0 = none	0 = never (0%)
	1 = mild	1 = occasionally (1-33%)
	2 = moderate	2 = often (33-67%)
	3 = severe	3 = usually (67-100%)

	ANXIETY (S)	ANXIETY (P)	AVOID (S)	AVOID (P)
Telephoning in public (P)	_____	_____	_____	_____
Participating in small groups (P)	_____	_____	_____	_____
Eating in public places (P)	_____	_____	_____	_____
Drinking with others in public places (P)	_____	_____	_____	_____
Talking to people in authority (S)	_____	_____	_____	_____
Acting, performing, or giving a talk in front of an audience (P)	_____	_____	_____	_____
Going to a party (S)	_____	_____	_____	_____
Working while being observed (P)	_____	_____	_____	_____
Writing while being observed (P)	_____	_____	_____	_____
Calling someone you don't know very well (S)	_____	_____	_____	_____
Talking with people you don't know very well (S)	_____	_____	_____	_____
Meeting strangers (S)	_____	_____	_____	_____
Urinating in a public bathroom (P)	_____	_____	_____	_____
Entering a room when others are already seated (P)	_____	_____	_____	_____
Being the center of attention (S)	_____	_____	_____	_____
Speaking up at a meeting (P)	_____	_____	_____	_____
Taking a test (P)	_____	_____	_____	_____
Expressing a disagreement or disapproval to people you don't know very well (S)	_____	_____	_____	_____
Looking at people you don't know very well in the eyes (S)	_____	_____	_____	_____
Giving a report to a group (P)	_____	_____	_____	_____
Trying to pick up someone (P)	_____	_____	_____	_____
Returning goods to a store (S)	_____	_____	_____	_____
Giving a party (S)	_____	_____	_____	_____
Resisting a high pressure salesperson (S)	_____	_____	_____	_____
Total Performance (P) Subscore	_____	_____	_____	_____
Total Social (S) Subscore	_____	_____	_____	_____
TOTAL SCORE	_____	_____	_____	_____

H. SOCIAL PHOBIA AND ANXIETY INVENTORY (SPAI)

OVERVIEW

The SPAI, developed by S Turner et al, is a 45-item, self-rated inventory that assesses cognition, somatic symptoms, and avoidance in a variety of social phobic and agoraphobic situations. The scale yields an overall score for severity of social phobia. The SPAI has two subscales, the social phobia and agoraphobia subscales. Subscale scores are derived by summing across all items for each scale. The difference score on the SPAI (formerly called the total score) is derived by subtracting the agoraphobia subscale score from the social phobia subscale scale. By subtracting the agoraphobia score from the social phobia score, a purer measure of social phobia is provided. The SPAI may be utilized as a screening device in outpatient or inpatient facilities, as well as schools, residential treatment settings, and correctional facilities. Additionally, the SPAI may be useful in employment settings to assist in evaluation of individuals who may have difficulty in positions requiring social interactions and social performance. The SPAI may be used with adolescents and adults.

GENERAL APPLICATIONS

The SPAI is used to evaluate severity of social phobia and to detect maladaptive social anxiety in adolescents and adults.

SELECTED PSYCHOMETRIC PROPERTIES

The SPAI has good internal consistency, with Cronbach's alphas from 0.95 to 0.96 for the social phobia scale, and alphas ranging from 0.85 to 0.95 for the agoraphobia scale. Test-retest reliability has been reported to be 0.86.

REFERENCES

Turner SM, Beidel DC, Dancu DV, et al, "An Empirically Derived Inventory to Measure Social Fears and Anxiety: The Social Phobia and Anxiety Inventory," *Psychol Assessment*, 1989, 1:35-40.

COPYRIGHT

Samuel M Turner, PhD
Deborah C Beidel, PhD
Constance V Dancu, PhD
Multi-Health Systems, Inc
P.O. Box 950
North Tonawanda, NY 14120-0950
Tel: 1-800-456-3003

SCALE GENERALLY DONE BY

Clinician or trained rater, including school officials and personnel officers.

TIME TO COMPLETE SCALE

20-30 minutes

REPRESENTATIVE STUDY UTILIZING SCALE

Osman A, Barrios FX, Aukes D, et al, "Psychometric Evaluation of the Social Phobia and Anxiety Inventory in College Students," *J Clin Psychol*, 1995, 51(2):235-43.

H. SOCIAL PHOBIA AND ANXIETY INVENTORY (SPAI) *(Continued)*

SAMPLE ENTRIES OF THE
SPAI - THE SOCIAL PHOBIA AND ANXIETY INVENTORY

Name: _____ Age: _____ Sex: M F Date: _____/_____/_____

Please use the scale listed opposite and circle the number which best reflects how frequently you experience these responses.

	New	Very Infrequent	Infrequent	Sometimes	Frequent	Very Frequent	Always
2. I feel anxious when entering social situations where there is a large group	0	1	2			5	6
6. I feel anxious when speaking in a small informal meeting	0	1	2		4	5	6
8. I feel so anxious in social situations that I leave the social gathering			2	3	4	5	6
23. I feel anxious when being criticized or rejected by:							
strangers	0	1	2	3	4	5	6
authority figures		1	2	3	4	5	6
opposite sex		1	2	3	4	5	6
people in general		1	2	3	4	5	6
32. I experience the following in a social situation							
sweating	0	1	2	3	4	5	6
blushing	0	1	2	3	4	5	6
shaking	0	1	2	3	4	5	6
frequent urge to urinate	0	1	2	3	4	5	6
heart palpitations	0	1	2	3	4	5	6
33. I feel anxious when I am home alone	0	1	2	3	4	5	6

SAMPLE

III. OBSESSIVE-COMPULSIVE SYMPTOMS

I. LEYTON OBSESSIONAL INVENTORY (LOI)

OVERVIEW

The Leyton Obsessional Inventory, developed by J Cooper, is a 69-question scale dealing with the subjective assessment of obsessional traits and symptoms. There is a detailed set of standard instructions required to administer the scale, and the procedures need supervision by the rater. A first stage yields "yes" or "no" answers for a number of obsessional symptoms and associated personality states (eg, checking behaviors). A second stage evaluates the degree of resistance experienced by the patient to the symptoms which are present (ranging from no resistance = 0, to severe feelings of resistance = 3). A third stage evaluates the degree of interference current symptoms are causing (ranging from no interference = 0, to a great deal of interference = 3). A strength of the scale includes its comprehensive evaluation of specific obsessional symptoms; however, a number of not uncommon symptoms, such as obscene or violent thoughts are not assessed.

GENERAL APPLICATIONS

The LOI evaluates presence and severity of obsessional symptoms.

SELECTED PSYCHOMETRIC PROPERTIES

The validity of the LOI is good, with little overlap in scoring between obsessional individuals and nonobsessional individuals. The product-moment correlation coefficient for the symptom score is 0.87 and the trait score is 0.91.

REFERENCES

Cooper J, "The Leyton Obsessional Inventory," *Psychol Med*, 1970, 1(1):48-64.

COPYRIGHT

Psychological Medicine
Cambridge University Press
40 W 20th Street
New York, NY 10011

SCALE GENERALLY DONE BY

Clinician or trained rater

TIME TO COMPLETE SCALE

15-20 minutes for nonobsessional individuals; 45-60 minutes for obsessional individuals

REPRESENTATIVE STUDY UTILIZING SCALE

Asbahr FR, Negrao AB, Gentil JA, et al, "Obsessive-Compulsive and Related Symptoms in Children and Adolescents With Rheumatic Fever With and Without Chorea: A Prospective 6-Month Study,"*Am J Psychiatry*, 1998, 155(8):1122-4.

III. OBSESSIVE-COMPULSIVE SYMPTOMS *(Continued)*

THE LEYTON OBSESSIONAL INVENTORY

APPENDIX I - Leyton Obsessional Card Inventory - Female Version

"Check" indicates that this word should be written on the back of the card; the operator deals with these three cards according to the "instructions for users". (**) indicates that a mark is put on the back of the card to show that it goes through to the resistance and interference stages.

SYMPTOM QUESTIONS

Thoughts

1. Are you often inwardly compelled to do certain things even though your reason tells you it is not necessary? (Check)

2. Do unpleasant or frightening thoughts or words ever keep going over and over in your mind? (Check)

3. Do you ever have persistent imaginings that your children or husband might be having an accident or that something might have happened to them? (**)

4. Have you ever been troubled by certain thoughts or ideas of harming yourself or persons in your family - thoughts which come and go without any particular reason? (**)

Checking

5. Do you often have to check things several times?

6. Do you ever have to check gas or water taps or light switches after you have already turned them off? (**)

7. Do you ever have to go back and check doors, cupboards, or windows to make sure that they are really shut? (**)

Dirt and Contamination

8. Do you hate dirt and dirty things?

9. Do you ever feel that if something has been used, touched, or knocked by someone else it is in some way spoiled for you? (**)

10. Do you dislike brushing against people or being touched in any way? (**)

11. Do you feel that even a slight contact with bodily secretions (such as sweat, saliva, urine, etc), is unpleasant or dangerous, or liable to contaminate your clothes or belongings? (**)

12. Do you worry if you go through a day without having your bowels open?

Dangerous Objects

13. Are you ever worried by the thoughts of pins, needles, or bits of hair that might have been left lying about? (**)

14. Do you worry about household things that might chip or splinter if they were to be knocked or broken? (**)

15. Does the sight of knives, hammers, hatchets, or other possibly dangerous things in your home ever upset you or make you feel nervous? (**)

Personal Cleanliness and Tidiness

16. Do you tend to worry a bit about personal cleanliness or tidiness?

17. Are you fussy about keeping your hands clean? (**)

18. Do you ever wash and iron clothes when they are not obviously dirty in order to keep them extra clean and fresh? (**)

19. Do you take care that the clothes you are wearing are always clean and neat, whatever you are doing? (**)

20. Do you like to put your personal belongings in set places or patterns? (**)

21. Do you take great care in hanging and folding your clothes at night? (**)

Household Cleanliness and Tidiness

22. Are you very strict about keeping the house always very clean and tidy? (**)
23. Do you dislike having a room untidy or not quite clean for even a short time? (**)
24. Do you sometimes get angry that children spoil your nice clean and tidy rooms?
25. Do you like furniture or ornaments to be in exactly the same place always? (**)
26. Do your easy chairs have cushions which you like to keep exactly in position?
27. If you notice any bits or specks on the floor or furniture do you have to remove them at once before you are due to clean round? (**)
28. Do you ever clean or dust the rooms that haven't had time to get dirty just to make sure that they are really clean? (**)
29. Do you ever have to dust, sweep, or wash things over again several times just to make sure they are really clean? (**)

Order and Routine

30. Do you have to keep to strict timetables or routines for doing ordinary things? (**)
31. Do you have to keep a certain order for undressing and dressing, or washing and bathing? (**)
32. Do you get a bit upset if you cannot do your housework at set times or in a certain order? (**)

Repetition

33. Do you ever have to do things over again a certain number of time before they seem quite right? (**)
34. Do you ever have to count things several times or go through numbers in your mind? (**)
35. Do you ever get behind with the housework because you have to do something over again several times? (**)

Overconscientiousness and Lack of Satisfaction

36. Are you a person who often has a guilty conscience over quite ordinary things?
37. Are you the sort of person who has to pay a great deal of attention to details? (**)
38. Are you ever overconscientious or very strict with yourself?
39. Do you ever waste time by doing a thing more thoroughly than is really necessary just to see if it is really finished? (**)
40. Even when you have done something carefully, do you often feel that it is somehow not quite right or complete? (**)
41. Do you feel unsettled or guilty if you haven't been able to do something exactly as you would like? (**)
42. Do you always fail to explain things properly, in spite of having planned beforehand exactly what to say?

Indecision

43. Do you have difficulty in making up your mind? (**)
44. Do you have to turn things over and over in your mind for a long time before being able to decide about what to do? (**)
45. Do you ask yourself questions or have doubts about a lot of things you do? (**)
46. Are there any particular things that you try to keep away from or that you avoid doing, because you know that you would be upset by them? (**) (Check)

III. OBSESSIVE-COMPULSIVE SYMPTOMS *(Continued)*

TRAIT QUESTIONS

Hoarding

47. Do you find it difficult to throw things away? (**)

48. Do you keep rather a lot of empty boxes, paper bags, old newspapers, or empty tins in case they come in useful one day? (**)

49. Does your stock of soap, detergents, or cleaning materials ever get large because you find yourself buying more than you actually use?

Cleanliness

50. Do you regard cleanliness as a virtue in itself?

Meanness

51. Do you get more pleasure from saving money than from spending it?

52. Are you more careful with money than most people you know?

53. Do you keep regular accounts of the money you spend every day?

Irritable and Morose

54. Do you usually look on the gloomy side of things?

55. Do people often get on your nerves and make you feel irritable?

56. When you feel critical of someone, do you usually say what you are thinking?

57. Do you get angry or irritated if people don't do things carefully or correctly?

Rigidity

58. Do you try to avoid changes in your house or work or in the way you do things?

59. Do you try to avoid changing your mind once you have made a decision about something?

60. Are you a person who likes to stick to principles and decisions whatever the opposition or difficulties?

61. Do you pride yourself on thinking things over very carefully before making decisions?

Health

62. Do you think that regular daily bowel movements are important for your health?

63. Do you often get scared that you might be developing some sort of serious illness or cancer?

Regularity

64. Are you very systematic and methodical in your daily life?

65. Do you like to get things done exactly right, down to the smallest detail?

66. Do you think it is important to follow rules and regulations exactly?

67. Do you like to have set times or orders for doing your household jobs?

Punctuality

68. Are you ever late because you just can't seem to get through everything in time? (**)

69. If you have to catch a train or keep an important appointment, do you have to plan out how to do it beforehand in great detail? (**)

CHANGES IN WORDING FOR MALE VERSION

18. Becomes: Do you ever ask to have clothes washed or cleaned that are not obviously dirty in order to keep them extra clean and fresh? (**)

22. Becomes: Are you strict about the house always being kept very clean and tidy?

28. Becomes: Do you often do any dusting or cleaning at home without being asked to do so? (**)

29. Becomes: Do you ever have to clean or wash things over again several times just to make sure they are really clean? (**)

32. Substitute "work" for "housework"

35. Substitute "work" for "housework"

49. Omit

67. Becomes: Do you like to have set times or orders for doing your work?

APPENDIX 2

Instructions for Use of Leyton Obsessional Card Inventory

1. Check that you have:
   a. Complete set of obsessional (1-69) and Cornell (70-121) cards, arranged in alternating blocks - namely, 1-23, 70-86, 24-47, 87-104, 48-69, 105-121.
   b. Five "Resistance Statement" cards marked 1 to 5 on the back.
   c. Four "Interference Statement" cards marked 1 to 4 on the back.
   d. One "Yes" and "No" postbox.
   e. A scoring sheet. (Simply a sheet with the numbers 1 to 121 laid out with enough space between for recording the Resistance and Interference symbols, and room for details of the subject and date.)

2. Make sure that the cards are in the correct order and the right way up. They should be arranged in numerical order, with the questions facing up. The number of the card should be written in the top right hand corner of the back of the card.

3. Put the subject's name, age, status, the date and time of starting, and your name on the top of the scoring sheet.

4. Arrange the seats of yourself and the subject so that you are either facing each other across a small table, or you are sitting one on each side of a corner.

5. Say to the subject: "I want to get your replies to a number of questions about your general health, and about how you feel in yourself about various things. We find that a good way to do this is to give you the questions each printed on a card, and for you to answer by putting them in the Yes and No box. Read each question carefully, and then make a fairly quick decision about whether to answer "yes" or "no". You may find yourself wanting to answer not exactly "yes" and not exactly "no", but in this case put it in the slot which is most nearly correct for you. Try to give your answer without asking any questions about what is written on the card. If you really are quite unable to decide, then guess. Try to do it fairly quickly without a long debate with yourself over each question. Everybody comes out differently on these questions, and there is no "right" or "wrong" number of "yes" or "no" answers - just answer the questions as they apply to you."

III. OBSESSIVE-COMPULSIVE SYMPTOMS *(Continued)*

6. Put the first half of the card pack in front of the subject with the question upwards, and ask them to put the cards in the appropriate boxes after turning the cards upside down - show them what you mean - so that the card comes through to the other side with its back facing you with the numbers the right way up.

7. Ask the subject to start, and ring on the score sheet all the "yes" answers. Keep those "yes" answers with "?" or "check" on the back, and discard the others.

8. Do not discuss the questions in detail with the subject. Answer questions by first merely repeating the question on the card, and by saying "I want to know how you feel about it - what does it mean to you. Just take the words as *you* use them. If you do not know or cannot decide, then just guess."

9. When all the questions have been answered, remove the postbox, and set out the "Resistance Statement" cards. Say to the subject, "Now I would like you to show me how you feel about some of the things to which you answered "yes". You may feel that to do these things is quite sensible and reasonable (point to card), or just habit, or you may feel that you do not want to do some of these things and in fact try to stop yourself doing them. Please look at these questions again, and place each one in front of the card which fits your feeling about it most nearly." Make sure that the subject has read and understood each statement card. Then give the subject the "yes" cards and ask him to place them face down with the numbers showing to the interviewer (as when posting them before), in front of the statements.

10. Look at the number of each "?" card as it is placed by the subject, and record his reply on the scoring sheet alongside the number of the question - for example, put S for sensible, H for habit, U for unnecessary, R for try to stop, and R+ for try very hard to stop.

11. Ask the subject to give the reason why s/he answered "yes" to each "check" card. If the example is not connected with an obsessional trait or symptom, discard it and cross out the "yes" mark on the score sheet, otherwise proceed as for the other query cards.

12. Collect up these cards again, and set out the "Interference Statement" cards and say to the subject, "Now I would like you to show if any of these things you do interfere with other things, or waste your time at all" - explain the card statements as above, and score them on the sheet in the same way - for instance, by putting alongside the question numbers D for interferes a great deal, M for interferes moderately, L for interferes a little, and nothing for no interference. The subject has now finished. Record the time. Collect up all the cards, and put them back in order, with questions upwards ready for the next time.

J. YALE-BROWN OBSESSIVE COMPULSIVE SCALE (Y-BOCS)

OVERVIEW

The Y-BOCS, developed by W Goodman et al, is a rating scale to evaluate the severity of illness in individuals with obsessive-compulsive disorder (OCD). For the most part, the ratings depend on patient self-report; however, the final rating incorporates the clinical judgement of the interviewer. This 10-item rating scale is designed for use as a semistructured interview, using the questions provided, in the listed order. Items are rated on a 0 to 4 scale (0 = none, 4 = extreme), and are based upon information obtained on report and observation during the interview. Prior to beginning the questions, the rater is instructed to explain to the patient the definition of obsessions (unwelcome and distressing ideas, thoughts, images, or impulses that repeatedly enter your mind) and of compulsions (behaviors or acts that you feel driven to perform although you may recognize them as senseless or excessive). The interviewer should also describe some examples of obsessions and compulsions, and be sure the patient understands both concepts. The first five items of the Y-BOCS are devoted to assessment of obsessions, while the last five items are devoted to assessment of compulsions. A Y-BOCS symptom check-list exists as an aid to identify current symptoms. Strengths of the Y-BOCS include its brevity and ease of administration, although its use is limited by being well studied only in populations with diagnosed OCD. Unlike many other scales that evaluate obsessional symptoms, the Y-BOCS is able to measure the severity of OCD symptoms that are not influenced by the type or number of obsessions or compulsions present.

GENERAL APPLICATIONS

The Y-BOCS is a widely used scale to assess severity and change over time in symptoms of obsessive compulsive disorder.

SELECTED PSYCHOMETRIC PROPERTIES

The authors have reported an interrater reliability of the Y-BOCS of 0.72-0.98. Intraclass correlation has been reported as 0.80.

REFERENCES

Goodman WK, Price LH, Rasmussen SA, et al, "The Yale-Brown Obsessive Compulsive Scale. I: Development, Use, and Reliability," *Arch Gen Psychiatry*, 1989, 46(11):1006-11.

Goodman WK, Price LH, Rasmussen SA, et al, "The Yale-Brown Obsessive Compulsive Scale. II: Validity," *Arch Gen Psychiatry*, 1989; 46(11):1012-6.

COPYRIGHT

Wayne K Goodman, MD
Department of Psychiatry
University of Florida
College of Medicine
Department of Psychiatry
PO Box 100256
Gainesville, FL 32610
Individuals wishing to purchase copies of the scale must contact Dr Goodman

J. YALE-BROWN OBSESSIVE COMPULSIVE SCALE (Y-BOCS)
(Continued)

SCALE GENERALLY DONE BY

Clinician or trained rater

TIME TO COMPLETE SCALE

20 minutes

REPRESENTATIVE STUDY UTILIZING SCALE

Von Ranson KM, Kaye WH, Weltzin TE, et al, "Obsessive-Compulsive Disorder Symptoms Before and After Recovery From Bulimia Nervosa," *Am J Psychiatry*, 1999, 156(11):1703-8.

YALE-BROWN OBSESSIVE COMPULSIVE SCALE (Y-BOCS)

(SAMPLE ENTRIES)

1. TIME OCCUPIED BY OBSESSIVE THOUGHTS

   Q. How much of your time is occupied by obsessive thoughts? [When obsessions occur as brief, intermittent intrusions, it may be difficult to assess time occupied by them in terms of total hours. In such cases, estimate time by determining how frequently they occur. Consider both the number of times the intrusions occur and how many hours of the day are affected. Ask]: How frequently do the obsessive thoughts occur? [Be sure to exclude ruminations and preoccupations which, unlike obsessions, are ego-syntonic and rational (but exaggerated).]

   - 0 = None
   - 1 = Mild, less than 1 hr/day or occasional intrusion
   - 2 = Moderate, 1 to 3 hrs/day or frequent intrusion
   - 3 = Severe, greater than 3 and up to 8 hrs/day or very frequent intrusion
   - 4 = Extreme, greater than 8 hrs/day or near constant intrusion

1b. OBSESSION-FREE INTERVAL (not included in total score)

   Q. On the average, what is the longest number of consecutive waking hours per day that you are completely free of obsessive thoughts? [If necessary, ask:] What is the longest block of time in which obsessive thoughts are absent?

   - 0 = No symptoms
   - 1 = Long symptom-free interval, more than 8 consecutive hours/day symptom-free
   - 2 = Moderately long symptom-free interval, more than 3 and up to 8 consecutive hours/day symptom-free
   - 3 = Short symptom-free interval, from 1 to 3 consecutive hours/day symptom-free
   - 4 = Extremely short symptom-free interval, less than 1 consecutive hour/day symptom-free

2. INTERFERENCE DUE TO OBSESSIVE THOUGHTS (not included in total score)

   Q. How much do your obsessive thoughts interfere with your social or work (or role) functioning? Is there anything that you don't do because of them? [If currently not working, determine how much performance would be affected if patients were employed.]

   - 0 = None
   - 1 = Mild, slight interference with social or occupational activities, but overall performance not impaired.
   - 2 = Moderate, definite interference with social or occupational performance, but still manageable
   - 3 = Severe, causes substantial impairment in social or occupational performance
   - 4 = Extreme, incapacitating

3. DISTRESS ASSOCIATED WITH OBSESSIVE THOUGHTS

   Q. How much distress do your obsessive thoughts cause you?
   [In most cases, distress is equated with anxiety; however, patients may report that their obsessions are "disturbing" but deny "anxiety." Only rate anxiety that seems triggered by obsessions, not generalized anxiety or anxiety associated with other conditions.]

   - 0 = None
   - 1 = Mild, not too disturbing
   - 2 = Moderate, disturbing, but still manageable
   - 3 = Severe, very disturbing
   - 4 = Extreme, near constant and disabling distress

IV. PANIC DISORDER

K. ACUTE PANIC INVENTORY (API)

OVERVIEW

The API is a 17-item scale developed by M Liebowitz et al, to evaluate the symptoms experienced by individuals during panic attacks. These are primarily somatic symptoms such as palpitations, rapid/difficult breathing, or sweating. Each item is rated on a 0 to 3 severity spectrum (0 = none, 3 = severe). There is an overall score, which is the sum of all rated items. Strengths of the scale include its brevity and ease of administration; however, the scale does not evaluate duration and number of panic attacks.

GENERAL APPLICATIONS

The API measures the characteristics and severity of panic attacks.

SELECTED PSYCHOMETRIC PROPERTIES

Limited psychometric data is available. The authors have reported that the scale is able to differentiate individuals with panic disorder from normals.

REFERENCES

Liebowitz MR, Fyer AJ, Gorman JM, et al, "Lactate Provocation of Panic Attacks. I. Clinical and Behavioral Findings," *Arch Gen Psychiat*, 1984, 41(8):764-70.

COPYRIGHT

Dr Michael Liebowitz
New York State Psychiatric Institute
722 W 168th St
New York, NY 10032

SCALE GENERALLY DONE BY

Clinician or trained rater

TIME TO COMPLETE SCALE

10-15 minutes

REPRESENTATIVE STUDY UTILIZING SCALE

Bandelow B, Wedekind D, Pauls J, et al, "Salivary Cortisol in Panic Attacks," *Am J Psychiatry*, 2000, 157(3):454-6.

ACUTE PANIC INVENTORY SCALE (API)

Symptom Rating Scale:
0 = No
1 = Slight
2 = Moderate
3 = Severe

Symptoms	#1	#2	#3	#4	#5	#6	#7	#8	#9
1. Do you feel faint?									
2. Are you afraid of dying?									
3. Are you afraid in general?									
4. Do you have palpitations?									
5. Is it hard for you to breathe or catch your breath?									
6. Do you have an urge to urinate?									
7. Do you have an urge to defecate?									
8. Do you feel dizzy or lightheaded?									
9. Do you feel confused at all?									
10. Do things and people seem unreal?									
11. Do you feel detached from part or all of your body?									
12. Is it hard for you to concentrate?									
13. Are you sweating at all?									
14. Is it difficult for you to speak?									
15. Would it be difficult for you to do your job (apart from being hooked up now)?									
16. Do you have any twitching, trembling, or inner shakiness?									
17. Do you feel nauseous, queasy?									
18. Are you afraid of going crazy?									
19. Are you afraid of losing control?									
20. Do you have any tingling?									
21. Are you experiencing any chest pain or discomfort?									
22. Do you have any difficulty in swallowing?									
23. Is your mouth dry?									
24. Do you feel weak?									
25. Do you have a desire to flee?									
26. Do you feel depressed?									
27. Do you feel you will embarrass or humiliate yourself?									

Anxiety and Apprehension Scales

BREATHLESS (Rating: 0-10)									
ANXIETY (Rating: 1-10)									
APPREHENSION (Rating: 1-10)									

L. SHEEHAN PATIENT-RATED ANXIETY SCALE (SPRAS)

OVERVIEW

The SPRAS, developed by D Sheehan, is a 35-item, patient-rated scale, which evaluates severity of symptoms in individuals with panic disorder. Items are rated on a 5-point spectrum ranging from "not at all" (least symptomatic) to "extremely" (most symptomatic). The scale is heavily weighted towards somatic symptoms of panic disorder such as choking sensation or lump in throat and episodes of diarrhea; however, there are also items that evaluate sleep problems, depression, mood swings, and obsessions and compulsions. There are 4 specific items which evaluate anxiety attacks: Situational anxiety, unexpected anxiety, unexpected limited symptoms attack, and anticipatory anxiety. Advantages of the scale include its ease of administration with no staff time required.

GENERAL APPLICATIONS

The SPRAS is a patient-rated scale to evaluate severity of panic disorder.

SELECTED PSYCHOMETRIC PROPERTIES

Interrater reliability and reliability over time (1-week intervals) have been reported to be acceptably high. The SPRAS is highly correlated with the HAM-A *on page 38*.

REFERENCES

Sheehan DV and Harnett-Sheehan K, "Psychometric Assessment of Anxiety Disorders," Ch 8, *Anxiety Psychobiolgoical and Clinical Perspectives*, Sartorius N, Andreoli V, Cassano G, et al, eds, Washington DC: Hemisphere Publishing Corp, 1990, 85-100.

Sheehan DV, "Appendix 2. The Sheehan Patient Rated Anxiety Scale," *J Clin Psychiatry*, 1999, 60(Suppl 18):63-4.

COPYRIGHT

David V Sheehan, MD, MBA
University of South Florida
Institute for Research in Psychiatry
3515 East Fletcher Avenue
Tampa, FL 33613-4788
Tel: 813-974-4544

SCALE GENERALLY DONE BY

Self-rated by patient

TIME TO COMPLETE SCALE

15 minutes

REPRESENTATIVE STUDY UTILIZING SCALE

Sheehan DV, Raj AB, Harnett-Sheehan K, et al, "The Relative Efficacy of High Dose Buspirone and Alprazolam in the Treatment of Panic Disorder. A Double-Blind Placebo Controlled Study," *Acta Psychiatrica Scand*, 1993, 88(1):1-11.

SHEEHAN PATIENT RATED ANXIETY SCALE

INSTRUCTIONS: Below is a list of problems and complaints that people sometimes have. This scale asks about how you have felt during THE PAST WEEK. Mark only one box for each problem, and do not skip any items.

DURING THE PAST WEEK, HOW MUCH DID YOU SUFFER FROM. . .	Not At All	A Little	Moderately	Markedly	Extremely
1. Difficulty in getting your breath, smothering, or overbreathing.	☐	☐	☐	☐	☐
2. Choking sensation or lump in throat.	☐	☐	☐	☐	☐
3. Skipping, racing, or pounding of your heart.	☐	☐	☐	☐	☐
4. Chest pain, pressure, or discomfort.	☐	☐	☐	☐	☐
5. Bouts of excessive sweating.	☐	☐	☐	☐	☐
6. Faintness, lightheadedness, or dizzy spells.	☐	☐	☐	☐	☐
7. Sensation of rubbery or "jelly" legs.	☐	☐	☐	☐	☐
8. Feeling off balance or unsteady like you might fall.	☐	☐	☐	☐	☐
9. Nausea or stomach problems.	☐	☐	☐	☐	☐
10. Feeling that things around you are strange, unreal, foggy, or detached from you.	☐	☐	☐	☐	☐
11. Feeling outside or detached from part or all of your body, or a floating feeling.	☐	☐	☐	☐	☐
12. Tingling or numbness in parts of your body.	☐	☐	☐	☐	☐
13. Hot flashes or cold chills.	☐	☐	☐	☐	☐
14. Shaking or trembling.	☐	☐	☐	☐	☐
15. Having a fear that you are dying or that something terrible is about to happen.	☐	☐	☐	☐	☐
16. Feeling you are losing control or going insane.	☐	☐	☐	☐	☐
17. SITUATIONAL ANXIETY ATTACK Sudden anxiety attacks with 4 or more of the symptoms listed previously that occur when you are in or about to go into a situation that is likely, from your experience, to bring on an attack.	☐	☐	☐	☐	☐

L. SHEEHAN PATIENT-RATED ANXIETY SCALE (SPRAS) *(Continued)*

SHEEHAN PATIENT RATED ANXIETY SCALE *(continued)*

DURING THE PAST WEEK, HOW MUCH DID YOU SUFFER FROM...	Not At All	A Little	Moderately	Markedly	Extremely
18. UNEXPECTED ANXIETY ATTACK Sudden unexpected anxiety attacks with 4 or more symptoms (listed previously) that occur with little or no provocation (ie, when you are NOT in a situation that is likely, from your experience, to bring on an attack).	☐	☐	☐	☐	☐
19. UNEXPECTED LIMITED SYMPTOM ATTACK Sudden unexpected spells with only one or two symptoms (listed previously) that occur with little or no provocation (ie, when you are NOT in a situation that is likely, from your experience, to bring on an attack).	☐	☐	☐	☐	☐
20. ANTICIPATORY ANXIETY EPISODE Anxiety episodes that build up as you anticipate doing something that is likely, from your experience, to bring on anxiety that is more intense than most people experience in such situations.	☐	☐	☐	☐	☐
21. Avoiding situations because they frighten you.	☐	☐	☐	☐	☐
22. Being dependent on others.	☐	☐	☐	☐	☐
23. Tension and inability to relax.	☐	☐	☐	☐	☐
24. Anxiety, nervousness, restlessness.	☐	☐	☐	☐	☐
25. Spells of increased sensitivity to sound, light, or touch.	☐	☐	☐	☐	☐
26. Attacks of diarrhea.	☐	☐	☐	☐	☐
27. Worrying about your health too much.	☐	☐	☐	☐	☐
28. Feeling tired, weak, and exhausted easily.	☐	☐	☐	☐	☐
29. Headaches or pains in neck or head.	☐	☐	☐	☐	☐
30. Difficulty in falling asleep.	☐	☐	☐	☐	☐
31. Waking in the middle of the night, or restless sleep.	☐	☐	☐	☐	☐
32. Unexpected waves of depression occurring with little or no provocatoin.	☐	☐	☐	☐	☐
33. Emotions and moods going up and down a lot in response to changes around you.	☐	☐	☐	☐	☐
34. Recurrent and persistent ideas, thoughts, impulses, or images that are intrusive, unwanted, senseless, or repugnant.	☐	☐	☐	☐	☐
35. Having to repeat the same action in a ritual (eg, checking, washing, counting repeatedly) when it's not really necessary.	☐	☐	☐	☐	☐

V. POST-TRAUMATIC STRESS DISORDER

M. CLINICIAN-ADMINISTERED PTSD SCALE (CAPS)

OVERVIEW

The Clinician-Administered PTSD Scale is a scale developed by researchers in the Veterans Affairs Medical Center System to assess the type and severity of DSM-III-R post-traumatic stress disorder symptoms. The basic CAPS consists of 17 items rated by the interviewer and covering the symptoms of PTSD according to the DSM criterions B, C, D. For criterion B, the persistent re-experience of events such as intrusive thoughts, dreams, flashbacks, psychological distress, and physiological reactivity to cues. For criterion C, the persistent avoidance of stimuli such as thoughts, activities, places; the inability to recall important aspects of the trauma; decreased interest in activities; feelings of detachment; restricted range of affect; pessimism about the future. For criterion D, the persistent symptoms of arousal shown as problems with sleeping, anger, concentration, hypervigilance, and an exaggerated startle response. For each of these items, the rater scores the frequency using a scale from 0 to 4 in which 0 is never, 1 is once or twice, 2 is once or twice a week, 3 is several times a week, and 4 is daily or almost every day. The rater will also score the same items, according to the intensity, using a scale from 0 to 4 in which 0 is no, 1 is mild, 2 is moderate, 3 is severe, and 4 is extreme. For criterion A, the patient is asked by the interviewer about the traumatic event. For criterion E, the patient is asked about the duration of the disturbance. For criterion F, the patient is asked about subjective distress with ratings from 0 to 4 according to the severity of the distress, the impairment in social functioning, and the impairment in occupational or other areas of functioning. The CAPS also has Global ratings that evaluate the global validity and the global severity of the symptoms. The CAPS will not only assess the type and severity of the PTSD symptoms but also can be scored according to the DSM diagnostic criteria providing a score signaling the presence or absence of the disorder. Despite the fact that the CAPS was developed to be utilized in military personnel, it is considered appropriate for the evaluation of other kinds of trauma. The full CAPS interview takes 50-60 minutes to complete by an interviewer with some clinical experience.

GENERAL APPLICATIONS

The CAPS is used to evaluate the type and severity of PTSD symptoms.

SELECTED PSYCHOMETRIC PROPERTIES

The CAPS interview is a psychometrically proven instrument that has been utilized in military and civilian populations exposed to different types of trauma. It has a high internal consistency with Cronbach's alphas ranging from 0.76 to 0.88. The CAPS correlates well with other measurements of PTSD including the Impact of Event Scale (IES) and the MMPI. The CAPS also appears sensitive to symptom improvement and has been utilized with different traumas, different populations, and clinical trials with different medications.

REFERENCES

Blake DD, Weathers FW, Nagy LM, et al, "A Clinician Rating Scale for Assessing Current and Lifetime PTSD: The CAPS-1," *Behav Therapist*, 1990, 13:187-8.

Malekzai AS, Niazi JM, Paige SR, et al, "Modification of CAPS-1 for Diagnosis of PTSD in Afghan Refugees," *J Trauma Stress*, 1996, 9(4):891-8.

V. POST-TRAUMATIC STRESS DISORDER *(Continued)*

COPYRIGHT

The CAPS was developed by the Veterans Administration, a governmental agency, therefore, it is in the public domain. The CAPS and its manual are available from the National Center for PTSD.
Terence M. Keane, PhD
National Center for PTSD
VA Boston Health Care System
150 South Huntington Avenue
Boston, MA 02130
e-mail: terry.keane@med.va.gov

SCALE GENERALLY DONE BY

Clinician or trained rater

TIME TO COMPLETE SCALE

50-60 minutes

REPRESENTATIVE STUDY UTILIZING SCALE

Elhai JD, Frueh BC, Davis JL, et al, "Clinical Presentations in Combat Veterans Diagnosed With Post-Traumatic Stress Disorder," *J Clin Psychol*, 2003, 59(3):385-97.

SAMPLE ENTRIES
of the

CLINICIAN-ADMINISTERED PTSD SCALE FOR DSM-IV
One Week Symptom Status Version
(CAPS-SX)

Criterion B. The traumatic event is persistently re-experienced in one (or more) of the following ways:

1. (B-1) recurrent and intrusive distressing recollections of the event, including images, thoughts, or perceptions. Note: In young children, repetitive play may occur in which themes or aspects of the trauma are expressed.

Frequency	*Intensity*	*Past week*
In the past week have you had unwanted memories of (EVENT)? What were they like? *(What did you remember?)* [IF NOT CLEAR:] *(Did they ever occur while you were awake, or only in dreams?)* [EXCLUDE IF MEMORIES OCCURRED ONLY DURING DREAMS] *How often?* 0　Never 1　Once 2　Two or three times 3　Four or five times 4　Daily or almost every day *Description/Examples*	**How much distress or discomfort did these memories cause you? Were you able to put them out of your mind and think about something else?** *(How hard did you have to try?)* **How much did they interfere with your life?** 0　None 1　Mild, minimal distress or disruption of activities 2　Moderate, distress clearly present but still manageable, some disruption of activities 3　Severe, considerable distress, difficulty dismissing memories, marked disruption of activities 4　Extreme, incapacitating distress, cannot dismiss memories, unable to continue activities *QV (specify)* _____	F _____ I _____

Criterion C. Persistent avoidance of stimuli associated with the trauma and numbing of general responsiveness (not present before the trauma), as indicated by three (or more) of the following:

10. (C-5) feeling of detachment or estrangement from others.

Frequency	*Intensity*	*Past week*
In the past week have you felt distant or cut off from other people? What was that like? How much of the time? When did you first start to feel that way? *(After the [EVENT]?)* 0　None of the time 1　Very little of the time (less than 10%) 2　Some of the time (approx. 20-30%) 3　Much of the time (approx. 50-60%) 4　Most or all of the time (more than 80%) *Description/Examples*	**How strong were your feelings of being distant or cut off from others?** *(Who do you feel closest to? How many people do you feel comfortable talking with about personal things?)* 0　No feelings of detachment or estrangement 1　Mild, may feel "out of synch" with others 2　Moderate, feelings of detachment clearly present, but still feels some interpersonal connection 3　Severe, marked feelings of detachment or estrangement from most people, may feel close to only one or two people 4　Extreme, feels completely detached or estranged from others, not close with anyone *QV (specify)* _____ ***Trauma-related?*** *1 definite 2 probably 3 unlikely* Current _____　　Lifetime _____	F _____ I _____

69

N. DAVIDSON TRAUMA SCALE (DTS)

OVERVIEW

The DTS, developed by J Davidson, is a well-recognized scale designed to measure the severity and frequency of symptoms of post-traumatic stress disorder (PTSD). The scale may be used as a screening tool for screening trauma victims, or to assess baseline status and treatment outcomes in individuals already diagnosed with PTSD. The scale is designed to evaluate PTSD symptoms from all types of trauma including accidents, sexual/criminal assault, combat, injury, theft, and bereavement. The DTS items are rated on a 0 to 4 spectrum (0 = not at all, 4 = daily/extreme). Each item corresponds to a DSM-IV symptom of PTSD, with each item being rated in terms of both severity and frequency. There are three symptom subscales which reflect the three symptom clusters of PTSD (intrusive thoughts, avoidance, and hyperarousal). Strengths of the DTS include its brevity and ease of administration.

GENERAL APPLICATIONS

The DTS is utilized as a screening and assessment tool for PTSD symptoms.

SELECTED PSYCHOMETRIC PROPERTIES

The DTS has been shown to have good predictive properties for response to treatment and is sensitive to treatment effect.

REFERENCES

Davidson JR, Book SW, Colket JT, et al, "Assessment of a New Self-Rating Scale for Post-Traumatic Stress Disorder," *Psychol Med*, 1997, 27(1):153-60.

COPYRIGHT

Jonathan RT Davidson, MD
Multi-Health Systems, Inc
P.O. Box 950
North Tonawanda, NY 14120-0950
Tel: 1-800-456-3003

SCALE GENERALLY DONE BY

Clinician or trained rater

TIME TO COMPLETE SCALE

10 minutes

REPRESENTATIVE STUDY UTILIZING SCALE

Fauerbach JA, Lawrence JW, Munster AM, et al, "Prolonged Adjustment Difficulties Among Those with Acute Post-Traumatic Distress Following Burn Injury," *J Behav Med*, 1999, 22(4):359-78.

SAMPLE ENTRIES OF THE

DAVIDSON TRAUMA SCALE

By Jonathan R.T. Davidson, MD

Name: _____ Age: _____ Sex: ☐ Male ☐ Female

Date: _____ / _____ / _____

Please identify the trauma that is most disturbing to you.

_____

Each of the following questions asks you about a specific symptom. For each question, consider how often in the last week the symptom troubled you and how severe it was. In the two boxes beside each question, write a number from 0 - 4 to indicate the frequency and severity of the symptom.	FREQUENCY	SEVERITY
	0 = Not At All	0 = Not At All Distressing
	1 = Once Only	1 = Minimally Distressing
	2 = 2-3 Times	2 = Moderately Distressing
	3 = 4-6 Times	3 = Markedly Distressing
	4 = Everyday	4 = Extremely Distressing

1. Have you ever had painful images, memories, or thoughts of the event?

2. Have you ever had distressing dreams of the event?

3. Have you felt as though the event was recurring? Was it as if you were reliving it?

4. Have you been upset by something that reminded you of the event?

5. Have you been physically upset by reminders of the event? (This includes sweating, trembling, racing heart, shortness of breath, nausea, or diarrhea)

6. Have you been avoiding any thoughts or feelings about the event?

O. MISSISSIPPI SCALE (MSS)

OVERVIEW

The Mississippi Scale (MSS), developed by Terence M Keane and collaborators, is a self-report instrument used to evaluate the severity of symptoms in Vietnam veterans suffering from Post-Traumatic Stress Disorder (PTSD). The scale has been modified for use with civilian trauma populations by changing the references to the military. The scale has 35 items categorized in four groups: Re-experiencing, Withdrawal and Numbing, Hyperarousal, and Self-Persecution. Three of these groups are closely related to the DSM criteria for PTSD. The subjects rate the items using a 5-point Likert-type scale going from 1 = not at all true to 5 = extremely true. The total score ranges from 35-175 with a score of 107 indicating the presence of a post-traumatic stress disorder in Vietnam veterans. The authors have made the clarification that there is no clear cut-off score for other populations. Despite the fact that a cut-off score has been determined for the diagnosis of PTSD in Vietnam veterans, the authors of the scale emphasize that this is not a diagnostic scale.

GENERAL APPLICATIONS

The MSS is a self-report instrument useful in the evaluation of the symptoms of PTSD.

SELECTED PSYCHOMETRIC PROPERTIES

The MSS has a high internal consistency with Cronbach's alpha of 0.86-0.94. The test-retest reliability was high. The MSS has high validity and correlates very well with other measurements of PTSD, such as the SCID-I and the MMPI PTSD scale. The MSS also discriminates between veterans with and without PTSD.

REFERENCES

Keane TM, Caddell JM, and Taylor KL, "Mississippi Scale for Combat-Related Post-Traumatic Stress Disorder: Three Studies in Reliability and Validity," *J Consult Clin Psychol*, 1988, 56(1):85-90.

Norris FH and Perilla JL, "The Revised Civilian Mississippi Scale for PTSD: Reliability, Validity, and Cross-Language Stability," *J Trauma Stress*, 1996, 9(2):285-98.

COPYRIGHT

Terence M Keane, PhD
National Center for PTSD
VA Boston Healthcare System
150 South Huntington Avenue
Boston, MA 02130
Tel: 617-232-9500, ext 4143
e-mail: terry.Keane@med.va.gov

SCALE GENERALLY DONE BY

Self-report scale

TIME TO COMPLETE SCALE

10-20 minutes

REPRESENTATIVE STUDY UTILIZING SCALE

Shalev AY, Peri T, Canetti L, et al, "Predictors of PTSD in Injured Trauma Survivors: A Prospective Study," *Am J Psychiatry*, 1996, 153(2):219-25.

MISSISSIPPI SCALE FOR COMBAT-RELATED POST-TRAUMATIC STRESS DISORDER

Please circle the number that best describes how you feel about each statement.

1. Before I entered the military, I had more close friends than I have now.

1	2	3	4	5
Not at all true	Slightly true	Somewhat true	Very true	Extremely true

2. I do not feel guilt over things that I did in the military.

1	2	3	4	5
Never true	Rarely true	Sometimes true	Usually true	Always true

3. If someone pushes me too far, I am likely to become violent.

1	2	3	4	5
Very unlikely	Unlikely	Somewhat unlikely	Very likely	Extremely likely

4. If something happens that reminds me of the military, I become very distressed and upset.

1	2	3	4	5
Never	Rarely	Sometimes	Frequently	Very frequently

5. The people who know me best are afraid of me.

1	2	3	4	5
Never	Rarely	Sometimes	Frequently	Very frequently

6. I am able to get emotionally close to others.

1	2	3	4	5
Never	Rarely	Sometimes	Frequently	Very frequently

7. I have nightmares of experiences in the military that really happened.

1	2	3	4	5
Never	Rarely	Sometimes	Frequently	Very frequently

8. When I think of some of the things I did in the military, I wish I were dead.

1	2	3	4	5
Never true	Rarely true	Sometimes true	Frequently true	Very frequently true

9. It seems as if I have no feelings.

1	2	3	4	5
Not at all true	Rarely true	Sometimes true	Frequently true	Very frequently true

O. MISSISSIPPI SCALE (MSS) *(Continued)*

10. Lately, I have felt like killing myself.

1	2	3	4	5
Not at all true	Slightly true	Somewhat true	Very true	Extremely true

11. I fall asleep, stay asleep and awaken only when the alarm goes off.

1	2	3	4	5
Never	Rarely	Sometimes	Frequently	Very frequently

12. I wonder why I am still alive when others died in the military.

1	2	3	4	5
Never	Rarely	Sometimes	Frequently	Very frequently

13. Being in certain situations makes me feel as though I am back in the military.

1	2	3	4	5
Never	Rarely	Sometimes	Frequently	Very frequently

14. My dreams at night are so real that I waken in a cold sweat and force myself to stay awake.

1	2	3	4	5
Never	Rarely	Sometimes	Frequently	Very frequently

15. I feel like I cannot go on.

1	2	3	4	5
Not at all true	Rarely true	Sometimes true	Very true	Almost always true

16. I do not laugh or cry at the same things other people do.

1	2	3	4	5
Not at all true	Rarely true	Somewhat true	Very true	Extremely true

17. I still enjoy doing many things that I used to enjoy.

1	2	3	4	5
Never true	Rarely true	Sometimes true	Very true	Always true

18. Daydreams are very real and frightening.

1	2	3	4	5
Never true	Rarely true	Sometimes true	Frequently true	Very frequently true

19. I have found it easy to keep a job since my separation from the military.

1	2	3	4	5
Not at all true	Slightly true	Somewhat true	Very true	Extremely true

20. I have trouble concentrating on tasks.

1	2	3	4	5
Never true	Rarely true	Sometimes true	Frequently true	Very frequently true

21. I have cried for no good reason.

1	2	3	4	5
Never true	Rarely true	Sometimes true	Frequently true	Very frequently true

22. I enjoy the company of others.

1	2	3	4	5
Never true	Rarely true	Sometimes true	Frequently true	Very frequently true

23. I am frightened by my urges.

1	2	3	4	5
Never true	Rarely true	Sometimes true	Frequently true	Very frequently true

24. I fall asleep easily at night.

1	2	3	4	5
Never true	Rarely true	Sometimes true	Frequently true	Very frequently true

25. Unexpected noises make me jump.

1	2	3	4	5
Never true	Rarely true	Sometimes true	Frequently true	Very frequently true

26. No one understands how I feel, not even my family.

1	2	3	4	5
Not at all true	Rarely true	Somewhat true	Very true	Extremely true

27. I am an easy-going, even-tempered person.

1	2	3	4	5
Never	Rarely	Sometimes	Usually	Very much so

28. I feel there are certain things that I did in the military that I can never tell anyone, because no one would ever understand.

1	2	3	4	5
Not at all true	Slightly true	Somewhat true	True	Very true

O. MISSISSIPPI SCALE (MSS) *(Continued)*

29. There have been times when I used alcohol (or other drugs) to help me sleep or to make me forget about things that happened while I was in the service.

1	2	3	4	5
Never	Infrequently	Sometimes	Frequently	Very frequently

30. I feel comfortable when I am in a crowd.

1	2	3	4	5
Never	Rarely	Sometimes	Usually	Always

31. I lose my cool and explode over minor everyday things.

1	2	3	4	5
Never	Rarely	Sometimes	Frequently	Very frequently

32. I am afraid to go to sleep at night.

1	2	3	4	5
Never	Rarely	Sometimes	Frequently	Almost always

33. I try to stay away from anything that will remind me of things which happened while I was in the military.

1	2	3	4	5
Never	Rarely	Sometimes	Frequently	Almost always

34. My memory is as good as it ever was.

1	2	3	4	5
Not at all true	Rarely true	Somewhat true	Usually true	Almost always

35. I have a hard time expressing my feelings, even to the people I care about.

1	2	3	4	5
Not at all true	Rarely true	Somewhat true	Usually true	Almost always

Reprinted by permission of Dr. Terence Keane.

P. POST-TRAUMATIC STRESS DIAGNOSTIC SCALE (PDS®)

OVERVIEW

The Post-Traumatic Stress Diagnostic Scale (PDS®) was developed by EB Foa and collaborators as an instrument to obtain a reliable diagnosis and to evaluate the symptoms of PTSD. The instrument is a self-report scale with 49 items organized in 4 sections. The first section has a list of different types of trauma, in section 2 the subject describes the type of trauma suffered, and part 3 has the symptoms according to the DSM-IV. These symptoms are rated according to frequency on a scale from 0-3. Part 4 rates the interference caused by the different symptoms in such areas as work, relationships with family, and recreational activities. The score is obtained by adding the scores of the 17 symptoms items.

GENERAL APPLICATIONS

The PDS® provides a diagnosis, profile of symptoms, symptom severity, and a level of impairment associated with PTSD.

SELECTED PSYCHOMETRIC PROPERTIES

The reliability provided by the authors is good. The internal consistency of the 17 items measuring symptom severity is excellent. The Cronbach's alphas were 0.92 for the total scale. Test-retest reliability is reported as satisfactory (kappa 0.74). The validity of the scale is good and the authors report a good correlation with the SCID-I and other PTSD scales with the problem that the PDS also correlates well with anxiety and depression scales.

REFERENCES

Foa EB, *Post-Traumatic Stress Diagnostic Scale: Manual*, Minneapolis, MN: National Computer Systems, 1995.

Foa EB, Cahman L, Jaycox L, et al, "The Validation of a Self-Report Measure of Post-Traumatic Stress Disorder: The Post-Traumatic Diagnostic Scale," *Psychol Assess*, 1997, 9:445-51.

COPYRIGHT

NCS Pearson, Inc
5601 Green Valley Drive
Bloomington, MN 55437
Tel: 952-681-3344

SCALE GENERALLY DONE BY

Self-report scale

TIME TO COMPLETE SCALE

10-15 minutes

REPRESENTATIVE STUDY UTILIZING SCALE

Ford BC, "Violence and Trauma: Predicting the Impact on the Well-Being of African American Women With Severe Mental Illness," *Violence Vict*, 2002, 17(2):219-32.

P. POST-TRAUMATIC STRESS DIAGNOSTIC SCALE (PDS®) *(Continued)*

SAMPLE ENTRIES OF THE
PDS®

Part 1

Many people have lived through or witnessed a very stressful and traumatic event at some point in their lives. Below is a list of traumatic events. Put a checkmark in the box next to ALL of the events that have happened to you or that you have witnessed.

(3) ☐ Nonsexual assault by a family member or someone you know (for example, being mugged, physically attacked, shot, stabbed, or held at gunpoint)

Part 2

(14) If you marked more than one traumatic event in Part 1, put a checkmark in the box below next to the event *that bothers you the most*. If you marked only ～e traumatic event in Part 1, mark the same one below.

☐ Accident
☐ Disaster
☐ Nonsexual assault/someone you know
☐ Nonsexual assault/stranger
☐ Sexual assault/someone you know
☐ Sexual assault/stranger
☐ Combat
☐ Sexual contact under 18 with s～eon～ ～nore years older
☐ Imprisonment
☐ Torture
☐ Life-threatening illness
☐ Other

In the box below, bri～ ～escribe ～ traumatic event you marked above.

Part 3

Below is a list of problems that people sometimes have after experiencing a traumatic event. Read each one carefully and circle the number (0-3) that best describes how often that problem has bothered you IN THE PAST MONTH. Rate each problem with respect to the traumatic event you described in Item 14.

0 Not at all or only one time
1 Once a week or less / once in a while
2 2 to 4 times a week / half the time
3 5 or more times a week / almost always

(28) **0 1 2 3** Trying to avoid activities, people, or places that remind you of the traumatic event

DEPRESSION

RATING SCALES

TABLE OF CONTENTS

A. BECK DEPRESSION INVENTORY (BDI)

OVERVIEW

The BDI, developed by A Beck, is a rating to measure the severity of depression. Unlike many other scales for depression, such as the HAM-D *on page 100* and the MADRS *on page 106*, the BDI is a self-rated scale, in which individuals rate their own symptoms of depression. The BDI is a 21-item scale which evaluates key symptoms of depression including mood, pessimism, sense of failure, self-dissatisfaction, guilt, punishment, self-dislike, self-accusation, suicidal ideas, crying, irritability, social withdrawal, indecisiveness, body image change, work difficulty, insomnia, fatigability, loss of appetite, weight loss, somatic preoccupation, and loss of libido. Individuals are asked to rate themselves on a 0 to 3 spectrum (0 = least, 3 = most), with a score range of 0 to 63. Total score is a sum of all items. There are two subscales of the BDI, including a cognitive-affective subscale and a somatic-performance subscale. The cognitive-affective subscale may be particularly useful for the evaluation of depression in the elderly or medically ill, and in those with substance abuse. Strengths of the BDI include its brevity and lack of clinician/staff time required for administration. When evaluating change in depression severity over time, ideally, the BDI should be paired with an observer-rated scale.

GENERAL APPLICATIONS

The BDI is a self-rated scale to evaluate depression severity.

SELECTED PSYCHOMETRIC PROPERTIES

The authors have reported that the average internal-consistency estimates of the total scores were 0.86 for psychiatric patients. The average correlation of the BDI score with clinical ratings of depression was >0.60 for both psychiatric patients and for normal adults.

REFERENCES

Beck AT, Steer RA, and Garbing MG, "Psychometric Properties of the Beck Depression Inventory: Twenty-Five Years of Evaluation," *Clin Psychol Rev*, 1988, 8:77-100.

Beck AT and Steer RA, *Manual for the Beck Depression Inventory*, San Antonio: Psychological Corporation, 1993.

COPYRIGHT

Aaron T Beck, MD
The Psychological Corporation
555 Academic Court
San Antonio, TX 78204-2498
Tel: 1-800-211-8378

SCALE GENERALLY DONE BY

Self-rated scale

TIME TO COMPLETE SCALE

5-10 minutes

REPRESENTATIVE STUDY UTILIZING SCALE

Hellerstein DJ, Batchelder ST, Little SA, et al, "Venlafaxine in the Treatment of Dysthymia: An Open-Label Study," *J Clin Psychiatry*, 1999, 60(12):845-9.

B. CARROLL DEPRESSION SCALE (CDS-R, CRS)

OVERVIEW

The Carroll Depression Scale, developed by B Carroll et al, is a 61-item instrument to evaluate severity of depression in adults. This includes diagnoses of major depression, dysthymic disorder, depression with melancholic features, and depression with atypical features. A revised form of the scale is currently available. The most current version of the CDS is a revision of the original 52-item CDS. Items are rated as "yes" or "no". There is also a brief form of the Carroll depression scale which is useful as a screening tool for depressive symptoms and which requires less than 5 minutes to administer. The CDS is offered by a commercial publisher, and a computerized version with manuals and scoring forms is also available.

GENERAL APPLICATIONS

The Carroll Depression Scale is appropriate for evaluating baseline depressive symptoms and treatment response over time. The brief version of the scale is used as a screening tool.

SELECTED PSYCHOMETRIC PROPERTIES

The CDS correlates well with other commonly utilized depression rating scales, such as the HAM-D *on page 100* and the BDI *on page 80*. Correlation of the CDS with the HAM-D has been reported to be good (r = 0.71), while correlation with the self-rated BDI was even better (r = 0.86). Individual items of the CDS have a median correlation of 0.55 with the total CDS score.

REFERENCES

Carroll BJ, Feinberg M, Smouse PE, et al, "The Carroll Rating Scale for Depression. I. Development, Reliability and Validation," *Br J Psychiatry*, 1981, 138:194-200.

COPYRIGHT

Bernard Carroll, PhD
Multi-Health Systems Incorporated
P.O. Box 950
North Tonawanda, NY 14120-0950
Tel: 1-800-456-3003

SCALE GENERALLY DONE BY

Self-rated by patient

TIME TO COMPLETE SCALE

20 minutes

REPRESENTATIVE STUDY UTILIZING SCALE

Senra C, "Evaluation and Monitoring of Symptom Severity and Change in Depressed Outpatients," *J Clin Psychol*, 1996, 52(3):317-24.

B. CARROLL DEPRESSION SCALE (CDS-R, CRS) *(Continued)*

SAMPLE ENTRIES OF THE
CDS-R

Bernard Carroll, MG, PhD, FRC Psych

Name: _____   Sex: ☐ Male ☐ Female

Date of Birth: _____ / _____ / _____   Today's Date: _____ / _____ / _____

<u>Instructions:</u> Complete all of the following statements by circling "YES   .O" ba   on how you
have felt during the PAST FEW DAYS.

1. I feel just as energetic as always	**YES**	**NO**
2. I am losing weight	**YES**	**NO**
3. I have dropped many of my intere ts and iv.	**YES**	**NO**
11. I wake up much earlier than I need the orning	**YES**	**NO**
12. Dying is the best solution r m	**YES**	**NO**
16. I am miser. a c l li e crying	**YES**	**NO**

C. CORNELL DYSTHYMIA RATING SCALE (CDRS)

OVERVIEW

The Cornell Dysthymia Rating Scale (CDRS), developed by B Mason et al, is designed to evaluate the milder symptoms of chronically depressed outpatients. This is in comparison to the more severe symptoms of depression found in individuals with major depressive disorder. Individuals with chronic, milder depression/dysthymia often lack the typical neurovegetative symptoms of major depression, but may experience such symptoms as poor self-esteem and social withdrawal, which may cause substantial impairment or diminished quality of life. The CDRS is a 20-item clinician rated scale, with well-defined anchor points for each item. Items are rated on a 0 to 4 spectrum (0 = not at all, 4 = severe). Raters are instructed to assess both frequency and severity of symptoms, initially from the two-week period prior to baseline, and then over the duration of each subsequent rating period.

GENERAL APPLICATIONS

The CDRS is used to evaluate baseline severity of dysthymia and change in symptoms over time.

SELECTED PSYCHOMETRIC PROPERTIES

As reported by the authors, the CDRS shows greater breadth in the range of individual item and sum score compared to the HAM-D in a sample of dysthymic patients rated with both scale. Convergent validity of the CDRS is good, with CDRS total scores significantly correlated with HAM-D scores at baseline ($r = 0.65$) and in terms of change scores ($r = 0.80$).

REFERENCES

Mason BJ, Kocsis JH, Leon AC, et al, "Measurement of Severity and Treatment Response in Dysthymia," *Psych Ann*, 1993, 23:625-31.

COPYRIGHT

Barbara J Mason, PhD
Alcohol Disorders Research Clinic
Department of Psychiatry and Behavioral Sciences
1400 NW 10th Avenue, Suite 307A (D-79)
Miami, FL 33136

SCALE GENERALLY DONE BY

Clinician or trained rater

TIME TO COMPLETE SCALE

20 minutes

REPRESENTATIVE STUDY UTILIZING SCALE

Hellerstein DJ, Batchelder ST, Little SA, et al, "Venlafaxine in the Treatment of Dysthymia: An Open-Label Study," *J Clin Psychiatry*, 1999, 60(12):845-9.

C. CORNELL DYSTHYMIA RATING SCALE (CDRS) *(Continued)*

CORNELL DYSTHYMIA RATING SCALE

INSTRUCTIONS: Rate each item for the previous week.

1. DEPRESSED MOOD:

Subjective feelings of depression based on verbal complaints of feeling depressed, sad, blue, gloomy, down in the dumps, empty, "don't care." Do not include such ideational aspects as discouragement, pessimism, and worthlessness or suicide attempts (all of which are to be rated separately).

- ☐ 0 - Not at all
- ☐ 1 - Slight, eg, only occasionally feels "sad" or "down"
- ☐ 2 - Mild, eg, often feels somewhat "depressed", "blue", or "downhearted"
- ☐ 3 - Moderate, eg, most of the time feels depressed
- ☐ 4 - Severe, eg, most of the time feels "very depressed" or "miserable"

2. LACK OF INTEREST OR PLEASURE:

Pervasive lack of interest in work, family, friends, sex, hobbies, and other leisure-time activities. Severity is determined by the number of important activities in which the subject has less interest or pleasure compared to nonpatients.

- ☐ 0 - All activities interesting/pleasurable
- ☐ 1 - 1 or 2 activities less interesting or pleasurable
- ☐ 2 - Several activities less interesting or pleasurable
- ☐ 3 - Most activities less interesting or pleasurable with 1 or 2 exceptions
- ☐ 4 - Total absence of pleasure in almost all activities

3. PESSIMISM:

Discouragement, pessimism, and hopelessness

- ☐ 0 - Not at all discouraged about the future
- ☐ 1 - Slight, eg, occasional feellings of mild discouragement about the future
- ☐ 2 - Mild, eg, often somewhat discouraged, but can usually be talked into feeling hopeful
- ☐ 3 - Moderate, eg, often feels quite pessimistic about the future and can only sometimes be talked into feeling hopeful
- ☐ 4 - Severe, eg, pervasive feelings of intense pessimism or hopelessness

4. SUICIDAL TENDENCIES:

Suicidal tendencies, including preoccupation with thoughts of death or suicide. Do not include mere fears of dying.

- ☐ 0 - Not at all
- ☐ 1 - Slight, eg, occasionally feels life is not worth living
- ☐ 2 - Mild eg, frequent thoughts that s/he would be better off dead or occasional thoughts of wishing s/he were dead
- ☐ 3 - Moderate, eg, often thinks of suicide, has thought of a specific method, or made an impulsive attempt not requiring medical attention
- ☐ 4 - Severe, eg, has made a planned attempt requiring medical intervention

5. LOW SELF-ESTEEM:

Negative evaluation of self, including feelings of inadequacy, failure, worthlessness

- ☐ 0 - Not at all
- ☐ 1 - Slight, eg, occasional feelings of inadequacy
- ☐ 2 - Mild, eg, often feels somewhat inadequate
- ☐ 3 - Moderate, eg, often feels like a failure
- ☐ 4 - Severe, eg, constant, pervasive feelings of worthlessness

6. GUILT:

Feelings of self-reproach or excessive, inappropriate guilt for things done or not done

- ☐ 0 - Not at all
- ☐ 1 - Slight, eg, occasional feelings of self-blame
- ☐ 2 - Mild, eg, often somewhat guilty about past actions, the significance of which s/he exaggerates, such as consequences of his/her illness
- ☐ 3 - Moderate, eg, often feels quite guilty about past actions or feelings of guilt which s/he can't explain
- ☐ 4 - Severe, eg, pervasive feelings of intense guilt or generalizes feelings of self-blame to many situations

7. HELPLESSNESS:

Feelings of passivity, lack of control, needing someone's assistance to get mobilized

- ☐ 0 - Not at all
- ☐ 1 - Slight and of doubtful clinical significance
- ☐ 2 - Mild, eg, of clinical significance, but only occasional and never very intense; effort to take initiative, but does so
- ☐ 3 - Moderate, eg, often aware of feeling quite helpless or occasionally feeling very helpless; missed opportunities by not taking initiative; needs a lot of coaxing or reassurance
- ☐ 4 - Marked, eg, most of the time feeling quite helpless or often feeling very helpless

8. SOCIAL WITHDRAWAL:

Lack of social contact with persons out of the home

- ☐ 0 - Not at all
- ☐ 1 - Possibly less sociable than the norm
- ☐ 2 - At times definitely avoids socializing
- ☐ 3 - Often avoids friends and social interactions
- ☐ 4 - Almost all the time avoids interpersonal contacts

9. INDECISIVENESS:

Difficulty making decisions

- ☐ 0 - Not at all
- ☐ 1 - Slight, eg, occasional difficulty making decisions
- ☐ 2 - Mild, eg, often has difficulty making decisions
- ☐ 3 - Moderate, eg, frequently ruminates excessively and feels unsure when decision making
- ☐ 4 - Severe, eg, usually unable to make even simple decisions in most situations

C. CORNELL DYSTHYMIA RATING SCALE (CDRS) *(Continued)*

10. LOW ATTENTION AND CONCENTRATION:

Distractible, unfocused, confused thinking, impaired short-term memory

- ☐ 0 - Not at all
- ☐ 1 - Occasional mild distractibility
- ☐ 2 - At times, definite difficulty concentrating
- ☐ 3 - Often has difficulty concentrating
- ☐ 4 - Almost all the time has significant difficulty paying attention and concentrating, eg, cannot retain what is read

11. PSYCHIC ANXIETY:

Subjective feelings of anxiety, fearfulness, or apprehension, excluding anxiety attacks, whether or not accompanied by somatic anxiety, and whether focused on specific concerns or not.

- ☐ 0 - Not at all
- ☐ 1 - Slight, eg, occasionally feels somewhat anxious
- ☐ 2 - At times, definitely feels anxious
- ☐ 3 - Moderate, eg, most of the time feels anxious
- ☐ 4 - Severe, eg, most of the time feels very anxious

12. SOMATIC ANXIETY:

Has been bothered by 1 or more physiological concomitants of anxiety other than during a panic attack. They include symptoms associated with panic attacks, as well as headaches, stomach cramps, diarrhea, or muscle tension. This item should be scored whether or not the subject has had panic attacks.

- ☐ 0 - Not at all or only during anxiety attacks
- ☐ 1 - Slight, eg, occasionally palms sweat excessively
- ☐ 2 - Mild, eg, often has 1 or more physical symptoms to a mild degree
- ☐ 3 - Moderate, eg, often has several symptoms or symptoms to a considerable degree
- ☐ 4 - Severe, eg, very frequently is bothered by 2 or more symptoms

13. WORRY:

Worrying, brooding, painful preoccupation and inability to get mind off unpleasant thoughts (may or may not be accompanied by depressive mood).

- ☐ 0 - Not at all
- ☐ 1 - Slight, eg, occasionally worries about some realistic problem
- ☐ 2 - Mild, eg, often worries excessively about a realistic problem or occasionally about some trivial problem
- ☐ 3 - Moderate, eg, very often worries excessively about a realistic problem and often worries about some trivial problem
- ☐ 4 - Severe, eg, most of the time is spent in worrying or brooding

14. IRRITABILITY OR EXCESSIVE ANGER:

Feelings of anger, resentment, or annoyance (directed externally) whether expressed overtly or not. Rate only the intensity and duration of the subjective mood.

- ☐ 0 - Not at all or clearly of no clinical significance
- ☐ 1 - Slight and of doubtful clinical significance
- ☐ 2 - Mild, eg, definitely more than called for by the situation but only occasional and never very intense
- ☐ 3 - Moderate, eg, often aware of snapping at others, feeling quite angry or occasionally very angry
- ☐ 4 - Marked, eg, most of the time aware of losing temper, yelling, or often feeling very angry

15. SOMATIC GENERAL:

Physical symptoms such as heaviness in limbs, back, or head, backaches, muscle aches

- ☐ 0 - Not at all
- ☐ 1 - Slight, eg, occasional backache
- ☐ 2 - Mild, eg, often has 1 or more physical symptoms to a mild degree
- ☐ 3 - Moderate, eg, often has 1 or more symptoms to a considerable degree
- ☐ 4 - Severe, eg, very frequently is bothered by 2 or more symptoms which can interfere with function

16. LOW PRODUCTIVITY:

Decreased effectiveness or productivity at school, work, or home, as compared with nonpatients

- ☐ 0 - Not at all
- ☐ 1 - Occasional decrease in functioning in 1 or 2 areas
- ☐ 2 - Frequent decrease in functioning in 1 or 2 areas
- ☐ 3 - Frequent decrease in functioning in several areas
- ☐ 4 - Decrease in functioning in almost all areas a great deal of the time

17. LOW ENERGY:

Subjective feeling of lack of energy or fatigue. (Do not confuse with lack of interest.)

- ☐ 0 - Not at all
- ☐ 1 - Probably less energy than normal
- ☐ 2 - At times, definitely more tired or less energy than normal
- ☐ 3 - Often feels tired or without energy
- ☐ 4 - Almost all the time feels very tired or without energy or spends a great deal of the time resting

18. LOW SEXUAL INTEREST, ACTIVITY:

- ☐ 0 - Not at all
- ☐ 1 - Possibly less than normal
- ☐ 2 - At times, definitely low
- ☐ 3 - Often low
- ☐ 4 - Almost all the time

19. INSOMNIA:

Sleep disturbance, including difficulty in getting to sleep, staying asleep, or sleeping too much. Take into account the estimated number of hours slept and subjective sense of adequacy of time spent sleeping. If subject is using medication, ask what he thinks it would be like without medication.

CHOOSE EITHER A OR B

A. DIFFICULTY GETTING TO SLEEP OR STAYING ASLEEP

- ☐ 0 - Not at all
- ☐ 1 - Slight, eg, occasional difficulty
- ☐ 2 - Mild, eg, often has some significant difficulty
- ☐ 3 - Moderate, eg, usually has considerable difficulty
- ☐ 4 - Marked, eg, almost always has great difficulty

B. SLEEPS TOO MUCH

- ☐ 0 - Not at all
- ☐ 1 - Slight, eg, occasional difficulty
- ☐ 2 - Mild, eg, often has some significant difficulty
- ☐ 3 - Moderate, eg, usually has considerable difficulty
- ☐ 4 - Marked, eg, almost always has great difficulty

C. CORNELL DYSTHYMIA RATING SCALE (CDRS) *(Continued)*

CHOOSE EITHER A OR B

A. WORSE IN MORNING

☐ 0 - Not worse in morning or variable

☐ 1 - Minimally, or questionably worse

20. DIURNAL MOOD VARIATION:

☐ 2 - Mildly worse

Extent to which, for at least 1 week, there is a constant fluctuation of depressed mood and other symptomatology coinciding with the first or second half of day. Generally, if the mood is worse in one part of the day, it will be better in the other. However, for occasional subjects who are better in the afternoon and worse both in the morning and evening, choose the one time that represents the greatest severity of symptoms.

☐ 3 - Moderately worse

☐ 4 - Considerably worse

B. WORSE IN EVENING

☐ 0 - Not worse in evening or variable

☐ 1 - Minimally or questionably worse

☐ 2 - Mildly worse

☐ 3 - Moderately worse

☐ 4 - Considerably worse

Rater's Name: _____   Cornell Dysthymia Score: _____

D. DEPRESSION OUTCOMES MODULE (DOM)

OVERVIEW

The Depression Outcomes Module, by G Smith et al, was developed with the assistance of a multidisciplinary group of individuals. The DOM evaluates patients with major depression and assesses their symptom severity and functioning over time. There are five components of the module: 1) The Patient Screen, 2) The Patient Baseline Assessment, 3) The Clinician Baseline Assessment, 4) The Patient Follow-up Assessment, and 5) The Medical Record Review form. Both symptoms and patient functional level are assessed. The patient screener consists of three questions and takes approximately one minute to complete.

The Patient Baseline Assessment, administered to patients who have a preliminary diagnosis of depression, has 80 items and covers verification of diagnostic criteria, measure of outcomes, and measures of prognostic variables. This includes general level of functioning, initial evaluation of depression severity, sociodemographic characteristic, number of days of hospitalization, and psychiatric history.

The Clinician Baseline Assessment has 20 items and evaluates diagnosis, prognostic characteristics, and treatment information such as psychotropic medication history. The Patient Follow-up Assessment has 83 items and provides information on treatment received since baseline. The Follow-up Assessment is intended to be repeated on a quarterly basis.

The Medical Record Review, intended to be done by a trained medical records clerk, has 11 items and is also intended to be repeated quarterly. The DOM has a user's manual and a computerized version has been developed. Strengths of the DOM include its usefulness in primary care as well as specialty mental health treatment settings.

GENERAL APPLICATIONS

The DOM measures the types of treatment received by patients with depression and evaluates outcomes of care.

SELECTED PSYCHOMETRIC PROPERTIES

The diagnostic portion of the DOM in patients has very high sensitivity (up to 100% in early studies), and a specificity of 77.8%. Depression severity correlated with clinician ratings of depression using the HAM-D, $r = 0.41$, $p < .01$. Intraclass correlation alpha for suicidality ranges from 0.56-0.70.

REFERENCES

Rost K, Smith GR, Burnam MA, et al, "Measuring the Outcomes of Care for Mental Health Problems: The Case of Depressive Disorders," *Med Care*, 1992, 30(Suppl 5):MS266-73.

Smith GR, Burnam MA, Burns BJ, et al, "The Depression Outcomes Module," University of Arkansas for Medical Sciences, Little Rock: Centers for Mental Healthcare Research, 1995.

D. DEPRESSION OUTCOMES MODULE (DOM) *(Continued)*

COPYRIGHT

G Richard Smith, Jr, MD
Centers for Mental Healthcare Research
Department of Psychiatry
University of Arkansas for Medical Sciences
5800 W. 10th St, Suite 605
Little Rock, AR 72204

SCALE GENERALLY DONE BY

Patient Baseline and Follow-up Assessment done by patient; Clinician Baseline done by clinician; and Medical Record Review done by trained clerical worker.

TIME TO COMPLETE SCALE

Patient Baseline and Follow-up Assessment each require 25 minutes; Clinician Assessment requires 5-10 minutes; and Medical Record Review requires 5-10 minutes

REPRESENTATIVE STUDY UTILIZING SCALE

Rost K, Williams C, Wherry J, et al, "The Process and Outcomes of Care for Major Depression in Rural Family Practice Settings," *J Rural Health*, 1995, 11(2):114-21.

DEPRESSION OUTCOMES MODULE:
PATIENT BASELINE ASSESSMENT

Name_____ Clinician_____

ID#_____ Site_____

Date Completed_____ Clinic Visit Date_____

INSTRUCTIONS:

This survey asks for your views about your feelings and your health. This information will be kept confidential and will help your doctors keep track of how you feel.

Answer every question by circling the appropriate number, 1, 2, 3, etc, checking off the appropriate answer, or writing a number where indicated. If you are unsure about how to answer a question, please give the best answer you can and make a comment in the **left margin.**

1. Do you have or have you had any of the following medical conditions?

	(Circle one number on each line)	YES	NO
a. Anemia		1	2
b. Arthritis or any kind of rheumatism		1	2
c. Asthma		1	2
d. Bronchitis		1	2
e. Cancer		1	2
f. Cataracts		1	2
g. Diabetes		1	2
h. Gall bladder trouble		1	2
i. Heart disease		1	2
j. High blood pressure		1	2
k. Kidney trouble		1	2
l. Lung disease		1	2
m. Migraine headaches		1	2
n. Repeated bladder disorders		1	2
o. Repeated seizures		1	2
p. Repeated stomach problems		1	2
q. Repeated trouble with neck, back, or spine		1	2
r. Stroke		1	2
s. Tuberculosis		1	2
t. Ulcer		1	2
u. Other		1	2

2. Have you ever spent any time as a patient in a hospital for mental or emotional problems?   1   2

3. Do any blood relatives (mother, father, sisters, or brothers) have a history of problems with depression or alcoholism?   1   2

4. How old were you the first time you had a period when you felt sad, blue, or depressed for **2 weeks or more?**

_____ less than 12 years old

_____ 12-18 years old

_____ 19-35 years old

_____ 36-64 years old

_____ 65 years or older

D. DEPRESSION OUTCOMES MODULE (DOM) *(Continued)*

5. Before the current episode, how many different times in your life have you had a period when you felt sad, blue, or depressed for **at least 2 weeks?**

   _____ 0

   _____ 1

   _____ 2

   _____ 3

   _____ 4 or more

   _____ I have always felt sad

		YES	NO
6.	Did this current period of feeling sad occur just after someone close to you had died?	1	2
6a.	Did you lose this person in the last two months?	1	2

7. How many people do you feel you can tell just about anything to, people you can count on for understanding or support?

   _____ people (if none, enter 0)

		(Circle one)	
		YES	NO
8.	**During the past 2 years,** have you felt depressed or sad **most days?**	1	2
9.	**During the past 2 years,** was there a period of **2 months or more** when you did **not** feel depressed or sad most days?	1	2

The following questions ask you how you have been feeling during the past 4 weeks.

10. **During the past 4 weeks,** how many days did your physical health or emotional problems keep you in bed **all or most of the day? (Your answer may range from 0 to 28 days.)**

   _____ days (if none, enter 0)

11. **During the past 4 weeks,** how many days did you cut down on the things you usually do for **one-half day or more** because of your physical health or emotional problems? **(Your answer may range from 0 to 28 days. Do not include days already counted in Question 10.)**

   _____ days (if none, enter 0)

		(Circle one)	
		YES	NO
12.	**During the past 4 weeks,** did you work at any time at a job or business not counting work around the house?	1	2
		(if no, skip to Question 14)	

13. **During the past 4 weeks,** how many days did you miss more than half of the day from your job or business because of illness or injury? **(Your answer may range from 0 to 28 days.)**

   _____ days (if none, enter 0)

14. **During the past 4 weeks,** to what extent did emotional problems interfere with your social activities?

   (Circle one)

Not at all	1
Slightly	2
Moderately	3
Quite a bit	4
Extremely	5

The following questions ask you about your daily living. Questions 15-17 are about your use of alcoholic beverages.

	(Circle one)	
	YES	**NO**
15. Did you ever think that you were an excessive drinker?	1	2

16. Have you ever drunk as much as a fifth of liquor in one day? That would be about 20 drinks, or 3 bottles of wine, or as much as 3 six-packs of beer in one day.

Yes, more than once	1
Yes, but only once	2
No	3

	(Circle one)	
	YES	**NO**
17. Has there ever been a period of 2 weeks when every day you were drinking 7 or more beers, 7 or more drinks, or 7 or more glasses of wine?	1	2
18. Have you ever used one of the drugs listed below on your own more than 5 times in your life? "On your own" means to get high or without a prescription, or more than was prescribed.	1	2

(If yes, circle drugs below. If no, skip to Question 21.)

a. **Marijuana** (hashish, pot, grass)

b. **Stimulants** (speed, amphetamines, crystal, methamphetamines)

c. **Sedatives** (barbiturates, sleeping pills, Quaaludes, Xanax, tranquilizers, Valium, Librium, red devils)

d. **Cocaine** (coke, crack)

e. **Heroin**

f. **Opiates** (Other than heroin; codeine, Demerol, morphine, methadone, Darvon, opium)

g. **Psychedelics** (LSD, mescaline, peyote, psilocybin, mushrooms, DMT)

h. **PCP**

i. **Inhalants** (glue, toluene, gasoline, paint)

j. **Other** (nitrous oxide, amyl nitrite)

	(Circle one)	
	YES	**NO**

Questions 19-20 are about any experiences you have had with the drugs and other substances listed above.

19. Did you ever find you needed larger amounts of these drugs to get an effect, or that you could no longer get high on the amount you used to use?	1	2
20. Did you ever have any emotional or psychological problems from using drugs - like feeling crazy or paranoid or depressed, or uninterested in things?	1	2

D. DEPRESSION OUTCOMES MODULE (DOM) *(Continued)*

The following questions ask you about how you have been feeling in the past 4 weeks.

21. How often **in the past 4 weeks** have you felt depressed, blue, or in low spirits for most of the day? **(Circle one)**

Not at all	1
1 to 3 days a week	2
Most days a week	3
Nearly every day for at least 2 weeks	4

22. How often **in the past 4 weeks** did you have days in which you experienced little or no pleasure in most of your activities?

Not at all	1
1 to 3 days a week	2
Most days a week	3
Nearly every day for at least 2 weeks	4

23. How often **in the past 4 weeks** has your appetite been either less than usual or greater than usual?

Not at all	1
1 to 3 days a week	2
Most days a week	3
Nearly every day for at least 2 weeks	4

24. **In the past 4 weeks,** have you gained or lost weight without trying to?

No	1
Yes, a little weight	2
Yes, some weight	3
Yes, a lot of weight	4

25. How often **in the past 4 weeks** have you had difficulty sleeping or trouble with sleeping too much?

Not at all	1
1 to 3 days a week	2
Most days a week	3
Nearly every day for at least 2 weeks	4

26. **In the past 4 weeks,** has your physical activity been slowed down or speeded up so much that people who know you could notice?

No	1
Yes, a little slowed or speeded up	2
Yes, somewhat slowed or speeded up	3
Yes, very slowed or speeded up	4

27. **In the past 4 weeks,** have you often felt more tired out or less energetic than usual?

No	1
Yes, a little tired out	2
Yes, somewhat tired out	3
Yes, very tired out	4

28. How often **in the past 4 weeks** have you felt worthless or been bothered by feelings of guilt?

    Not at all   1

    1 to 3 days a week   2

    Most days a week   3

    Nearly every day for at least 2 weeks   4

29. **In the past 4 weeks,** have you often had trouble thinking, concentrating, or making decisions?

    No   1

    Yes, a little trouble thinking   2

    Yes, some trouble thinking   3

    Yes, a lot of trouble thinking   4

30. How often have you thought about death or suicide **in the past 4 weeks?**

    Not at all   1

    1 to 3 days a week   2

    Most days a week   3

    Nearly every day for at least 2 weeks   4

31. **In the past 4 weeks,** have you thought a lot about a specific way to commit suicide?

    No   1

    Yes   2

32. In general, would you say your health is: **(Circle one)**

    Excellent   1

    Very good   2

    Good   3

    Fair   4

    Poor   5

33. **Compared to one year ago,** how would you rate your health in general now?   **(Circle one)**

    Much better now than one year ago   1

    Somewhat better now than one year ago   2

    About the same   3

    Somewhat worse now than one year ago   4

    Much worse now than one year ago   5

The following items are about activities you might do during a typical day. Does your health now limit you in these activities? If so, how much?

(Circle one number on each line)	Yes, limited a lot	Yes, limited a little	No, not limited at all
34. Vigorous activities, such as running, lifting heavy objects, participating in strenuous sports	1	2	3
35. Moderate activities, such as moving a table, pushing a vacuum cleaner, bowling, or playing golf	1	2	3
36. Lifting or carrying groceries	1	2	3

D. DEPRESSION OUTCOMES MODULE (DOM) *(Continued)*

(Circle one number on each line)	Yes, limited a lot	Yes, limited a little	No, not limited at all
37. Climbing several flights of stairs	1	2	3
38. Climbing one flight of stairs	1	2	3
39. Bending, kneeling, or stooping	1	2	3
40. Walking more than a mile	1	2	3
41. Walking several blocks	1	2	3
42. Walking one block	1	2	3
43. Bathing or dressing yourself	1	2	3

During the past 4 weeks, have you had any of the following problems with your work or other regular daily activities as a result of your physical health?

(Circle one number on each line)	YES	NO
44. Cut down the amount of time you spent on work or other activities	1	2
45. Accomplished less than you would like	1	2
46. Were limited in the kind of work or other activities	1	2
47. Had difficulty performing the work or other activities (for example, it took extra effort)	1	2

During the past 4 weeks, have you had any of the following problems with your work or other regular daily activities as a result of any emotional problems (such as feeling depressed or anxious)?

(Circle one number on each line)	YES	NO
48. Cut down the amount of time you spent on work or other activities	1	2
49. Accomplished less than you would like	1	2
50. Didn't do work or other activities as carefully as usual	1	2

51. **During the past 4 weeks,** to what extent has your physical health or emotional problems interfered with your normal social activities with family, friends, neighbors, or groups?

	(Circle one number)
Not at all	1
Slightly	2
Moderately	3
Quite a bit	4
Extremely	5

52. How much bodily pain have you had during **the past 4 weeks?**   **(Circle one number)**

None	1
Very mild	2
Mild	3
Moderate	4
Severe	5
Very severe	6

53. **During the past 4 weeks,** how much did pain interfere with your normal work (including both work outside the home and housework?)   **(Circle one number)**

Not at all	1
A little bit	2
Moderately	3
Quite a bit	4
Extremely	5

These questions are about how you feel and how things have been with you **during the past 4 weeks**. For each question, please give the one answer that comes closest to the way you have been feeling.

How much of the time **during the past 4 weeks**.....

(Circle one number on each line)

	All of the time	Most of the time	A good bit of the time	Some of the time	A little of the time	None of the time
54. Did you feel full of pep?	1	2	3	4	5	6
55. Have you been a very nervous person?	1	2	3	4	5	6
56. Have you felt so down in the dumps that nothing could cheer you up?	1	2	3	4	5	6
57. Have you felt calm and peaceful?	1	2	3	4	5	6
58. Did you have a lot of energy?	1	2	3	4	5	6
59. Have you felt downhearted and blue?	1	2	3	4	5	6
60. Did you feel worn out?	1	2	3	4	5	6
61. Have you been a happy person?	1	2	3	4	5	6
62. Did you feel tired?	1	2	3	4	5	6

63. **During the past 4 weeks,** how much of the time **has your physical health or emotional problems** interfered with your social activities (like visiting with friends, relatives, etc)?   **(Circle one number)**

All of the time	1
Most of the time	2
Some of the time	3
A little of the time	4
None of the time	5

D. DEPRESSION OUTCOMES MODULE (DOM) *(Continued)*

How TRUE or FALSE is each of the following statements for you?

(Circle one number on each line)

	Definitely true	Mostly true	Don't know	Mostly false	Definitely false
64. I seem to get sick a little easier than other people.	1	2	3	4	5
65. I am as healthy as anybody I know.	1	2	3	4	5
66. I expect my health to get worse.	1	2	3	4	5
67. My health is excellent.	1	2	3	4	5

Please answer YES or NO for each question by circling "1" or "2" on each line.

	YES	NO
68. In the past year, have you had 2 weeks or more during which you felt sad, blue, or depressed; or when you lost all interest or pleasure in things that you usually cared about or enjoyed?	1	2
69. Have you had 2 years or more in your life when you felt depressed or sad most days, even if you felt okay sometimes?	1	2
70. Have you felt depressed or sad much of the time in the past year?	1	2

71. What is your birth date?

Month_____ Day _____ Year _____

For the following questions, please circle one number.

72. What is your sex?
    - Male 1
    - Female 2

73. Which of the following best describes your racial background?
    - American Indian or Alaskan Native 1
    - Asian/Oriental or Pacific Islander 2
    - Black/African-American 3
    - White/Caucasian 4
    - Spanish/Hispanic 5
    - Other 6

74. Which of the following best describes your current marital status?
    - Married/Cohabitating 1
    - Widowed 2
    - Separated 3
    - Divorced 4
    - Never married 5

75. What is the highest grade you completed in school?
    - 8th grade or less 1
    - Some high school 2
    - High school graduate 3
    - Some college 4
    - College graduate 5
    - Any postgraduate work 6

76. How many people <u>other than yourself</u> live in your household?
    (fill in the blanks)

      Number of adults: _____

      Number of children: _____

77. Which of the following categories best describes your household's total income before taxes last year? Please include income from all sources such as salaries and wages, Social Security, retirement income, investments, and other sources.

Less than $20,000	1
$20,000 - $39,999	2
$40,000 - $59,999	3
$60,000 - $79,999	4
$80,000 or more	5

78. What is your zip code? ____/____/____/____/____

79. Who completed this form?

I filled it out with no help	1
I filled it out with help from family or friends	2
I filled it out with help from a healthcare provider	3
Family or friends	4
Healthcare provider	5

E. HAMILTON RATING SCALE FOR DEPRESSION (HAM-D, HRSD)

OVERVIEW

The Hamilton Rating Scale for Depression (HAM-D, HRSD), developed by M Hamilton, is the most widely utilized rating scale to assess symptoms of depression. A review of leading psychiatric journals in 1994 demonstrated that the HAM-D was the assessment instrument of choice when rating depressive symptoms in 66% of published research studies. The HAM-D is an observer-rated scale consisting of 17 to 21 items (including two 2-part items, weight and diurnal variation). Ratings are made on the basis of the clinical interview, plus any additional available information such as nursing or family member report. The items are rated on either a 0 to 4 spectrum (0 = none/absent and 4 = most severe) or a 0 to 2 spectrum (0 = absent/none and 2 = severe). A modification of the scale, with anchor points, was published in the ECDEU manual (Guy, 1976). Although the author intended the scale to be utilized only in patients with primary depression, in real-life settings the scale is sometimes used to evaluate depressive symptoms in patients with other disorders, such as schizophrenia or bipolar disorder. The HAM-D heavily emphasizes somatic symptoms of depression and works best for the assessment of individuals with relatively severe illness. The HAM-D also relies quite heavily on the clinical interviewing skills and experience of the rater in evaluating individuals with depressive illness. As most patients score zero on rare items in depression (depersonalization, obsessional and paranoid symptoms), the total score on the HAM-D generally consists of only the sum of the first 17 items. The strengths of the HAM-D include its excellent validation/research base, and ease of administration. Its use is limited in individuals who have psychiatric disorders other than primary depression. If the HAM-D is utilized in the assessment of individuals with schizophrenia, it should always be paired with a scale that is more specific to schizophrenic symptoms (eg, the BPRS *on page 130* or the PANSS *on page 158*). The HAM-D has been translated into nearly all European languages, and is used all over the world.

GENERAL APPLICATIONS

The HAM-D is used to assess severity of depression.

SELECTED PSYCHOMETRIC PROPERTIES

Interrater reliability for the total score ranges from 0.87 to 0.95. This may be improved upon slightly with two experienced raters working together. Validity of the scale appears high.

REFERENCES

Hamilton M, "A Rating Scale for Depression," *J Neurol Neurosurg Psychiatr*, 1960, 23:56-62.

Hamilton M, "Development of a Rating Scale for Primary Depressive Illness," *Br J Soc Clin Psychol*, 1967, 6(4):278-96.

Hamilton M, "Hamilton Psychiatric Rating Scale for Depression," *ECDEU Assessment Manual for Psychopharmacology*, Guy W, ed, Washington DC: U.S. Department of Health, Education, and Welfare, 1976, 179-92.

Snaith RP, "Present Use of the Hamilton Depression Rating Scale: Observation on Method of Assessment in Research of Depressive Disorders," *Br J Psychiatry*, 1996, 168(5):594-7.

COPYRIGHT

Dr John Waterhouse
Crichton Royal Hospital
Banken Road
Dumfries DG1 4TG, Scotland
The British Psychological Society
Turpin Distribution Services Ltd
Blackhorse Road
Letchworth
Herts SG6 1HN, UK

SCALE GENERALLY DONE BY

Clinician or trained rater

TIME TO COMPLETE SCALE

20-30 minutes

REPRESENTATIVE STUDY UTILIZING SCALE

Franchini L, Zanardi R, Gasperini M, et al, "Two-Year Maintenance Treatment With Citalopram, 20 mg, in Unipolar Subjects With High Recurrence Rate," *J Clin Psychiatry*, 1999, 60(12):861-5.

E. HAMILTON RATING SCALE FOR DEPRESSION (HAM-D, HRSD)
(Continued)

HAMILTON PSYCHIATRIC RATING SCALE FOR DEPRESSION

INSTRUCTIONS: For each item, select the one "cue" which best characterizes the patient.

Depressed Mood *(sadness, hopeless, helpless, worthless)*

0 = Absent

1 = These feeling states indicated only on questioning

2 = These feeling states spontaneously reported verbally

3 = Communicates feeling states nonverbally (ie, through facial expression, posture, voice, and tendency to weep)

4 = Patient reports **virtually only** these feeling states in his spontaneous verbal and nonverbal communication

Feelings of Guilt

0 = Absent

1 = Self-reproach, feels he has let people down

2 = Ideas of guilt or rumination over past errors or sinful deeds

3 = Present illness is a punishment. Delusions of guilt.

4 = Hears accusatory or denunciatory voices and/or experiences threatening visual hallucinations

Suicide

0 = Absent

1 = Feels life is not worth living

2 = Wishes he were dead or any thoughts of possible death to self

3 = Suicide ideas or gesture

4 = Attempts at suicide (any serious *attempt* rates 4)

Insomnia Early

0 = No difficulty falling asleep

1 = Complains of occasional difficulty falling asleep (eg, more than 30 minutes)

2 = Complains of nightly difficulty falling asleep

Insomnia Middle

0 = No difficulty

1 = Patient complains of being restless and disturbed during the night

2 = Waking during the night - any getting out of bed rates 2 *(except for purposes of voiding)*

Insomnia Late

0 = No difficulty

1 = Waking in early hours of the morning but goes back to sleep

2 = Unable to fall asleep again if he gets out of bed

Work and Activities

0 = No difficulty

1 = Thoughts and feelings of incapacity, fatigue or weakness related to activities; work or hobbies

2 = Loss of interest in activity; hobbies or work - either directly reported by patient, or indirect in listlessness, indecision and vacillation *(feels he has to push self to work or activities)*

3 = Decrease in actual time spent in activities or decrease in productivity. In hospital, rate 3 if patient does not spend at least 3 hours daily in activities *(hospital job or hobbies)* exclusive of ward chores.

4 = Stopped working because of present illness. In hospital, rate 4 if patient engages in no activities except ward chores, or if patient fails to perform ward chores unassisted.

Retardation (slowness of thought and speech; impaired ability to concentrate; decreased motor activity)

0 = Normal speech and thought

1 = Slight retardation at interview

2 = Obvious retardation at interview

3 = Interview difficult

4 = Complete stupor

Agitation

0 = None

1 = Fidgetiness

2 = Playing with hands, hair, etc

3 = Moving about, can't sit still

4 = Hand wringing, nail biting, hair-pulling, biting of lips

Anxiety Psychic

0 = No difficulty

1 = Subjective tension and irritability

2 = Worrying about minor matters

3 = Apprehensive attitude apparent in face or speech

4 = Fears expressed without questioning

Anxiety Somatic

0 = Absent

1 = Mild

2 = Moderate

3 = Severe

4 = Incapacitating

Physiological concomitants of anxiety *(eg, dry mouth, wind, indigestion, diarrhea, cramps, belching, palpitations, headaches, hyperventilation, sighing, urinary frequency, sweating)*

Somatic Symptoms - Gastrointestinal

0 = None

1 = Loss of appetite but eating without staff encouragement; heavy feelings in abdomen

2 = Difficulty eating without staff urging; requests or requires laxatives or medication for bowels or medication for GI symptoms

E. HAMILTON RATING SCALE FOR DEPRESSION (HAM-D, HRSD)
(Continued)

Somatic Symptoms - General

0 = None
1 = Heaviness in limbs, back, or head; backaches, headache, muscle aches; loss of energy
   and fatigability
2 = Any clear-cut symptom rates 2

Genital Symptoms *(loss of libido, menstrual disturbance)*

0 = Absent
1 = Mild
2 = Severe

Hypochondriasis

0 = Not present
1 = Self-absorption (bodily)
2 = Preoccupation with health
3 = Frequent complaints, requests for help, etc
4 = Hypochondriacal delusions

Loss of Weight (rate either A or B)

A. *When rating by history:*
   0 = No weight loss
   1 = Probable weight loss associated with present illness
   2 = Definite (according to patient) weight loss
   3 = Not assessed

B. *On weekly ratings by ward psychiatrist, when actual weight changes are measured:*
   0 = Less than 1 lb weight loss in week
   1 = Greater than 1 lb weight loss in week
   2 = Greater than 2 lb weight loss in week
   3 = Not assessed

Insight

0 = Acknowledges being depressed and ill
1 = Acknowledges illness but attributes cause to bad food, climate, overwork, virus, need
   for rest, etc
2 = Denies being ill at all

Diurnal Variation

A. *Note whether symptoms are worse in morning or evening. If NO diurnal variation, mark
   none.*
   0 = No variation
   1 = Worse in AM
   2 = Worse in PM

B. *When present, mark the severity of the variation. Mark "None" if NO variation.*
   0 = None
   1 = Mild
   2 = Severe

Depersonalization and Derealization *(feelings of unreality, nihilistic ideas)*

0 = Absent
1 = Mild
2 = Moderate
3 = Severe
4 = Incapacitating

Paranoid Symptoms

0 = None
1 = Suspicious
2 = Ideas of reference
3 = Delusions of reference and persecution

Obsessional and Compulsive Symptoms

0 = Absent
1 = Mild
2 = Severe

F. MONTGOMERY-ASBERG DEPRESSION RATING SCALE (MADRS)

OVERVIEW

The MADRS, developed by SA Montgomery and M Asberg, is a rating scale for the assessment of depression, which was drawn from a larger scale, the Comprehensive Psychopathological Rating Scale (CPRS) *on page 134*. The MADRS consists of 10 items that are all core symptoms of depression. Nine of the items are based upon patient report, and one is on the rater's observation of the patients. Items of the MADRS are rated on a 0 to 6 scale (0 = no abnormality, 6 = severe). Unlike the more commonly utilized HAM-D, the MADRS does not focus predominately on the somatic symptoms of depression, but rather focuses on symptoms such as sadness, tension, lassitude, pessimistic thoughts, and suicidal thoughts. The MADRS is frequently utilized in medication therapy clinical trials to evaluate the effects of psychotropic medication on symptoms of depressive illness.

GENERAL APPLICATIONS

The MADRS is used to assess symptoms of depression, particularly in response to treatment over time.

SELECTED PSYCHOMETRIC PROPERTIES

The MADRS scores correlate well with scores on the HAM-D. Interrater reliability of the scale with different pairs of raters has been reported to be 0.89 to 0.97 by the authors. Interrater reliability between raters of different disciplines (psychiatrist/nurse) has also been demonstrated to be good.

REFERENCES

Montgomery S, Asberg M, Jornestedt L, et al, "Reliability of the CPRS Between the Disciplines of Psychiatry, General Practice, Nursing, and Psychology in Depressed Patients," *Acta Psychiatr Scand Suppl*, 1978, 271:29-32.

Montgomery SA and Asberg M, "A New Depression Scale Designed to be Sensitive to Change," *Br J Psychiatry*, 1979, 134:382-9.

COPYRIGHT

The Royal College of Psychiatrists
The British Journal of Psychiatry
17 Belgrave Square, SW1X 8PG

SCALE GENERALLY DONE BY

Psychiatrists, psychologists, nurses, and trained raters

TIME TO COMPLETE SCALE

20 minutes

REPRESENTATIVE STUDY UTILIZING SCALE

Feighner JP and Overo K, "Multicenter, Placebo-Controlled, Fixed-Dose Study of Citalopram in Moderate-to-Severe Depression," *J Clin Psychiatry*, 1999, 60(12):824-30.

MADRS

The rating should be based on a clinical interview moving from broadly phrased questions about symptoms to more detailed ones which allow a precise rating of severity. The rater must decide whether the rating lies on the defined scale steps (0, 2, 4, 6) or between them (1, 3, 5).

It is important to remember that it is only on rare occasions that a depressed patient is encountered who cannot be rated on the items in the scale. If definite answers cannot be elicited from the patient, all relevant clues as well as information from other sources should be used as a basis for the rating in line with customary clinical practice.

The scale may be used for any time interval between ratings, be it weekly or otherwise, but this must be recorded.

Item List

1. Apparent sadness
2. Reported sadness
3. Inner tension
4. Reduced sleep
5. Reduced appetite
6. Concentration difficulties
7. Lassitude
8. Inability to feel
9. Pessimistic thoughts
10. Suicidal thoughts

1. Apparent Sadness

Representing despondency, gloom, and despair (more than just ordinary transient low spirits), reflected in speech, facial expression, and posture. Rate by depth and inability to brighten up.

0 No sadness
1
2 Looks dispirited but does brighten up without difficulty
3
4 Appears sad and unhappy most of the time
5
6 Looks miserable all the time; extremely despondent

2. Reported Sadness

Representing reports of depressed mood, regardless of whether it is reflected in appearance or not. Includes low spirits, despondency, or the feeling of being beyond help and without hope. Rate according to intensity, duration, and the extent to which the mood is reported to be influenced by events.

0 Occasional sadness in keeping with the circumstances
1
2 Sad or low but brightens up without difficulty
3
4 Pervasive feelings of sadness or gloominess. The mood is still influenced by external circumstances.
5
6 Continuous or unvarying sadness, misery, or despondency

F. MONTGOMERY-ASBERG DEPRESSION RATING SCALE (MADRS)
(Continued)

3. Inner Tension

Representing feelings of ill-defined discomfort, edginess, inner turmoil, mental tension mounting to either panic, dread, or anguish. Rate according to intensity, frequency, duration, and the extent of reassurance called for.

  0 Placid; only fleeting inner tension

  1

  2 Occasional feelings of edginess and ill-defined discomfort

  3

  4 Continuous feelings of inner tension or intermittent panic which the patient can only master with some difficulty

  5

  6 Unrelenting dread or anguish; overwhelming panic

4. Reduced Sleep

Representing the experience of reduced duration or depth of sleep compared to the subject's own normal pattern when well.

  0 Sleeps as usual

  1

  2 Slight difficulty dropping off to sleep or slightly reduced, light or fitful sleep

  3

  4 Sleep reduced or broken by at least two hours

  5

  6 Less than two or three hours sleep

5. Reduced Appetite

Representing the feeling of a loss of appetite compared with when well. Rate by loss of desire for food or the need to force oneself to eat.

  0 Normal or increased appetite

  1

  2 Slightly reduced appetite

  3

  4 No appetite; food is tasteless

  5

  6 Needs persuasion to eat at all

6. Concentration Difficulties

Representing difficulties in collecting one's thoughts mounting to incapacitating lack of concentration. Rate according to intensity, frequency, and degree of incapacity produced.

  0 No difficulties in concentrating

  1

  2 Occasional difficulties in collecting one's thoughts

  3

  4 Difficulties in concentrating and sustaining thought which reduces ability to read or hold a conversation

  5

  6 Unable to read or converse without great difficulty

7. Lassitude

Representing a difficulty getting started or slowness initiating and performing everyday activities.

0   Hardly any difficulty in getting started; no sluggishness

1

2   Difficulties in starting activities

3

4   Difficulties in starting simple routine activities which are carried out with effort

5

6   Complete lassitude; unable to do anything without help

8. Inability to Feel

Representing the subjective experience of reduced interest in the surroundings, or activities that normally give pleasure. The ability to react with adequate emotion to circumstances or people is reduced.

0   Normal interest in the surroundings and in other people

1

2   Reduced ability to enjoy usual interests

3

4   Loss of interest in the surroundings; loss of feelings for friends and acquaintances

5

6   The experience of being emotionally paralyzed; inability to feel anger, grief, or pleasure; and a complete or even painful failure to feel for close relatives and friends

9. Pessimistic Thoughts

Representing thoughts of guilt, inferiority, self-reproach, sinfulness, remorse, and ruin.

0   No pessimistic thoughts

1

2   Fluctuating ideas of failure, self-reproach, or self-depreciation

3

4   Persistent self-accusations, or definite but still rational ideas of guilt or sin; increasingly pessimistic about the future

5

6   Delusions of ruin, remorse, or unredeemable sin; self-accusations which are absurd and unshakable

10. Suicidal Thoughts

Representing the feeling that life is not worth living, that a natural death would be welcome, suicidal thoughts, and preparations for suicide. Suicidal attempts should not, in themselves, influence the rating.

0   Enjoys life or takes it as it comes

1

2   Weary of life; only fleeting suicidal thoughts

3

4   Probably better off dead; suicidal thoughts are common, and suicide is considered as a possible solution, but without specific plans or intentions

5

6   Explicit plans for suicide when there is an opportunity; active preparations for suicide

G. RASKIN DEPRESSION RATING SCALE

OVERVIEW

The Raskin Depression Scale, developed by A Raskin et al, is a simple, clinician-rated scale to assess nonpsychotic, nonbipolar, depressed patients. Originally designed to identify and screen hospitalized patients suitable for inclusion into research studies to evaluate treatments of depression, the Raskin scale may be used to assess baseline symptoms of depression, and change in depressive symptoms over time. Sources of information may include patient self-report, nursing report of patient behavior, and information obtained during patient interview. There are three items on the Raskin scale which evaluate a patient's verbal report of depressive symptoms, depressed behavior, and secondary symptoms of depression which cover a variety of somatic complaints. Items are rated on a 1 to 5 scale (1 = not at all, 5 = very much). Strengths of the Raskin scale include its brevity and quick administration. Due to the scale's lack of specificity, it is usually paired with another more specific rating scale to assess depression severity, such as the HAM-D *on page 100*.

GENERAL APPLICATIONS

The Raskin scale is used to assess baseline severity of depression and change over time. It is sometimes used in pharmacology studies as a screen for eligibility for baseline degree of depression severity.

SELECTED PSYCHOMETRIC PROPERTIES

The authors have reported that patients who score a "9" or greater on the Raskin scale have the equivalent of a moderate amount of depression. It is recommended that a variety of rating scales be utilized to assess the specific domains of depressive illness.

REFERENCES

Raskin A, Schulterbrandt J, Reating N, et al, "Replication of Factors of Psychopathology in Interview, Ward Behavior, and Self-Report Ratings of Hospitalized Depressives," *J Nerv Ment Dis*, 1969, 148(1):87-98.

COPYRIGHT

Not applicable

SCALE GENERALLY DONE BY

Psychiatrist, psychologist, or trained rater

TIME TO COMPLETE SCALE

10-15 minutes

REPRESENTATIVE STUDY UTILIZING SCALE

Bennie EH, Mullin JM, and Martindale JJ, "A Double-Blind Multicenter Trial Comparing Sertraline and Fluoxetine in Outpatients With Major Depression," *J Clin Psychiatry*, 1995, 56(6):229-37.

RASKIN DEPRESSION SCALE

Rate each of the following according to the degrees of severity below:

1 = Not at all
2 = Somewhat
3 = Moderately
4 = Considerably
5 = Very much

I. _____ Verbal report: Feels blue, talks of feeling helpless or worthless, complains of loss of interest, may wish to be dead, reports of crying spells

II. _____ Behavior: Looks sad, cries easily, speaks in a sad voice, psychomotor retardation, lacking energy

III. _____ Secondary symptoms of depression: Insomnia/hypersomnia, dry mouth, GI complaints, suicide attempt recently, change in appetite, cognitive problems

H. ZUNG DEPRESSION SCALE (SDS and DSI)

OVERVIEW

The Zung Depression Scale (SDS), developed by W Zung, is a 20-item, self-rated scale for the assessment of depression in adults. The Zung is rated on a 1 to 4 spectrum (1 = none, 4 = severe) and includes a variety of somatic symptoms such as sleep disturbance, weight loss, constipation, tachycardia, fatigue, and decreased appetite. There is a clinician-rated analogue, the Depression Status Inventory (DSI), also developed by Zung, which contains the same 20 items as the patient-rated scale. The DSI provides a global measure of the intensity of depressive symptoms. The ECDEU manual contains versions of both the SDS and DSI. Strengths of the Zung scale, as with the BDI *on page 80*, include its brevity and ease of administration. The Zung scale may have a limited ability to detect change over time. It has been suggested that the Zung scale may be best suited as a screening tool for depression in clinical populations.

GENERAL APPLICATIONS

Assessment of depression in adults.

SELECTED PSYCHOMETRIC PROPERTIES

Scoring on the SDS significantly differentiates patients with depressive disorders from those with schizophrenia, anxiety disorders, personality disorders, and transient situational disturbances. The author has reported a Pearson product moment correlation of 0.87 between the Zung patient-rated scale and the DSI.

REFERENCES

Zung WW, "A Self-Rating Depression Scale," *Arch Gen Psychiat*, 1965, 12:63-70.

Zung WW, "The Depression Status Inventory: An Adjunct to the Self-Rating Depression Scale," *J Clin Psychol*, 1972, 28(4):539-43.

Zung WW, "Self-Rating Depression Scale (SDS)," *ECDEU Assessment Manual for Psychopharmacology*, Guy W, ed, Washington DC: U.S. Department of Health, Education, and Welfare, 1976, 333-6.

COPYRIGHT

ECDEU versions - not applicable

SCALE GENERALLY DONE BY

SDS: Self-rated
DSI: Rated by clinician or trained rater

TIME TO COMPLETE SCALE

10 minutes

REPRESENTATIVE STUDY UTILIZING SCALE

Miura H, Kitagami T, and Ohta T, "Application of the Zung Self-Rating Depression Scale to Patients Before and After Introduction to Haemodialysis," *Psychiatry Clin Neurosci*, 1999, 53(3):381-5.

Department of Health, Education and Welfare
Public Health Service
National Institute of Mental Health

ZUNG SDS

(ECDEU Version)

INSTRUCTIONS:

Listed below are 20 statements. Please read each one carefully and decide how much of the statement describes how you have been feeling during the past week. Decide whether the statement applies to you for NONE OR A LITTLE OF THE TIME, SOME OF THE TIME, A GOOD PART OF THE TIME, OR MOST OR ALL OF THE TIME. Mark the appropriate column for each statement.

STATEMENT	NONE OR A LITTLE OF THE TIME	SOME OF THE TIME	A GOOD PART OF THE TIME	MOST OR ALL OF THE TIME
1. I feel downhearted and blue				
2. Morning is when I feel the best				
3. I have crying spells or feel like it				
4. I have trouble sleeping at night				
5. I eat as much as I used to				
6. I still enjoy sex				
7. I notice that I am losing weight				
8. I have trouble with constipation				
9. My heart beats faster than usual				
10. I get tired for no reason				
11. My mind is as clear as it used to be				
12. I find it easy to do the things I used to do				
13. I am restless and can't keep still				
14. I feel hopeful about the future				
15. I am more irritable than usual				
16. I find it easy to make decisions				
17. I feel that I am useful and needed				
18. My life is pretty full				
19. I feel that others would be better off if I were dead				
20. I still enjoy the things I used to do				

H. ZUNG DEPRESSION SCALE (SDS and DSI) *(Continued)*

DEPRESSION STATUS INVENTORY (DSI)

(ECDEU Version)

The data upon which the judgments are based comes from the interview with the patient. The items in the scale are to be quantified by using the information available to the rater. This includes both clinical observation and the material reported by the patient.

1 = None; 2 = Mild; 3 = Moderate; 4 = Severe

Depressed Mood

_____ Do you ever feel sad or depressed

Crying Spells

_____ Do you have crying spells or feel like it?

Diurnal Variation (symptoms worse in morning)

_____ Is there any part of the day when you feel worse? Best?

Sleep Disturbance

_____ Frequent and early AM wakings

Decreased Appetite

_____ How is your appetite?

Weight Loss

_____ Have you lost any weight?

Decreased Libido

_____ Do you enjoy looking, talking, or being with attractive men/women?

Constipation

_____ Do you have trouble with constipation?

Tachycardia

_____ Have you had times when your heart was beating faster than usual?

Fatigue

_____ How easily do you get tired?

Psychomotor Agitation

_____ Do you find yourself restless and can't sit still?

Psychomotor Retardation

_____ Do you feel slowed down in doing the things you usually do?

Confusion

_____ Do you ever feel confused and have trouble thinking?

Emptiness

_____ Do you feel life is empty for you?

Hopelessness

_____ How hopeful do you feel about the future?

Indecisiveness

_____ How are you at making decisions?

Irritability

_____ How easily do you get irritated?

Dissatisfaction

_____ Do you still enjoy the things you used to?

Personal Devaluation

_____ Do you ever feel useless and not wanted?

Suicidal Ruminations

_____ Have you had thoughts about doing away with yourself?

BIPOLAR DISORDER

ASSESSMENT SCALES

TABLE OF CONTENTS

A. BECH-RAFAELSEN MANIA SCALE

OVERVIEW

The Bech-Rafaelsen scale, developed by P Bech and OJ Rafaelsen, is an 11-item scale to evaluate severity of manic symptoms. It was initially intended to be combined with the HAM-D to cover pertinent items of the whole mood spectrum. (Later the authors developed a scale to assess melancholic symptoms). Each item is rated on a five-point spectrum in which 1 = mild, and 4 = severe or extreme. There are well-defined anchor points for each item. The last item rates work/activity ability of the patient, split into first rating assessment, and follow-up assessment. Strengths of the Bech-Rafaelsen scale include its brevity and ease of administration, however, it is not as commonly used as the YMRS *on page 126.*

GENERAL APPLICATIONS

The Bech-Rafaelsen Mania Rating Scale evaluates severity of manic symptoms at baseline and over time.

PSYCHOMETRIC PROPERTIES

The authors have reported interrater reliability of 0.97 to 0.98 when administered by psychiatrists.

REFERENCES

Bech P, Bolwig TG, Kramp P, et al, "The Bech-Rafaelsen Mania Scale and the Hamilton Depression Scale," *Acta Psychiatr Scand*, 1979, 59(4):420-30.

COPYRIGHT

Munksgaard
Norre Sogade 35, PO Box 2148
1016 Copenhagen K, Denmark
Tel: +45 77 33 33 33

SCALE GENERALLY DONE BY

Clinician or trained rater

TIME TO COMPLETE SCALE

15-20 minutes

REPRESENTATIVE STUDY UTILIZING SCALE

Grunze H, Erfurth A, Marcuse A, et al, "Tiagabine Appears Not to Be Efficacious in the Treatment of Acute Mania," *J Clin Psychiatry*, 1999, 60(11):759-62.

MANIA RATING SCALE (Bech & Rafaelsen)

LIST OF DEFINITIONS

1. Activity (Motor)

0   Normal motor activity, adequate facial expression
1   Slightly increased motor activity, lively facial expression
2   Somewhat excessive motor activity, lively gestures
3   Outright excessive motor activity, on the move most of the time. Rises one or several times during interview.
4   Constantly active, restlessly energetic. Even if urged, patient cannot sit still.

2. Activity (Verbal)

0   Normal verbal activity
1   Somewhat talkative
2   Very talkative, no spontaneous intervals in the conversation
3   Difficult to interrupt
4   Impossible to interrupt, completely dominates conversation

3. Flight of Thoughts

0   Cohesive speech, no flight of thoughts
1   Lively descriptions, explanations and elaborations without losing connection with the topic of conversation. The speech is still cohesive.
2   Now and again it is difficult for the patient to stick to the topic, as the patient is distracted by random associations (often rhymes, clangs, puns, pieces of verse or music).
3   The line of thought is regularly disrupted by diversionary associations
4   It is difficult to impossible to follow the patient's line of thought, as the patient constantly jumps from one topic subject to another

4. Voice/Noise Level

0   Natural volume of voice
1   Speaks loudly without being noisy
2   Voice discernible at a distance, and somewhat noisy
3   Vociferous, voice discernible at a long distance, is noisy, singing
4   Shouting, screaming, or using other sources of noise due to hoarseness

5. Hostility/Destructiveness

0   No signs of impatience or hostility
1   Somewhat impatient or irritable, but control is maintained
2   Markedly impatient or irritable. Provocation badly tolerated.
3   Provocative, makes threats, but can be calmed down
4   Overt physical violence. Physically destructive.

A. BECH-RAFAELSEN MANIA SCALE *(Continued)*

6. Mood (Feelings of Well-being)

0   Neutral mood
1   Slightly elevated mood, optimistic, but still adapted to situation
2   Moderately elevated mood, joking, laughing
3   Markedly elevated mood, exuberant both in manner and speech
4   Extremely elevated mood, quite irrelevant to situation

7. Self-esteem

0   Normal self-esteem
1   Slightly increased self-esteem, slightly boasting
2   Moderately increased self-esteem, boasting; frequent use of superlatives
3   Bragging, unrealistic ideas
4   Grandiose ideas which cannot be corrected

8. Contact

0   Normal contact
1   Slightly meddling, putting his oar in
2   Moderately meddling and arguing
3   Dominating, arranging, directing, but still in context with the setting
4   Extremely dominating and manipulating, without context with the setting

9. Sleep (Average of Last 3 Nights)

0   Habitual duration of sleep
1   Duration of sleep reduced by 25%
2   Duration of sleep reduced by 50%
3   Duration of sleep reduced by 75%
4   No sleep

10. Sexual Interest

0   Habitual sexual interest and activity
1   Slight increase in sexual interest and activity
2   Moderate increase in sexual interest and activity
3   Marked increase in sexual interest and activity, as shown in manner and speech
4   Completely and inadequately occupied by sexuality

11. Work

A. *At first rating of the patient*

0   Normal work activity
1   Slightly increased drive, but work quality is slightly reduced, as motivation is changing, and the patient somewhat distractible
2   Increased drive, but motivation clearly fluctuating. The patient has difficulties in judging own work quality and the quality is indeed lowered. Often quarrels at work.
3   Work capacity clearly reduced, and from time to time the patient loses control; has to stop work and be sick-listed. If the patient is hospitalized, he can participate for some hours per day in ward activities.
4   The patient is (or ought to be) hospitalized and unable to participate in ward activities.

B. *At weekly ratings*

0   a) The patient has resumed work at his/her normal activity level
     b) When the patient will have no trouble in resuming normal work

1   a) The patient is working, but the effort is somewhat reduced due to changing motivation
     b) It is doubtful whether the patient can resume normal work on a full scale due to distractibility and changing motivation

2   a) The patient is working, but at a clearly reduced level (eg, due to episodes of nonattendance)
     b) The patient is still hospitalized or sick-listed. He is only able to resume work if special precautions are taken; close supervision and/or reduced time.

3   The patient is still hospitalized or sick-listed and is unable to resume work. In hospital, he participated for some hours per day in ward activities.

4   The patient is still fully hospitalized and generally unable to participate in ward activities.

B. MANIC-STATE RATING SCALE (MSRS)

OVERVIEW

The MSRS, also called the Beigel scale, is a clinician rated, 26-item rated scale to assess manic symptoms. Developed by A Beigel et al, at the National Institute of Mental Health, the scale was originally developed for use on a inpatient ward and may be rated by nursing staff based upon patient behaviors, or upon patient interview. The 26 items are each given a frequency score on a 0 to 5 scale and an intensity score on a 1 to 5 scale. The individual item score is the product of these ratings. Eleven of the items evaluate elation-grandiosity and paranoid-destructiveness. There are no anchor points for the severity ratings. Strengths of the MSRS include its utility for individuals who may have difficulty with interviews, although the length of the scale may be a limitation. A 28-item version has been developed for interview use (Blackburn, 1977).

GENERAL APPLICATIONS

The MSRS is a scale to evaluate severity of manic symptoms.

PSYCHOMETRIC PROPERTIES

The authors have demonstrated high reliability and validity of the MSRS. Interrater reliability for each item has been reported to range from 0.89 to 0.99.

REFERENCES

Bech P, Bolwig TG, Dein E, et al, "Quantitative Rating of Manic States. Correlation Between Clinical Assessment and Biegel's Objective Rating Scale," *Acta Psychiatr Scand*, 1975, 52(1):1-6.

Beigel A, Murphy DL, and Bunney WE Jr, "The Manic-State Rating Scale: Scale Construction, Reliability, and Validity," *Arch Gen Psychiat*, 1971, 25:256-62.

Blackburn IM, Loudon JB, and Ashworth CM, "A New Scale for Measuring Mania," *Psychol Med*, 1977, 7(3):453-8.

COPYRIGHT

Not applicable

SCALE GENERALLY DONE BY

Inpatient ward staff, nurses, or trained raters

TIME TO COMPLETE SCALE

15 minutes

REPRESENTATIVE STUDY UTILIZING SCALE

Lerer B, Moore N, Meyendorff E, et al, "Carbamazepine Versus Lithium in Mania: A Double-Blind Study," *J Clin Psychiatry*, 1987, 48(3):89-93.

THE MANIC-STATE RATING SCALE

Part A Frequency (How much of the time?)							Part B Intensity (How intense is it?)				
None	Infrequent	Some	Much	Most	All		Very Minimal	Minimal	Moderate	Marked	Very Marked
0	1	2	3	4	5	The Patient	1	2	3	4	5
						1. Looks depressed.					
						2. Is talking.					
						3. Moves from one place to another.					
						4. Makes threats.					
						5. Has poor judgment.					
						6. Dresses inappropriately.					
						7. Looks happy and cheerful.					
						8. Seeks out others.					
						9. Is distractible.					
						10. Has grandiose ideas.					
						11. Is irritable.					
						12. Is combative or destructive.					
						13. Is delusional.					
						14. Verbalizes depressive feelings.					
						15. Is active.					
						16. Is argumentative.					
						17. Talks about sex.					
						18. Is angry.					
						19. Is careless about dress and grooming.					
						20. Has diminished impulse control.					
						21. Verbalizes feelings of well-being.					
						22. Is suspicious.					
						23. Makes unrealistic plans.					
						24. Demands contact with others.					
						25. Is sexually preoccupied.					
						26. Jumps from one subject to another.					

C. MOOD DISORDERS QUESTIONNAIRE (MDQ)

OVERVIEW

The Mood Disorder Questionnaire (MDQ) is a useful screening instrument for bipolar spectrum disorder in a psychiatric outpatient population. The MDQ is a self-report, single-page, paper and pencil inventory, which screens for a lifetime history of a manic or hypomanic syndrome (Hirschfeld, 2000). The scale, derived from DSM-IV criteria and clinical experience, consists of 13 items rated on a 4-point scale (ranging from "no problem" to "serious problem") and two additional items, which evaluate level of functional impairment due to manic/hypomanic symptoms. Each "yes" response is scored as one point, and points are totaled (range 0 to 13). The authors have reported that a score of 7 or higher is the optimal cut-off point to screen positively for bipolar spectrum disorder. Respondents must also check "yes" for the item asking about symptom time period and endorse a severity of "moderate" or "serious." The MDQ may be easily scored by a physician, nurse, or a trained rater. Bipolar spectrum disorders can often go unrecognized and undiagnosed because of the wide range of symptoms seen in individuals with these disorders. The MDQ is a brief and easy-to-use tool that has been developed relatively recently (Hirschfeld, 2000) to address the issue of under recognition of bipolar spectrum illness.

GENERAL APPLICATIONS

The MDQ is a screening instrument for bipolar spectrum disorder.

SELECTED PSYCHOMETRIC PROPERTIES

The authors report a sensitivity of 0.73 and a specificity of 0.90. This compares well to sensitivities and specificities of instruments used to screen psychiatric disorders which have a mean sensitivity of 0.84 and a specificity of 0.72 (Hirschfeld 2000, Mulrow 1985).

REFERENCES

Hirschfeld RM, Williams JB, Spitzer RL, et al, "Development and Validation of a Screening Instrument for Bipolar Spectrum Disorder: The Mood Disorder Questionnaire," *Am J Psychiatry*, 2000, 157(11):1873-5.

Mulrow CD, Williams JW Jr, Gerety MB, et al, "Case-Finding Instruments for Depression in Primary Care Settings," *Ann Intern Med*, 1995, 122(12):913-21.

COPYRIGHT

Not applicable

SCALE GENERALLY DONE BY

Self-rated scale

TIME TO COMPLETE SCALE

5 minutes

REPRESENTATIVE STUDY UTILIZING SCALE

Calabrese JR, Hirschfeld RA, Reed M, et al, "Impact of Bipolar Disorders in a U.S. Community Sample," *J Clin Psychiatry,* (in press).

MOOD DISORDERS QUESTIONNAIRE (MDQ)

1. Has there ever been a period of time when you were not your usual self and........

   ...you felt so good or so hyper that other people thought you were not your normal   Yes   No
   self or you were so hyper that you got into trouble?

   ...you were so irritable that you shouted at people or started fights or arguments?   Yes   No

   ...you felt much more self-confident than usual?   Yes   No

   ...you got much less sleep than usual and found you didn't really miss it?   Yes   No

   ...you were much more talkative or spoke faster than usual?   Yes   No

   ...thoughts raced through your head or you couldn't slow your mind down?   Yes   No

   ...you were so easily distracted by things around you that you had trouble   Yes   No
   concentrating or staying on track?

   ...you had much more energy than usual?   Yes   No

   ...you were much more active or did many more things than usual?   Yes   No

   ...you were much more social or outgoing than usual; for example, you telephoned   Yes   No
   friends in the middle of the night?

   ...you were much more interested in sex than usual?   Yes   No

   ...you did things that were unusual for you or that other people might have thought   Yes   No
   were excessive, foolish, or risky?

   ...spending money got you or your family into trouble?   Yes   No

2. If you checked YES to more than one of the above, have several of these ever   Yes   No
   happened during the same period of time?

3. How much of a *problem* did any of these cause you - like being unable to work;
   having family, money, or legal troubles; getting into arguments or fights?

   No problem   Minor problem   Moderate problem   Serious problem

D. YOUNG MANIA RATING SCALE (YMRS)

OVERVIEW

The YMRS, developed by RC Young et al, is probably the most frequently utilized rating scale to assess manic symptoms. The scale has 11 items and is based upon the patient's subjective report of his or hers clinical condition over the previous 48 hours. Additional information is based upon clinical observations made during the course of the clinical interview. The items are selected based upon published descriptions of the core symptoms of mania. The YMRS follows the style of the Hamilton Rating Scale for Depression (HAM-D *on page 100*), with each item given a severity rating. There are four items that are graded on a 0 to 8 scale (irritability, speech, thought content, and disruptive/aggressive behavior), while the remaining seven items are graded on a 0 to 4 scale. These four items are given twice the weight of the others to compensate for poor cooperation from severely ill patients. There are well described anchor points for each grade of severity. The authors encourage the use of whole or half point ratings once experience with the scale is acquired. Strengths of the YMRS include its brevity, widely accepted use, and ease of administration. The usefulness of the scale is limited in populations with diagnoses other than mania.

GENERAL APPLICATIONS

The YMRS is a rating scale to evaluate manic symptoms at baseline and over time in individuals with mania.

PSYCHOMETRIC PROPERTIES

Interrater reliability of the total YMRS has been reported to be 0.93 by the authors, with interrater reliability coefficients for each individual item ranging from 0.67 to 0.95. The YMRS correlates well with other accepted mania rating scale such as the Manic-State Rating Scale (MSRS) *on page 122*.

REFERENCES

Young RC, Biggs JT, Ziegler VE, et al, "A Rating Scale for Mania: Reliability, Validity, and Sensitivity," *Br J Psychiatry*, 1978, 133:429-35.

COPYRIGHT

The Royal College of Psychiatrists
The British Journal of Psychiatry
17 Belgrave Square SW1X 8PG

SCALE GENERALLY DONE BY

Clinician or other trained rater with expertise with manic patients.

TIME TO COMPLETE SCALE

15-30 minutes

REPRESENTATIVE STUDY UTILIZING SCALE

Hirschfeld RM, Allen MH, McEvoy JP, et al, "Safety and Tolerability of Oral Loading Divalproex Sodium in Acutely Manic Bipolar Patients," *J Clin Psychiatry*, 1999, 60(12):815-8.

YOUNG MANIA RATING SCALE

Guide for Scoring Items:

The purpose of each item is to rate the severity of that abnormality in the patient. When several keys are given for a particular grade of severity, the presence of only one is required to qualify for that rating.

The keys provided are guides. One can ignore the keys if that is necessary to indicate severity, although this should be the exception rather than the rule.

Scoring between the points given (whole or half points) is possible and encouraged after experience with the scale is acquired. This is particularly useful when severity of a particular item in a patient does not follow the progression indicated by the keys.

1. Elevated Mood

0   Absent
1   Mildly or possibly increased on questioning
2   Definite subjective elevation; optimistic, self-confident; cheerful; appropriate to content
3   Elevated, inappropriate to content; humorous
4   Euphoric; inappropriate laughter; singing

2. Increased Motor Activity-Energy

0   Absent
1   Subjectively increased
2   Animated; gestures increased
3   Excessive energy; hyperactive at times; restless (can be calmed)
4   Motor excitement; continuous hyperactivity (cannot be calmed)

3. Sexual Interest

0   Normal; not increased
1   Mildly or possibly increased
2   Definite subjective increase on questioning
3   Spontaneous sexual content; elaborates on sexual matters; hypersexual by self-report
4   Overt sexual acts (toward patients, staff, or interviewer)

4. Sleep

0   Reports no decrease in sleep
1   Sleeping less than normal amount by up to one hour
2   Sleeping less than normal by more than one hour
3   Reports decreased need for sleep
4   Denies need for sleep

5. Irritability

0   Absent
2   Subjectively increased
4   Irritable at times during interview; recent episodes of anger or annoyance on ward
6   Frequently irritable during interview; short, curt throughout
8   Hostile, uncooperative; interview impossible

D. YOUNG MANIA RATING SCALE (YMRS) *(Continued)*

6. Speech (Rate and Amount)

0   No increase
2   Feels talkative
4   Increased rate or amount at times, verbose at times
6   Push; consistently increased rate and amount; difficult to interrupt
8   Pressured; uninterruptible, continuous speech

7. Language-Thought Disorder

0   Absent
1   Circumstantial; mild distractibility; quick thoughts
2   Distractible, loses goal of thought; changes topics frequently; racing thoughts
3   Flight of ideas; tangentiality; difficult to follow; rhyming, echolalia
4   Incoherent; communication impossible

8. Content

0   Normal
2   Questionable plans, new interests
4   Special project(s); hyper-religious
6   Grandiose or paranoid ideas; ideas of reference
8   Delusions; hallucinations

9. Disruptive-Aggressive Behavior

0   Absent, cooperative
2   Sarcastic; loud at times, guarded
4   Demanding; threats on ward
6   Threatens interviewer; shouting; interview difficult
8   Assaultive; destructive; interview impossible

10. Appearance

0   Appropriate dress and grooming
1   Minimally unkempt
2   Poorly groomed; moderately disheveled; overdressed
3   Disheveled; partly clothed; garish make-up
4   Completely unkempt; decorated; bizarre garb

11. Insight

0   Present; admits illness; agrees with need for treatment
1   Possibly ill
2   Admits behavior change, but denies illness
3   Admits possible change in behavior, but denies illness
4   Denies any behavior change

PSYCHOSIS
RATING SCALES

TABLE OF CONTENTS

A. BRIEF PSYCHIATRIC RATING SCALE (BPRS)

OVERVIEW

The BPRS, developed by JE Overall and DR Gorham, is a very widely used, relatively brief scale that measures major psychotic and nonpsychotic symptoms in individuals with a major psychiatric disorder, particularly schizophrenia. The 18-item BPRS is perhaps the most researched instrument in psychiatry. Various versions of the scale exist, with the intention of improving reliability and validity. Sixteen symptom constructs were originally listed for rating on a seven-point scale (1 = not present, 7 = most severe), which document the intensity of symptoms in relatively independent areas. A version also exists with ratings on a 0 to 6 scale. The rating is based upon observations made by the clinician/rater during a 15- to 30-minute interview (items which measure tension, emotional withdrawal, mannerisms and posturing, motor retardation, and uncooperativeness), and subject verbal report (items which measure conceptual disorganization, unusual thought content, anxiety, guilt feelings, grandiosity, depressive mood, hostility, somatic concern, hallucinatory behavior, suspiciousness, and blunted affect). Subsequent additions to the scale were two additional items of excitement and disorientation.

The limitations of the BPRS include somewhat ambiguous criteria for the various levels of severity, with potential for overlap in some of the items that are most broadly defined. Strengths of the scale include its brevity, ease of administration, wide use, and well-researched status.

GENERAL APPLICATIONS

The BPRS is appropriate for evaluating baseline psychopathology, clinical outcome, and treatment response, with the frequency of repeat administrations at the discretion of the clinical investigator. The scale was developed primarily for inpatient populations, but it may also be utilized for outpatients.

SELECTED PSYCHOMETRIC PROPERTIES

Reliability coefficients of 0.56 to 0.87 have been reported by the authors. Reliability may be improved by having two clinicians work together, one of whom conducts the interview, while the other obtains supplementary information. The raters make independent ratings, but responses are discussed between the two raters. Another approach involves discussion of each item with a "consensus" rating.

REFERENCES

Hedlund JL and Vieweg BW, "The Brief Psychiatric Rating Scale (BPRS): A Comprehensive Review," *J Operat Psychiatr*, 1980, 11:48-65.

Overall JE and Gorham DR, "The Brief Psychiatric Rating Scale," *Psychol Rep*, 1962, 10:799-812.

Overall JE and Gorham DR, "The Brief Psychiatric Rating Scale (BPRS): Recent Developments in Ascertainment and Scaling," *Psychopharmacol Bull*, 1988, 24:97-9.

Overall JE and Gorham DR, "The Brief Psychiatric Scale," *ECDEU Assessment Manual for Psychopharmacology*, Guy W, ed, Rockville, MD: U.S. Department of Health, Education, and Welfare, 1976, 157-69.

COPYRIGHT

Not applicable

SCALE GENERALLY DONE BY

Psychiatrists, psychologists, other trained raters

TIME TO COMPLETE SCALE

15-30 minutes

REPRESENTATIVE STUDY UTILIZING SCALE

Evans JD, Heaton RK, Paulsen JS, et al, "Schizoaffective Disorder: A Form of Schizophrenia or Affective Disorder?" *J Clin Psychiatry*, 1999, 60(12):874-82.

A. BRIEF PSYCHIATRIC RATING SCALE (BPRS) *(Continued)*

THE BRIEF PSYCHIATRIC RATING SCALE (BPRS)

This form consists of 18-symptom constructs, each to be rated on a 7-point scale of severity, ranging from "not present" to "extremely severe". If a specific symptom is not rated, mark "0" = Not Assessed. Enter the score for the description which best describes the patient's condition.

> 0 = not assessed
> 1 = not present
> 2 = very mild
> 3 = mild
> 4 = moderate
> 5 = moderately severe
> 6 = severe
> 7 = extremely severe

1. _____ **Somatic Concern:** Degree of concern over present bodily health. Rate the degree to which physical health is perceived as a problem by the patient, whether complaints have a realistic basis or not.

2. _____ **Anxiety:** Worry, fear, or overconcern for present or future. Rate solely on the basis of verbal report of patient's own subjective experiences. Do not infer anxiety from physical signs or from neurotic defense mechanisms.

3. _____ **Emotional Withdrawal:** Deficiency in relating to the interviewer and to the interviewer situation. Rate only the degree to which the patient gives the impression of failing to be in emotional contact with other people in the interview situation.

4. _____ **Conceptual Disorganization:** Degree to which the thought processes are confused, disconnected, or disorganized. Rate on the basis of integration of the verbal products of the patient; do not rate on the basis of patient's subjective impression of his own level of functioning.

5. _____ **Guilt Feelings:** Overconcern or remorse for past behavior. Rate on the basis of the patient's subjective experiences of guilt as evidenced by verbal report with appropriate affect; do not infer guilt feelings from depression, anxiety, or neurotic defenses.

6. _____ **Tension:** Physical and motor manifestations of tension, nervousness, and heightened activation level. Tension should be rated solely on the basis of physical signs and motor behavior and not on the basis of subjective experiences of tension reported by the patient.

7. _____ **Mannerisms and Posturing:** Unusual and unnatural motor behavior, the type of motor behavior which causes certain mental patients to stand out in a crowd of normal people. Rate only abnormality of movements; do not rate simple heightened motor activity here.

8. _____ **Grandiosity:** Exaggerated self-opinion, conviction of unusual ability or powers. Rate only on the basis of patient's statements about himself or self in relation to others, not on the basis of his demeanor in the interview situation.

9. _____ **Depressive Mood:** Despondency in mood, sadness. Rate only degree of despondency; do not rate on the basis of inferences concerning depression based upon general retardation and somatic complaints.

10. _____ **Hostility:** Animosity, contempt, belligerence, disdain for other people outside the interview situation. Rate solely on the basis of the verbal report of feelings and actions of the patient toward others; do not infer hostility from neurotic defenses, anxiety, nor somatic complaints. Rate attitude toward interviewer under "uncooperativeness".

THE BRIEF PSYCHIATRIC RATING SCALE (BPRS) *(continued)*

11. _____ **Suspiciousness:** Belief, delusional or otherwise, that others have now or have had in the past, malicious or discriminatory intent toward the patient. On the basis of verbal report, rate only those suspicions which are currently held whether they concern past or present circumstances.

12. _____ **Hallucinatory Behavior:** Perceptions without normal external stimulus correspondence. Rate only those experiences which are reported to have occurred within the last week and which are described as distinctly different from the thought and imagery processes of normal people.

13. _____ **Motor Retardation:** Reduction in energy level evidenced by slowed movements. Rate on the basis of observed behavior of the patient only; do not rate on the basis of patient's subjective impression of own energy level.

14. _____ **Uncooperativeness:** Evidence of resistance, unfriendliness, resentment, and lack of readiness to cooperate with interviewer. Rate only on the basis of the patient's attitude and responses to the interviewer, and interview situation; do not rate on the basis of reported resentment or uncooperativeness outside the interview situation.

15. _____ **Unusual Thought Content:** Unusual, odd, strange, or bizarre thought content. Rate here the degree of unusualness, not the degree of disorganization of thought processes.

16. _____ **Blunted Affect:** Reduced emotional tone, apparent lack of normal feeling or involvement.

17. _____ **Excitement:** Heightened emotional tone, agitation, increased reactivity.

18. _____ **Disorientation:** Confusion or lack of proper association for person, place, or time.

B. COMPREHENSIVE PSYCHOPATHOLOGICAL RATING SCALE (CPRS)

OVERVIEW

The CPRS was developed by an interdisciplinary task group, and is intended to measure changes in psychopathology over time. The scale contains 67 items, including one global rating, and one item documenting the reliability of the interview. The majority (40 items) are based upon reported symptoms. The scale is graded from 0-3 for each item (0 = no symptoms, 4 = extreme), and the use of half steps is encouraged to improve sensitivity. Rating is based upon a clinical interview. The strengths of the CPRS include its emphasis on items that are sensitive to change, and its clear description of items. Disadvantages include a relatively long administration time period.

GENERAL APPLICATIONS

The CPRS is a scale to assess changes in psychopathology in serious mental illness.

SELECTED PSYCHOMETRIC PROPERTIES

Interrater reliability for the CPRS has been reported to be at least 0.78 or higher for most items.

REFERENCES

Asberg M, Montgomery SA, Perris C, et al, "A Comprehensive Psychopathological Rating Scale," *Acta Psychiatr Scand Suppl*, 1978, 271:5-27.

Jacobsson L, von Knorring L, Mattsson B, et al, "The Comprehensive Psychopathological Rating Scale - CPRS in Patients With Schizophrenic Syndromes. Interrater Reliability and in Relation to Marten's S-Scale," *Acta Psychiatr Scand Suppl*, 1978 271:39-44.

COPYRIGHT

Munksgaard
Norre Sogade 35, PO Box 2148
1016 Copenhagen K, Denmark

SCALE GENERALLY DONE BY

Mental health clinicians

TIME TO COMPLETE SCALE

45-60 minutes

REPRESENTATIVE STUDY UTILIZING SCALE

van Os J, Gilvarry C, Bale R, et al, "To What Extent Does Symptomatic Improvement Result in Better Outcome in Psychotic Illness? UK700 Group," *Psychol Med*, 1999, 29(5):1183-95.

The Comprehensive Psychopathological Rating Scale (CPRS)

Instructions to the rater:

The rating should be based on a flexible clinical interview where the subject is initially encouraged to describe in his own words, and in as much detail as possible, the symptoms that are relevant to him. The interviewer should then decide which items in the scale have not been fully covered and phrase questions in as broad and neutral manner as possible to allow the subject to elaborate these areas. If this is not sufficient for the rating, more specific questions may be needed. The first interview in a series intended to measure change is, to some extent, a training session for both the rater and the subject. It may, therefore, be useful to let the interview cover a much longer time span than will eventually be rated, to make sure that the subject fully understands the questions and to let the rater familiarize himself with the subject's history. This will make it easier for the rater to phrase the pertinent questions in later interviews. We have found it useful and would recommend that a separate sheet is used for each new rating.

ITEM LIST

Reported	Observed
1. Sadness	41. Apparent sadness
2. Elation	42. Elevated mood
3. Inner tension	43. Hostility
4. Hostile feelings	44. Labile emotional responses
5. Inability to feel	45. Lack of emotional responses
6. Pessimistic thoughts	46. Autonomic disturbances
7. Suicidal thoughts	47. Sleepiness
8. Hypochondriasis	48. Distractibility
9. Worrying over trifles	49. Withdrawal
10. Compulsive thoughts	50. Perplexity
11. Phobias	51. Blank spells
12. Rituals	52. Disorientation
13. Indecision	53. Pressure of speech
14. Lassitude	54. Reduced speech
15. Fatiguability	55. Specific speech defects
16. Concentration difficulties	56. Flight of ideas
17. Failing memory	57. Incoherent speech
18. Reduced appetite	58. Perseveration
19. Reduced sleep	59. Overactivity
20. Increased sleep	60. Slowness of movement
21. Reduced sexual interest	61. Agitation
22. Increased sexual interest	62. Involuntary movements
23. Autonomic disturbances	63. Muscular tension
24. Aches and pains	64. Mannerisms and postures
25. Muscular tension	65. Hallucinatory behavior
26. Loss of sensation or movement	66. Global rating of illness
27. Derealization	67. Assumed reliability of the rating
28. Depersonalization	
29. Feeling controlled	
30. Disrupted thoughts	
31. Ideas of persecution	
32. Ideas of grandeur	
33. Delusional mood	
34. Ecstatic experiences	
35. Morbid jealousy	
36. Other delusions	
37. Commenting voices	
38. Other auditory hallucinations	
39. Visual hallucinations	
40. Other hallucinations	

B. COMPREHENSIVE PSYCHOPATHOLOGICAL
RATING SCALE (CPRS) *(Continued)*

REPORTED PSYCHOPATHOLOGY

1 *Sadness*

Representing subjectively experienced mood, regardless of whether it is reflected in appearance or not. Includes depressed mood, low spirits, despondency, and the feeling of being beyond help and without hope. Rate according to intensity, duration, and the extent to which the mood is influenced by events. Elated mood is scored zero on this item.

0   Occasional sadness may occur in the circumstances.

1   Predominant feelings of sadness, but brighter moments occur.

2   Pervasive feelings of sadness or gloominess. The mood is hardly influenced by external circumstances.

3   Continuous experience of misery or extreme despondency.

2 *Elation*

Representing subjectively experienced mood, regardless of whether it is reflected in demeanor or not. Includes reports of well-being, high spirits, and unvarying exuberance. Rate according to intensity, duration, and the extent to which the mood is influenced by external circumstances. Distinguish from ecstatic experiences (34). Depressed mood is scored zero.

0   Occasional cheerfulness may occur in the circumstances.

1   Predominant feelings of well-being and high spirits, but lower moods occur.

2   Pervasive feelings of well-being and high spirits. The mood is hardly influenced by the circumstances. Longer periods of abundant good humor.

3   Unvarying exuberance, supreme well-being, intense exhilaration.

3 *Inner tension*

Representing feelings of ill-defined discomfort, edginess, inner turmoil, mental tension mounting to panic, dread, and anguish. Rate according to intensity, frequency, duration, and the extent of reassurance called for. Distinguish from sadness (1), worrying (9), and muscular tension (25).

0   Placid. Only fleeting inner tension.

1   Occasional feelings of edginess and ill-defined discomfort.

2   Continuous feelings of inner tension, or intermittent panic which the patient can only master with some difficulty.

3   Unrelenting dread or anguish. Overwhelming panic.

4 *Hostile feelings*

Representing anger, hostility, and aggressive feelings regardless of whether they are acted on or not. Rate according to intensity, frequency, and the amount of provocation tolerated. Inability to feel angry is scored zero on this item (Cf. inability to feel, 5)

0   Not easily angered.

1   Easily angered. Reports hostile feelings, which are easily dissipated.

2   Reacts to provocation with excessive anger or hostility.

3   Persistent anger, rage, or intense hatred which is difficult or impossible to control.

5 *Inability to feel*

Representing the subjective experience of reduced interest in the surroundings, or activities that normally give pleasure. The ability to react with adequate emotion to circumstances or people is reduced. Distinguish from lassitude (14).

0   Normal interest in the surroundings and in other people.

1   Reduced ability to enjoy usual interests. Reduced ability to feel anger.

2   Loss of interest in the surroundings. Loss of feelings for friends and acquaintances.

3   The experience of being emotionally paralyzed, inability to feel anger or grief, and a complete or even painful failure to feel for close relatives and friends.

6 *Pessimistic thoughts*

Representing thoughts of guilt, inferiority, self-reproach, sinfulness, remorse, and ruin

0   No pessimistic thoughts.

1   Fluctuating ideas of failure, self-reproach, or self-depreciation.

2   Persistent self-accusations, or definite but still rational ideas of guilt or sin. Increasingly pessimistic about the future.

3   Delusions of ruin, remorse, and unredeemable sin. Absurd self-accusation.

7 *Suicidal thoughts*

Representing the feeling that life is not worth living, that a natural death would be welcome, suicidal thoughts, and preparation for suicide. Suicidal attempts should not in themselves influence the rating.

0   Enjoys life or takes it as it comes.

1   Weary of life. Only fleeting suicidal thoughts.

2   Much better off dead. Suicidal thoughts are common, and suicide is considered as a possible solution, but without specific plans or intention.

3   Explicit plans for suicide when there is an opportunity. Active preparations for suicide.

8 *Hypochondriasis*

Representing exaggerated preoccupation or unrealistic worrying about ill health or disease. Distinguish from worrying over trifles (9), aches and pains (24), and loss of sensation or movement (26).

0   No particular preoccupation with ill health.

1   Reacting to minor bodily dysfunction with foreboding. Exaggerated fear of disease.

2   Convinced that there is some disease, but can be reassured, if only briefly.

3   Incapacitating or absurd hypochondriacal convictions (body rotting away, bowels have not worked for months).

B. COMPREHENSIVE PSYCHOPATHOLOGICAL RATING SCALE (CPRS) *(Continued)*

9 *Worrying over trifles*

Representing apprehension, and undue concern over trifles, which is difficult to stop and out of proportion to the circumstances. Distinguish from inner tension (3), pessimistic thoughts (6), hypochondriasis (8), compulsive thoughts (10), phobias (11), and indecision (13),

    0 No particular worries.

    1 Undue concern, worrying that can be shaken off.

    2 Apprehensive and bothered about trifles or minor daily routines.

    3 Unrelenting and often painful worrying. Reassurance is ineffective.

10 *Compulsive thoughts*

Representing disturbing or frightening thoughts or doubts which are experienced as silly or irrational, but keep coming back against one's will. Distinguish from hypochondriasis (8), worrying over trifles (9), and disrupted thoughts (30).

    0 No repetitive thoughts.

    1 Occasional compulsive thoughts which are not disturbing.

    2 Frequent disturbing compulsive thoughts.

    3 Incapacitating or obnoxious obsessions, occupying one's entire mind.

11 *Phobias*

Representing feelings of unreasonable fear in specific situations (eg, buses, supermarkets, crowds, feeling enclosed, being alone) which are avoided if possible.

    0 No phobias.

    1 Feelings of vague discomfort in particular situations which can be mastered without help or by taking simple precautions like avoiding rush hours when possible.

    2 Certain situations consistently provoke marked discomfort, and are avoided without impairing social performance.

    3 Incapacitating phobias which severely restrict activities (eg, completely unable to leave home).

12 *Rituals*

Representing a compulsive repeating of particular acts or rituals which are regarded as unnecessary or absurd and resisted initially but cannot be suppressed without discomfort. The rating is based on the time spent on rituals and the degree of social incapacity.

    0 No compulsive behavior.

    1 Slight or occasional compulsive checking.

    2 Clear-cut compulsive rituals which do not interfere with social performance.

    3 Extensive rituals or checking habits that are time-consuming and incapacitating.

13 *Indecision*

Representing vacillation and difficulty in choosing between simple alternatives. Distinguish from worrying over trifles (9), and compulsive thoughts (10).

    0   No indecisiveness.

    1   Some vacillation but can still make a decision when necessary.

    2   Indecisiveness or vacillation which restricts or prevents action, makes it difficult to answer simple questions or make simple choices.

    3   Extreme indecisiveness even in situations where conscious deliberation is not normally required, such as whether to sit or stand, enter or stay outside.

14 *Lassitude*

Representing a difficulty getting started or slowness initiating and performing everyday activities. Distinguish from indecision (13) and fatiguability (15).

    0   Hardly any difficulty in getting started. No sluggishness.

    1   Difficulties in starting activities.

    2   Difficulties in starting simple routine activities which are carried out only with effort.

    3   Complete inertia; unable to start activity without help.

15 *Fatiguability*

Representing the experience of tiring more easily than usual. When lassitude (14) is extreme, this item is difficult to evaluate. If impossible, do not rate. Distinguish from lassitude (14).

    0   Ordinary staying power. Not easily fatigued.

    1   Tires easily but does not have to take a break more often than usual.

    2   Easily wearied. Frequently forced to pause and rest.

    3   Exhaustion interrupts almost all activities or even makes them impossible.

16 *Concentration difficulties*

Representing difficulties in collecting one's thoughts mounting to incapacitating lack of concentration. Rate according to intensity, frequency, and degree of incapacity produced. Distinguish from failing memory (17), and disrupted thoughts (30).

    0   No difficulties in concentrating

    1   Occasional difficulties in collecting one's thoughts.

    2   Difficulties in concentrating and sustaining thought which interfere with reading or conversation.

    3   Incapacitating lack of concentration.

17 *Failing memory*

Representing subjective disturbances of recall compared with previous ability. Distinguish from concentration difficulties (16).

    0   Memory as usual.

    1   Occasional increased lapses of memory.

    2   Reports of socially inconvenient or disturbing loss of memory.

    3   Complaints of complete inability to remember.

B. COMPREHENSIVE PSYCHOPATHOLOGICAL RATING SCALE (CPRS) *(Continued)*

18 *Reduced appetite*

Representing the feeling of a loss of appetite compared with when well.

    0   Normal or increased appetite.
    1   Slightly reduced appetite.
    2   No appetite. Food is tasteless. Need to force oneself to eat.
    3   Must be forced to eat. Food refusal.

19 *Reduced sleep*

Representing a subjective experience of reduced duration or depth of sleep compared to the subject's own normal pattern when well.

    0   Sleeps as usual.
    1   Slight difficulty dropping off to sleep or slightly reduced, light, or fitful sleep.
    2   Sleep reduced or broken by at least 2 hours.
    3   Less than two or three hours' sleep.

20 *Increased sleep*

Representing a subjective experience of increased duration or depth of sleep, compared to the subject's own normal pattern when well.

    0   No extra sleep.
    1   Sleeps deeper or longer than usual.
    2   Several hours extra sleep.
    3   Spends a great part of the day asleep in spite of normal or increased sleep at night.

21 *Reduced sexual interest*

Representing descriptions of a reduced sexual interest or a reduction of sexual activity (this should always be judged against the subject's usual sexual habits when well). Habitual impotence or frigidity should be ignored when assessing interest. Distinguish from inability to feel (5). Increased sexual interest is rated 0.

    0   No reduction of sexual interest.
    1   Sexual interest is admitted to be reduced, but activity is unimpaired.
    2   Definite reduction of sexual interest. Ordinary sexual activities are reduced or nonexistent.
    3   Complete sexual indifference.

22 *Increased sexual interest*

Representing descriptions of a stronger sexual interest than usual, which may be reflected in an increase in sexual activities or fantasies. (This should always be judged against the subject's usual sexual habits when well.)

    0   No increase in sexual interest.
    1   Increase in sexual interest or fantasies not reflected in activities.
    2   Definite increase in sexual interest or activities, or intrusive sexual fantasies.
    3   Totally preoccupied with sexual fantasies. Very marked increase in sexual activities.

23 *Autonomic disturbances*

Representing descriptions of palpitations, breathing difficulties, dizziness, increased sweating, cold hands and feet, dry mouth, indigestion, diarrhea, frequent micturition. Distinguish from inner tension (3), aches and pains (24), and loss of sensation or movement (26).

0   No autonomic disturbances.

1   Occasional autonomic symptoms which occur under emotional stress.

2   Frequent or intense autonomic disturbances which are experienced as discomforting or socially inconvenient.

3   Very frequent autonomic disturbances which interrupt other activities or are incapacitating.

24 *Aches and pains*

Representing reports of bodily discomfort, aches, and pains. Rate according to intensity, frequency and duration, and also request for relief. Disregard any opinion of organic cause. Distinguish from hypochondriasis (8), autonomic disturbance (23), and muscular tension (25).

0   Absent or transient aches.

1   Occasional definite aches and pains.

2   Prolonged and inconvenient aches and pains. Requests for effective analgesics.

3   Severely interfering or crippling pains.

25 *Muscle tension*

Representing the description of increased tension in the muscles and a difficulty in relaxing physically. Distinguish from aches and pains (24).

0   No increase in muscular tension.

1   Some occasional increase in muscular tension, more evident in demanding situations.

2   Considerable difficulty in finding a comfortable position when sitting or laying. Disturbing muscular tension.

3   Painful muscular tension. Completely incapable of relaxing physically.

26 *Loss of sensation or movement*

Representing impairment or loss of particular motor or sensory functions. Disregard any organic basis. Distinguish from hypochondriasis (8), autonomic disturbances (23), and aches and pains (24).

0   No impairment of sensory or motor functions.

1   Slight and transient impairment which does not disturb ordinary activities.

2   Clear-cut impairment or loss of some function, but manages daily activities without help.

3   Severely incapacitating and persistent sensorimotor loss which necessitates help, such as blindness, inability to walk or speak.

B. COMPREHENSIVE PSYCHOPATHOLOGICAL
RATING SCALE (CPRS) *(Continued)*

27 *Derealization*

Representing a change in the quality of awareness of the surroundings, which may appear artificial. Also includes deja-vu, deja-vecu, and changed intensity of perceptions. Distinguish from depersonalization (28).

    0   No change in awareness.

    1   Occasional episodes of deja-vu phenomena or derealization.

    2   Frequent episodes of derealization.

    3   Very frequent or persistent derealization.

28 *Depersonalization*

Representing a change in the quality of awareness of oneself combined with feelings of unreality, bodily change, detachment, or radical change of person. Distinguish from inability to feel (5), derealization (27), feeling controlled (29).

    0   No experience of change.

    1   Occasional or vague feelings of change in oneself.

    2   Feelings of change of person which are intrusive.

    3   Continuous experience of a radical change of one's person.

29 *Feeling controlled*

Representing the experience of being in the literal sense influenced or controlled from without, and the experience that feelings, impulses, or volitions are imposed from without. Also rated under this heading is the experience of being able to control others in a similar manner. Distinguish from disrupted thoughts (30), and ideas of persecution (31).

    0   Ordinary influence from social forces.

    1   Vague or unconvincing report of being unnaturally influenced from without.

    2   Occasional but clear experiences of being controlled from without (eg, by means of hypnosis).

    3   Continuous experiences that feelings or impulses do not derive from oneself, but are forced into one (eg, by means of rays).

30 *Disrupted thoughts*

Representing the experience of a sudden stoppage of thoughts (thought blocking), or thoughts being put into one's head (insertion), or being taken out (withdrawal), or listened to or broadcast. Distinguish from compulsive thoughts (10), and concentration difficulties (16).

    0   No thought interruptions.

    1   Vague or unconvincing reports of episodes of interruptions to thought.

    2   Occasional but clear thought blocking or occasional episodes of thought insertion or withdrawal. Feeling that thoughts are being read.

    3   Disturbing or disabling thought interruptions. Thought broadcasting.

31 *Ideas of persecution*

Representing suspiciousness, exaggerated self-consciousness, the conviction of being talked about or watched or persecuted with malicious intent.

0 No undue suspiciousness or self-consciousness.

1 Vague feelings of being observed. Occasional suspicions of malice.

2 Pervasive feelings of being talked about, threatened, or persecuted.

3 Unalterable conviction of being the victim of systematic persecution. Delusional misinterpretation of ordinary events or "cues". Conviction of being referred to beyond the realm of likelihood (eg, television or in newspapers).

32 *Ideas of grandeur*

Representing exaggerated opinion of self-importance, capabilities or good health. Distinguish from elation (2), and ecstatic experiences (34).

0 No ideas of grandeur.

1 Self assured, with an inflated sense of one's own importance.

2 Clearly exaggerated opinion of self-importance and capabilities. Grandiose, facile, and unrealistic plans for the future.

3 Absurd, delusional ideas of grandeur.

33 *Delusional mood*

Representing strong, unreasonable premonitions, the feeling or sudden conviction that trivial events or things have a profound and bizarre significance. Distinguish from derealization (27), and ecstatic experiences (34).

0 Only ordinary superstitions. No delusional mood.

1 Vague premonitions that something personal and unknown is about to happen.

2 A strong feeling that generally trivial events have a special significance (delusional mood).

3 The sudden unshakable conviction, appearing out of the blue, that a particular set of events has a profound and often bizarre meaning (autochronous delusions).

34 *Ecstatic experiences*

Representing experiences of mystic rapture, bliss, or ecstatic happiness which may involve sudden illumination, insight into religious matters, or union with God. Distinguish from elation (2), and ideas of grandeur (32).

0 No ecstatic experiences.

1 Occasional inexplicable feelings of happiness with metaphysical overtones.

2 Frequent experiences of bliss rapture connected with feelings of sudden insight into metaphysical matters.

3 Marked, or continuous feelings of bliss or mystic rapture, "oceanic feelings", mystical union with God.

B. COMPREHENSIVE PSYCHOPATHOLOGICAL
RATING SCALE (CPRS) *(Continued)*

35 *Morbid jealousy*

Representing an absorbing preoccupation with the possible unfaithfulness of a sexual partner.

    0   No undue suspicions toward the partner.

    1   Vague feelings of insecurity and suspicions about the partner's faithfulness.

    2   Searches for and misinterprets "evidence" of unfaithfulness.

    3   Morbid ideas of jealousy dominate life and actions. Threatens the partner and tries to extract "confessions".

36 *Other delusions*

Representing any other delusions than those above (pessimistic thoughts (6), hypochondriasis (8), feeling controlled (29), ideas of persecution (31), ideas of grandeur (32), delusional mood (33), morbid jealousy (35)).

    0   No other delusions.

    1   Vague and unconvincing descriptions.

    2   Definitely pathological ideas, approaching delusional strength.

    3   Absurd delusions which may be reflected in behavior.

37 *Commenting voices*

Representing the experience of hearing one's own thoughts spoken or repeated aloud or hearing voices, commenting or arguing about one in the third person. Distinguish from other auditory hallucinations (38).

    0   No hallucinated commenting voices.

    1   Vague or unconvincing reports of commenting voices.

    2   Definite, but not disabling, hallucinated voices.

    3   Frequent, disabling hallucinated voices.

38 *Other auditory hallucinations*

Representing all hallucinated sounds or voices except commenting voices (37). Also includes auditory hallucinations in keeping with the predominant mood such as depression or elation.

    0   No auditory hallucinations, except for hypnagogic phenomena (on going to sleep).

    1   Misinterpretations of auditory stimuli. Vague or unconvincing reports of auditory hallucinations.

    2   Definite hallucinations which may be persistent but not intrusive.

    3   Loud or unpleasant hallucinations. Forceful commands.

39 *Visual hallucinations*

Representing a misinterpretation of a visual stimulus (illusion) or a false visual perception without any actual outside stimulus (hallucination).

    0   No false visual experiences, except for possible hypnagogic phenomena.

    1   Occasional illusions.

    2   Frequent illusions or occasional visual hallucinations.

    3   Clear, frequent, or persistent hallucinations.

40 *Other hallucinations*

Representing hallucinations of taste, smell, or bodily sensation. Specify the senses, and base the rating on the most severe.

    0   No hallucinations.

    1   Vague or unconvincing reports of hallucinations.

    2   Occasional, but definite, hallucinations.

    3   Clear, frequent, or persistent hallucinations.

OBSERVED PSYCHOPATHOLOGY

41 *Apparent sadness*

Representing despondency, gloom, and despair (more than just ordinary transient low spirits) reflected in speech, facial expression, and posture. Rate by depth and inability to brighten up.

    0   No sadness.

    1   Looks dispirited, but brightens up occasionally.

    2   Appears sad and unhappy all of the time.

    3   Extreme and continuous gloom and despondency.

42 *Elated mood*

Representing an elated and exuberant state (excludes ordinary transient high spirits). Includes evident increased well-being, self-confidence, elation, and hilarity shown in speech, choice of subject, facial expression, posture, and activity. Rate according to intensity and inability to respond seriously when demanded.

    0   Normal cheerfulness.

    1   Self-confident and somewhat expansive, but can change to seriousness when demanded.

    2   Expansive hilarity with exaggerated self-confidence and mirth that is out of tune. Unable to respond seriously.

    3   Displays persistent extreme exuberance, exhilaration, and absurd hilarity.

43 *Hostility*

Representing irritability, angry looks, words, or actions. Rate by intensity and frequency, and the small amount of provocation that elicits the response and the time taken to quieten.

    0   No evident hostility.

    1   Querulous, touchy, and irritable on provocation. Occasional angry glances.

    2   Pugnacious, quarrelsome, very aggressive gestures, but can be calmed down.

    3   Threatening behavior or actual physical violence.

44 *Labile emotional responses*

Representing rapidly changing moods (eg, sudden elation to sadness) with a tendency to display intense emotional responses. Should not be confused with the preponderant mood. Rate by speed and frequency of change.

    0   No sudden mood changes.

    1   Occasional and understandable rapid mood changes.

    2   Frequent sudden or exaggerated mood changes.

    3   Very rapid changes between intense opposite moods.

B. COMPREHENSIVE PSYCHOPATHOLOGICAL RATING SCALE (CPRS) *(Continued)*

45 *Lack of appropriate emotion*

Representing blunting of affects as shown by lack of emotional expression, or the occurrence of incongruous emotional displays which are clearly out of keeping with the situation. Distinguish from apparent sadness (41), and elated mood (42).

    0   Appropriate affect in keeping with mood.

    1   Apparent lack of concern, slightly odd displays of emotion.

    2   Responds in a clearly inappropriate way on sensitive issues, or appears not to respond at all.

    3   Only clearly bizarre emotional response, or total emotional indifference.

46 *Autonomic disturbances*

Representing signs of autonomic dysfunction, hyperventilation, or frequent sighing, blushing, sweating, cold hands, enlarged pupils, dry mouth, and fainting.

    0   No observed autonomic disturbances.

    1   Occasional or slight autonomic disturbances, such as blushing or blanching, or sweating under stress.

    2   Obvious autonomic disturbances on several occasions even when not under stress.

    3   Autonomic disturbances which disrupt the interview.

47 *Sleepiness*

Representing evident diminished ability to stay awake as seen in facial expression, speech, or posture. Distinguish from withdrawal (49), perplexity (50), and slowness of movement (60).

    0   Fully awake.

    1   Looks sleepy. Yawns occasionally.

    2   Tends to fall asleep when left in peace.

    3   Falls asleep during interview or is difficult to wake.

48 *Distractibility*

Representing attention easily diverted by irrelevant external stimuli. Distinguish from withdrawal (49), perplexity (50), blank spells (51), flight of ideas (56), and hallucinatory behavior (65).

    0   Adequately sustained attention.

    1   Attention occasionally distracted by irrelevant stimuli (eg, background noises).

    2   Easily distracted.

    3   Continually distracted by incidental events and objects which make interviewing difficult or impossible.

49 *Withdrawal*

Representing grossly restricted attention and apparent unawareness of people or surroundings. Distinguish from sleepiness (47), perplexity (50), blank spells (51), and reduced speech (54).

    0   Apparently well aware of the surroundings.

    1   Occasional withdrawal, but attention can be brought back without difficulty.

    2   Appears absent and withdrawn and is only brought back to the interview with difficulty.

    3   Completely withdrawn. Appears not to react to words or touch.

50 *Perplexity*

Representing bewilderment, a difficulty in comprehending any situation, and interpreting the context. Distinguish from sleepiness (47), distractibility (48), and withdrawal (49).

0   No perplexity.
1   Puzzled. Occasional difficulty understanding what should be simple questions.
2   Appears bewildered. Simple questions must be repeated to be understood. Occasional answers unrelated to the question.
3   Obviously perplexed and bewildered. Speech and behavior clearly inappropriate, as if in a dream.

51 *Blank spells*

Representing sudden stoppages and inattention while speaking, which last for a few seconds or longer. It is often accompanied by immobility and apparent thought blocking. Distinguish from reduced speech (54), specific speech defects (55), incoherent speech (57).

0   No blank spells.
1   Occasional lapses which could be interpreted as wandering of the mind.
2   Obvious blank spells even when not under particular stress.
3   Frequent or long blank spells which interfere with conversation.

52 *Disorientation*

Representing failure of orientation in time and place.

0   Fully oriented.
1   Minimal disorientation as to day or date.
2   Marked disorientation for date or some disorientation in time.
3   Markedly disoriented for time and place.

53 *Pressure of speech*

Representing pressure to talk, increased flow of speech, and undue loquaciousness. Reduced speech is scored zero on this item. Distinguish from flight of ideas (56), and incoherent speech (57).

0   Ordinary speech without undue loquaciousness.
1   Rapid, verbose speech. Gives detailed answers.
2   Garrulous and very difficult to interrupt.
3   Leads the interview. Words come tumbling out. Cannot be interrupted.

54 *Reduced speech*

Representing reticent or slowed speech with long delays or pauses. Pressure of speech is scored zero on this item. Distinguish from withdrawal (49), perplexity (50), blank spells (51), specific speech defects (55).

0   Ordinary speech without undue pauses.
1   Takes time to produce brief answers.
2   Extremely brief monosyllabic answers with long delays. Hardly any spontaneous comments and, when they occur, they are slow.
3   Monosyllabic answers are only produced with great effort. Almost or completely mute.

B. COMPREHENSIVE PSYCHOPATHOLOGICAL RATING SCALE (CPRS) *(Continued)*

55 *Specific speech defects*

Representing, for example, stuttering, dysarthria, and aphasia - specify the type, and any obvious reason.

    0   No specific difficulties with speech.

    1   Occasional speech defects, especially when upset.

    2   Very evident speech defects which are intrusive, but do not interfere with communication.

    3   Persistent and disturbing speech defects which markedly interfere with communication.

56 *Flight of ideas*

Representing a rapid flow of ideas shown in speech. There is a continuity of thought, even if it is difficult or even impossible to catch up, in contrast to incoherent speech (57).

    0   Ordinary flow of ideas.

    1   Free and lively associations with tendency to drift in the discussion.

    2   Rapid flow of ideas which can be followed. Frequent changes of subject which interfere with conversation.

    3   The rapid changes of subject, and the richness and speed of associations make conversation extremely difficult or impossible.

57 *Incoherent speech*

Representing circumlocutory disorganized or apparently illogical speech with inexplicable shifts from topic to topic, distortion and fragmenting of syntax, and words. Distinguish from flights of ideas (56).

    0   Coherent and understandable speech.

    1   Pedantic and slightly circumlocutory speech. Some idiosyncratic but comprehensible use of words or phrases, especially under stress.

    2   Illogical association between words or phrases even when not under stress. "Knights move" shifts.

    3   Obviously disjointed and illogical speech. Fragmentation of phrases or words or bizarre neologisms, which seriously interfere with communication.

58 *Perseveration*

Representing a tendency to get stuck, to repeat sentences or actions such as repeating the answer to a previous question to subsequent questions, and to constantly return to the same topic; or being unable to interrupt a thought or action.

    0   No perseveration.

    1   The same phrase is occasionally repeated. Returns to the same question several times.

    2   Repeats the same phrase, but can be persuaded to give more adequate answers. Difficulties in interrupting a line of thought or an action once started.

    3   Perseverating phrases or behavior makes communication difficult or impossible.

59 *Overactivity*

Representing an increase in frequency and extent of voluntary movement (facial movements, gait, accompanying movements, and gestures) and an increased speed in their initiation and completion. Distinguish from agitation (61), and involuntary movements (62).

0   Ordinary change between activity and rest.
1   Lively gestures and hurried gait but can rest.
2   Obviously expansive and rapid movements and gestures. Abrupt reactions. Leaves the chair occasionally during the interview.
3   Continuous wildly exaggerated motor activity. Cannot be persuaded to sit or lie down.

60 *Slowness of movement*

Representing a decrease in frequency and extent of voluntary movements. Facial movements, gait, accompanying movements and gestures retarded and sluggish.

0   Ordinary change between rest and activity.
1   Minimal gestures and facial movements.
2   Almost no spontaneous motor activity. Slow and labored movement.
3   Has to be led to the interview. No spontaneous movements. Immobile face. Stupor.

61 *Agitation*

Representing "purposeless" motor activity such as hand-wringing, picking at objects and clothes, inability to sit still. Distinguish from overactivity (59), involuntary movements (62), and mannerisms (64).

0   No agitation.
1   Difficult to keep hands still. Changes position several times during the interview. Fiddles with objects.
2   Obviously restless. Vacant and obtrusive picking at objects. Half-rises occasionally.
3   Cannot be persuaded to sit except for brief periods. Incessant purposeless wandering.

62 *Involuntary movements*

Representing the following involuntary movements - tics, tremor, choreoathetotic movements, dyskinesias, dystonias, and torticollis. Specify the type. Distinguish from overactivity (59), agitation (61), and mannerisms (64).

0   No involuntary movements.
1   Occasional involuntary movements when under stress.
2   Obvious and frequent involuntary movements, accentuated when under stress. Manages not to let them interfere with ordinary motor activity.
3   Continuous involuntary movements which seriously interfere with ordinary activities.

B. COMPREHENSIVE PSYCHOPATHOLOGICAL RATING SCALE (CPRS) *(Continued)*

63 *Muscular tension*

Representing observed muscular tension as shown in facial expression, posture, and movements.

0 Appears relaxed.

1 Slightly tense face and posture.

2 Moderately tense posture and face (easily seen in jaw and neck muscles). Does not seem to find a relaxed position when sitting. Stiff and awkward movements.

3 Strikingly tense. Often sits hunched and crouched, or tense and rigidly upright at the end of the chair.

64 *Mannerisms and postures*

Representing repeated or stereotypic complex movements or postures, such as grimacing, stylized movements, odd postures, catalepsy. The rating is based on frequency and degree of interference with other activities. Distinguish from perseveration (58), agitation (61), and involuntary movements (62) especially tics.

0 No mannerisms.

1 Occasional or doubtful grimaces or stylized movement.

2 Mannerisms, grimaces, or postures which are obvious, but do not interfere.

3 Pronounced mannerisms or posture which take over from ordinary motor activity.

65 *Hallucinatory behavior*

Representing odd behavior suggestive of hallucinations (eg, turning around suddenly, shouting, or apparently answering voices, retreating from presumed visual hallucinations). Should be rated regardless of whether hallucinations are admitted or not. Distinguish from involuntary movements (62), and mannerisms and posturing (64).

0 No hallucinatory behavior.

1 Odd behavior like talking to oneself, which might represent hallucinatory behavior, but is thought not to be.

2 Convincing hallucinatory behavior.

3 Bizarre or frequent hallucinatory behavior which interferes with the interview.

66 *Global rating of illness*

0 None. Absence of illness.

1 Minimal or doubtful illness which does not interfere.

2 Moderate and definite illness.

3 Severe or incapacitating illness.

67 *Assume reliability of the rating*

0 Very poor.

1 Fair.

2 Good.

3 Very good.

C. MANCHESTER SCALE

OVERVIEW

The Manchester scale, also referred to as the Krawiecka and Goldberg scale, is a brief scale to evaluate change in clinical status for individuals with psychotic conditions, such as schizophrenia. The scale is meant to be utilized by physicians who know the evaluated patient well. The scale consists of eight items which are graded on a 0 to 4 point scale (0 = some evidence symptom is present, but not pathological, 4 = severe symptoms). The scale is based upon a standard clinical interview, with emphasis upon the rated items. Additional information, such as knowledge of patient's previous condition, should also be utilized. Both positive and negative symptoms are assessed. The items evaluated include depression, anxiety, delusions and hallucinations, incoherence, flattened affect, poverty of speech, and psychomotor retardation. Strengths of the Manchester scale include its brevity, clear guidelines for use, and ease of administration. Disadvantages are lack of items that cover features of mania, and some lack of sensitivity for severity rating of certain symptoms (rating of 3 denotes moderate, rating of 4 denotes severe). The authors have produced a training videotape for this scale.

GENERAL APPLICATIONS

The Manchester scale is a brief instrument to assess change in clinical status of chronically psychotic patients.

SELECTED PSYCHOMETRIC PROPERTIES

The authors have demonstrated good interrelater reliability of the Manchester scale, with correlation coefficients ranging from 0.65 to 0.87.

REFERENCES

Krawiecka M, Goldberg D, and Vaughan M, "A Standardized Psychiatric Assessment Scale for Rating Chronic Psychiatric Patients," *Acta Psychiatr Scand*, 1977, 55(4):299-308.

COPYRIGHT

Munksgaard
Norre Sogade 35, PO Box 2148
1016 Copenhagen K, Denmark

SCALE GENERALLY DONE BY

Clinician or trained rater who knows patient well

TIME TO COMPLETE SCALE

10-15 minutes

REPRESENTATIVE STUDY UTILIZING SCALE

Kirov GK, Murray RM, Seth RV, et al, "Observations on Switching Patients With Schizophrenia to Risperidone Treatment. Risperidone Switching Study Group," *Acta Psychiatr Scand*, 1997, 95(5):439-43.

C. MANCHESTER SCALE *(Continued)*

MANCHESTER SCALE

GUIDELINES FOR THE USE OF THE FIVE-POINT SCALES

In making these ratings, the psychiatrist is expected to use his clinical judgment to make overall assessments about the patients in each particular area. For example, in making the rating for depression, the rater should be expressing his own clinical assessment of the severity of depression, based on both the patient's demeanor and behavior during the interview and the history that the patient has given concerning depression. It should be emphasized that a morbid rating (2, 3, or 4) for depression does not imply that the principal diagnosis made will necessarily be an affective illness.

General Rules for the Five-Point Scale

Rating "0" Absent: The item is, for all practical purposes, absent.

Rating "1" Mild: Although there is some evidence for the item in question, it is not considered pathological.

Rating "2" Moderate: The item is present in a degree just sufficient to be regarded as pathological.

Rating "3" Marked:
Rating "4" Severe: See individual definitions

DEPRESSION

This does not only include the actual behavior observed at interview - dejected pose, sad appearance, despondent manner - but should be a clinical rating which expresses the overall assessment of depression, and the contribution that this abnormality of affect is making to the abnormal mental state being rated. Whether there is a discrepancy between depression observed at interview and depressed mood reported as having been experienced in the past week, the rating made should be the greater of the two ratings.

Rating "0" Absent: Normal manner and behavior at interview. No depressive phenomena elicited.

Rating "1" Mild: Although there may be some evidence of depression - occasional gloominess, lack of verve, etc - the rater does not consider that it is pathological, or takes it to be an habitual trait not amounting to clinically significant depression.

Rating "2" Moderate: The patient is thought to be clinically depressed, but to a mild degree
or
Occasional depressed feelings which either cause significant distress or are looked upon by the patient as a significant departure from his usual self, in the past week.

Rating "3" Marked: The patient is thought to be clinically depressed, in marked degree
or
Frequent depressed feelings as described in "2" in the past week, or occasional extreme distress caused by depression.

Rating "4" Severe: The patient is thought to be clinically depressed in extreme degree. Major depressive phenomena should be present; strongly held suicidal ideas, uncontrollable weeping, etc
or
Depression has caused extreme distress frequently in the past week.

ANXIOUS

In addition to direct evidence of anxiety observed by the rater at interview, this rating should express the rater's view of the contribution which morbid anxiety is making to the mental state under consideration. (There may be some physiological signs of sympathetic overactivity, moist palms, mild tremor, blotchy patches on skin, etc.) Where anxiety is of such a degree that there is associated motor agitation, this will be rated on this key as not less than "3". Where there is a discrepancy between anxiety as observed at interview and anxiety expressed in the previous week, the rating made should be the greater of the two ratings.

Rating "0" Absent: Normal mood at interview.

Rating "1" Mild: Such tenseness as the patient displays is thought either to be an habitual trait not amounting to pathological proportions or is thought to be a reasonable response to the interview situation.

Rating "2" Moderate: The patient is thought to display a mild degree of clinically significant anxiety or tension.
or
Anxiety sufficient to cause significant distress has occurred occasionally in the past week.

Rating "3" Marked: The patient is thought to display a marked degree of clinically significant anxiety or tension. He may be apprehensive about the interview and need reassurance, but there are only minor disruptions of the interview due to anxiety. There may be associated motor agitation of mild degree.
or
Anxiety sufficient to cause significant distress has occurred frequently in the past week, *or* anxiety has caused extreme distress for the individual concerned occasionally in the past week.

Rating "4" Severe: The patient is thought to display an extreme degree of clinically significant anxiety or tension. He may be unable to relax, or there may be major disruptions of the interview due to anxiety. There may be associated motor agitation of marked degree, or a fearful preoccupation with impending events.
or
Anxiety has caused extreme distress for the individual concerned frequently in the past week.

FLATTENED, INCONGRUOUS AFFECT

Flatness refers to an impairment in the range of available emotional responses; the patient is unable to convey the impact of events while relating his history, and cannot convey warmth or affection while speaking about those near to him.

Rating "0" Absent: Normal mood at interview.

Rating "1" Mild: The patient may be laconic, taciturn, or unresponsive in discussing emotionally charged topics, but the rater considers that this is an habitual trait rather than a sign of illness.

Rating "2" Moderate: Clinically significant impairment of emotional response of mild degree. Definite lack of emotional tone discussing important topics; *or* occasional but undoubted incongruous emotional responses during the interview.

Rating "3" Marked: Clinically significant impairment of emotional response of marked degree. No warmth or affection shown. Cannot convey impact of events when giving history, no concern expressed about future.
or
Frequent incongruous responses of mild degree or occasional gross incongruity.

C. MANCHESTER SCALE *(Continued)*

Rating "4" Severe: Clinically significant impairment of emotional response of extreme degree; no emotional response whatever elicited.
or
Gross frequent incongruity; fatuous, supercilious, giggling, etc, in such a way as to disturb interview.

PSYCHOMOTOR RETARDATION

Rating "0" Absent: Normal manner and speech during interview. Questions answered fairly promptly; air of spontaneity and changes of expression.

Rating "1" Mild: Although there may be evidence of slowness or poor spontaneity, the rater considers that this is either an habitual trait or that it does not amount to clearly pathological proportions.

Rating "2" Moderate: The rater detects slowness or lack of spontaneity at interview and attributes this to psychiatric illness; it is just clinically detectable. Delays in answering questions would merit this rating providing that the rater considers that it is part of a morbid mental state rather than an habitual trait of the patient.

Rating "3" Marked: Psychomotor retardation attributable to psychiatric illness is easily detectable at interview and is thought to make a material contribution to the abnormalities of the patient's present mental state.

Rating "4" Severe: Psychomotor retardation is present in extreme degree for the individual concerned.

COHERENTLY EXPRESSED DELUSIONS

Rating "0" Absent: No abnormality detected at interview.

Rating "1" Mild: Eccentric beliefs and trivial misinterpretations; that bad weather is caused by nuclear tests; superstitions, religious sects, etc.

Rating "2" Moderate: Over-valued ideas and ideas of reference, or undoubted misinterpretations. Special meanings.

Rating "3" Marked: Undoubted delusions or delusional perceptions are described as having occurred in the past month, but the patient denies that he still holds the beliefs at present.
or
Delusional ideas are expressed but they are not strongly held or incorrigible.

Rating "4" Severe: Undoubted delusions are present and are still held by the patient.

HALLUCINATIONS

The rater must, therefore, decide whether hallucinations have occurred in the past week; if so, whether they are true - or pseudohallucinations, and how frequently they have occurred.

Rating "0" Absent: No evidence of hallucinations.

Rating "1" Mild: The hallucinatory experiences reported to the rater are not definitely morbid, hypnogogic hallucinations, eidetic images and illusions.

Rating "2" Moderate: Pseudohallucinations of hearing and vision; hallucinations associated with insight (eg, those following bereavement).

Rating "3" Marked: True hallucinations have been present in the past week, but have occurred infrequently.

Rating "4" Severe: True hallucinations have occurred frequently in the past week.

154

INCOHERENCE AND IRRELEVANCE OF SPEECH

Rating "0" Absent: No evidence of thought disorder.

Rating "1" Mild: Although replies are sometimes odd, the abnormalities fall short of those required for thought disorder; it is always possible to understand the connection between ideas.

Rating "2" Moderate: Occasional evidence of thought disorder elicited, but patient is otherwise coherent.

Rating "3" Marked: Frequent evidence of thought disorder but meaningful communication is possible with the patient.
or
Several episodes of incoherent speech occur.

Rating "4" Severe: Replies difficult to follow owing to lack of directing associations. Speech frequently incoherent, without a discernible thread of meaning.

POVERTY OF SPEECH, MUTE

Rating "0" Absent: Speech normal in quantity and form.

Rating "1" Mild: Patient only speaks when spoken to; tends to give brief replies.

Rating "2" Moderate: Occasional difficulties or silences but most of interview proceeds smoothly.
or
Conversation impeded by vagueness, hesitancy, or brevity of replies.

Rating "3" Marked: Monosyllabic replies; often long pauses or failure to answer at all.
or
Reasonable amount of speech, but answers slow and hesitant, lacking in content, or repetitions and wandering, that meaningful conversation was almost impossible.

Rating "4" Severe: Mute throughout interview, or speaks only two or three words.
or
Constantly murmuring under breath (prosectic catatonia).

D. NURSES' OBSERVATION SCALE FOR INPATIENT EVALUATION (NOSIE)

OVERVIEW

The NOSIE, developed by G Honigfeld and CJ Klett, is a 30-item scale designed to assess the behavior of patients on an inpatient unit. The rating is based upon continuous observation. The NOSIE was developed in 1965 and is still used with a moderate degree of frequency. The scale is rated according to the frequency of occurrence of the 30 designated behaviors during the previous 3 days (1 = never, 5 = always). The ratings are based upon direct observations of behavior and do not require interpretation nor inference. The advantages of the NOSIE are that it is quick, simple to administer, and may be used to assess patients that may be too ill to participate in more interactive rating scales, including nonverbal individuals.

GENERAL APPLICATIONS

The NOSIE is used to assess behavioral pathology in hospitalized individuals with serious mental illness. The scale is frequently utilized to assess change in behaviors from baseline, and can be utilized with the most severely ill psychiatric populations.

SELECTED PSYCHOMETRIC PROPERTIES

Interrater reliability has been demonstrated by intraclass correlations for pairs of ratings of 0.73 to 0.74 for manifest and depressive psychosis.

REFERENCES

Honigfeld G and Klett CJ, "The Nurses' Observation Scale for Inpatient Evaluation: The New Scale for Measuring Improvement in Chronic Schizophrenia," *J Clin Psychol*, 1965, 21:65-71.

Honigfeld G, Gillis RD, and Klett CJ, "NOSIE: Nurses' Observation Scale for Inpatient Evaluation," *ECDEU Assessment Manual for Psychopharmacology*, Guy W, ed, Rockville, MD: U.S. Department of Health, Education, and Welfare, 1976, 265-73.

COPYRIGHT

Not applicable

SCALE GENERALLY DONE BY

Inpatient nursing staff or trained rater

TIME TO COMPLETE SCALE

5-10 minutes

REPRESENTATIVE STUDY UTILIZING SCALE

Swett C and Mills T, "Use of the NOSIE to Predict Assaults Among Acute Psychiatric Patients. Nurse's Observational Scale for Inpatient Evaluation," *Psychiatr Serv*, 1997, 48(9):1177-80.

NURSES' OBSERVATION SCALE FOR INPATIENT EVALUATION (NOSIE)

For each of the 30 items below, rate this patient's behavior during the last THREE DAYS ONLY

1 = never
2 = sometimes
3 = often
4 = usually
5 = always

1. _____ Is sloppy

2. _____ Is impatient

3. _____ Cries

4. _____ Show interest in activities around him

5. _____ Sits, unless directed into activity

6. _____ Gets angry or annoyed easily

7. _____ Hears things that are not there

8. _____ Keeps his clothes neat

9. _____ Tries to be friendly to others

10. _____ Becomes easily upset if something doesn't suit him

11. _____ Refused to do the ordinary things expected of him

12. _____ Is irritable and grouchy

13. _____ Has trouble remembering

14. _____ Refuses to speak

15. _____ Laughs or smiles at funny comments or events

16. _____ Is messy in his eating habits

17. _____ Starts up a conversation with others

18. _____ Says he feels blue or depressed

19. _____ Talks about his interests

20. _____ Sees things that are not there

21. _____ Has to be reminded what to do

22. _____ Sleeps, unless directed into activity

23. _____ Says that he is no good

24. _____ Has to be told to follow hospital routine

25. _____ Has difficulty completing even simple tasks on his own

26. _____ Talks, mutters, or mumbles to himself

27. _____ Is slow moving and sluggish

28. _____ Giggles or smiles to himself without any apparent reason

29. _____ Quick to fly off the handle

30. _____ Keeps himself clean

E. POSITIVE AND NEGATIVE SYMPTOM SCALE FOR SCHIZOPHRENIA (PANSS)

OVERVIEW

The PANSS, developed by SR Kay et al is a 30-item rating scale that is specifically developed to assess individuals with schizophrenia and is used very widely in research settings. The PANSS is an adaptation from earlier psychopathology scales, including the BPRS *on page 130*. Although the items of the BPRS are embedded in the PANSS, they do not fully correspond to all BPRS items. The BPRS may be scored from the interview for the PANSS. Additionally, the PANSS closely corresponds to the SANS and the SAPS (see SANS *on page 161* and SAPS *on page 166*). The PANSS is based upon the premise that schizophrenia has two distinct syndromes, a positive and a negative syndrome. The positive syndrome includes productive features, such as delusions and hallucinations, while the negative syndrome includes those features which are lacking/poorly developed in individuals with schizophrenia, such as social withdrawal and flattened or blunted affect.

The PANSS consists of a semistructured clinical interview and any available supporting clinical information, such as family members or hospital staff report. There are 30 items which rate along a seven point continuum (1 = absent, 7 = extreme). The assessment provides separate scores in nine clinical domains including a positive syndrome, a negative syndrome, depression, a composite index, and general psychopathology. Ratings are generally based upon information relating to the past week.

To improve the standardization of the interview, a fully structured interview, the Structured Clinical Interview for the PANSS (SCI-PANSS) has been developed. The PANSS is available in Afrikaans, Bulgarian, Croatian, Czech, Danish, Dutch, Estonian, Finnish, German, Greek, Hebrew, Hungarian, Icelandic, Italian, Norwegian, Polish, Portugese, Romania, Russian, Slovakian, Spanish, and Swedish.

GENERAL APPLICATIONS

The PANSS evaluates the clinical profile of a patient with schizophrenia and provides assessment of treatment response.

SELECTED PSYCHOMETRIC PROPERTIES

Alpha-coefficient analysis has indicated high internal reliability and homogeneity among PANSS items, with coefficients ranging from 0.73 to 0.83 (p <.001) for each of the scales. The split-half reliability of the General Psychopathology Scale was demonstrated to be 0.80 (p <.001) by the authors. The authors have also demonstrated the discriminant and convergent validity of the PANSS dimensional assessment in relation to independent clinical, genealogical, psychometric, and historical measures.

REFERENCES

Kay SR, Opler LA, and Fiszbein A, "Significance of Positive and Negative Syndromes in Chronic Schizophrenia," *Br J Psychiatry*, 1986, 149:439-48.

Kay SR, Fiszbein A, and Opler LA, "The Positive and Negative Syndrome Scale (PANSS) for Schizophrenia," *Schizophr Bull*, 1987, 13(2):261-76.

Kay SR, Opler LA, and Lindenmayer JP, "Reliability and Validity of the Positive and Negative Syndrome Scale for Schizophrenics," *Psychiatry Res*, 1988, 23(1):99-110.

COPYRIGHT

Multi-Health Systems, Inc
P.O. Box 950
North Tonawanda, NY 14120-0950
Tel: 1-800-456-3003

SCALE GENERALLY DONE BY

Personnel trained in psychiatric interviewing techniques, with experience in working with populations with schizophrenia.

TIME TO COMPLETE SCALE

30-40 minutes

REPRESENTATIVE STUDY UTILIZING SCALE

Chouinard G, Jones B, Remington G, et al, "A Canadian Multicenter Placebo-Controlled Study of Fixed Doses of Risperidone and Haloperidol in the Treatment of Chronic Schizophrenic Patients," *J Clin Psychopharmacol*, 1993, 13(1):25-40.

E. POSITIVE AND NEGATIVE SYMPTOM SCALE
FOR SCHIZOPHRENIA (PANSS) *(Continued)*

SAMPLE ITEMS OF THE
PANSS QuikScore™

Write the appropriate number in the box adjacent to each symptom using the following scale.

1 = Absent
2 = Minimal
3 = Mild
4 = Moderate
5 = Moderately severe
6 = Severe
7 = Extreme

P1. DELUSIONS

P2. CONCEPTUAL DISORGANIZATION

P3. HALLUCINATORY BEHAVIOR

N1. BLUNTED AFFECT

N2. EMOTIONAL WITHDRAWAL

N3. POOR RAPPORT

F. SCALE FOR ASSESSMENT OF NEGATIVE SYMPTOMS (SANS)

OVERVIEW

The SANS is a 25-item scale, developed by N Andreasen, which is designed to assess negative symptoms in individuals with schizophrenia. The SANS is intended to be used with the Scale for Assessment of Positive Symptoms (see SAPS *on page 166*), also by Andreasen. The SANS items are rated on the basis of a clinical interview, direct observation, and any additional sources of information, including clinical staff or family member reports. The SANS evaluates five domains of the negative symptom complex, including alogia, affective flattening, avolition-apathy, anhedonia-asociality, and attention. The scale is rated on a 0 to 5 spectrum (0 = not present, 5 = severe). Ratings from the SAPS and SANS are divided into three symptom dimensions which include psychoticism, negative symptoms, and disorganization. The psychoticism dimension covers the global ratings of hallucinations and delusions; the negative dimension covers global ratings of affective flattening, alogia, avolition-apathy, and anhedonia-asociality; while the disorganization dimension covers global ratings of bizarre behavior, formal thought disorder, and inappropriate affect. Although the SANS was developed to assess negative symptoms in schizophrenia, it must be noted that the individual items on the SANS may be scored high for individuals with other types of serious mental illness, such as depression or drug-induced psychotic disorders. Strengths of the SANS include its relative ease of administration and well-researched reliability. Studies involving the SANS have been conducted in the United States, Japan, Italy, and Spain.

GENERAL APPLICATIONS

The SANS is utilized to assess baseline clinical status and change over time in individuals with schizophrenia. It is recommended that it be administered with the SAPS.

SELECTED PSYCHOMETRIC PROPERTIES

The SANS has been demonstrated to have good internal consistency, with Cronbach's alpha values from 0.67 to 0.90 for the five subscales. The SANS has also been found to correlate well the BPRS negative symptom items and with the negative symptom items on the PANSS.

REFERENCES

Andreasen N, "The Scale for the Assessment of Negative Symptoms (SANS)," University of Iowa, Department of Psychiatry, Iowa City, Iowa. 1981.

Andreasen N, "Modified Scale for the Assessment of Negative Symptoms," *NIMH Treatment Strategies in Schizophrenia Study*, U.S. Department of Health and Human Services, Public Health Administration, 1984, ADM 9-102, 9/85.

Andreasen N, "The Scale for the Assessment of Negative Symptoms (SANS). Conceptual and Theoretical Foundations," *Br J Psychiatry Suppl*, 1989, (7):49-58.

Miller DD, Arndt S, and Andreasen NC, "Alogia, Attentional Impairment, and Inappropriate Affect: Their Status in the Dimensions of Schizophrenia," *Compr Psychiatry*, 1993, 34(4):221-6.

Thiemann S, Csernansky JG, and Berger PA, "Rating Scales in Research: The Case of Negative Symptoms," *Psychiatry Res*, 1987, 20(1):47-55.

F. SCALE FOR ASSESSMENT OF NEGATIVE
SYMPTOMS (SANS) *(Continued)*

COPYRIGHT

N Andreasen
The University of Iowa
Department of Psychiatry
200 Hawkins Drive
Iowa City, Iowa 52242-1057

SCALE GENERALLY DONE BY

Clinicians with training in mental health or a trained rater

TIME TO COMPLETE SCALE

15-20 minutes

REPRESENTATIVE STUDY UTILIZING SCALE

Pallanti S, Quercioli L, Rossi A, et al, "The Emergence of Social Phobia During Clozapine Treatment and Its Response to Fluoxetine Augmentation," *J Clin Psychiatry*, 1999, 60(12):819-23.

SANS

0 = None   1 = Questionable   2 = Mild   3 = Moderate   4 = Marked   5 = Severe

AFFECTIVE FLATTENING OR BLUNTING

1. *Unchanged Facial Expression*   0   1   2   3   4   5

   The patient's face appears wooden, changes less
   than expected as emotional content of discourse
   changes.

2. *Decreased Spontaneous Movements*   0   1   2   3   4   5

   The patient shows few or no spontaneous movements,
   does not shift position, move extremities, etc.

3. *Paucity of Expressive Gestures*   0   1   2   3   4   5

   The patient does not use hand gestures, body position,
   etc, as an aid to expressing his ideas.

4. *Poor Eye Contact*   0   1   2   3   4   5

   The patient avoids eye contact or "stares through"
   interviewer even when speaking.

5. Affective Nonresponsivity   0   1   2   3   4   5

   The patient fails to smile or laugh when prompted.

6. *Lack of Vocal Inflections*   0   1   2   3   4   5

   The patient fails to show normal vocal emphasis
   patterns, is often monotonic.

7. *Global Rating of Affective Flattening*   0   1   2   3   4   5

   This rating should focus on overall severity of
   symptoms, especially unresponsiveness, eye contact,
   facial expression, and vocal inflections.

INAPPROPRIATE AFFECT

8. Inappropriate Affect   0   1   2   3   4   5

   The patient's affect is inappropriate or incongruous,
   not simply flat or blunted.

F. SCALE FOR ASSESSMENT OF NEGATIVE SYMPTOMS (SANS) *(Continued)*

SANS *(continued)*

0 = None   1 = Questionable   2 = Mild   3 = Moderate   4 = Marked   5 = Severe

ALOGIA

9. *Poverty of Speech*   0 1 2 3 4 5

The patient's replies to questions are restricted in
<u>amount,</u> tend to be brief, concrete, and unelaborated.

10. *Poverty of Content of Speech*   0 1 2 3 4 5

The patient's replies are adequate in amount, but tend
to be vague, overconcrete, or overgeneralized, and
convey little information.

11. *Blocking*   0 1 2 3 4 5

The patient indiicates, either spontaneously or with
prompting, that his train of thought was interrupted.

12. *Increased Latency of Response*   0 1 2 3 4 5

The patient takes a long time to reply to questions;
prompting indicates the patient is aware of the question.

13. *Global Rating of Alogia*   0 1 2 3 4 5

The core features of alogia are poverty of speech and
poverty of content.

AVOLITION - APATHY

14. *Grooming and Hygiene*   0 1 2 3 4 5

The patient's clothes may be sloppy or soiled, and he
may have greasy hair, body odor, etc.

15. *Impersistence at Work or School* 0 1 2 3 4 5

The patient has difficulty seeking or maintaining
employment, completing school work, keeping house, etc.
If an inpatient, cannot persist at ward activities, such as
OT, playing cards, etc.

16. *Physical Anergia*   0 1 2 3 4 5

The patient tends to be physically inert. He may sit
for hours and does not initiate spontaneous activity.

17. *Global Rating of Avolition - Apathy*   0 1 2 3 4 5

Strong weight may be given to one or two
prominent symptoms if particularly striking.

SANS (*continued*)

0 = None   1 = Questionable   2 = Mild   3 = Moderate   4 = Marked   5 = Severe

ANHEDONIA - ASOCIALITY

18. *Recreational Interests and Activities*   0 1 2 3 4 5

The patient may have few or no interests. Both the
quality and quantity of interests should be taken into
account.

19. *Sexual Activity*   0 1 2 3 4 5

The patient may show a decrease in sexual interest
and activity, or enjoyment when active.

20. *Ability to Feel Intimacy and Closeness*   0 1 2 3 4 5

The patient may display an inability to form close or
intimate relationships, especially with the opposite
sex and family.

21. *Relationships with Friends and Peers*   0 1 2 3 4 5

The patient may have few or no friends and may
prefer to spend all of his time isolated.

22. *Global Rating of Anhedonia-Asociality*   0 1 2 3 4 5

This rating should reflect overall severity, taking into
account the patient's age, family status, etc.

ATTENTION

23. *Social Inattentiveness*   0 1 2 3 4 5

A patient appears uninvolved or unengaged. He
may seem "spacy".

24. *Inattentiveness During Mental Status Testing*   0 1 2 3 4 5

Tests of "serial 7s" (at least 5 subtractions) and
spelling "world" backwards:
Score: 2 = 1 error; 3 = 2 errors; 4 = 3 errors

25. *Global Rating of Attention*   0 1 2 3 4 5

This rating should assess the patient's overall
concentration, clinically and on tests.

G. SCALE FOR ASSESSMENT OF POSITIVE SYMPTOMS (SAPS)

OVERVIEW

The SAPS is a 34-item scale, developed by N Andreasen, for the assessment of positive symptoms in individuals with schizophrenia. It is meant to be utilized in conjunction with the Scale for Assessment of Negative Symptoms (SANS *on page 161*), also by Andreasen. The SAPS is administered via a general clinical interview, plus a series of standardized questions. Additionally, any available supporting information, such as staff reports, should be utilized. The SAPS evaluates positive symptoms in great detail (eg, hallucinations are rated under six items). Positive symptom areas assessed include hallucinations, delusions, bizarre behavior, and formal thought disorder. Items are scored on a 0 to 5 (0 = no abnormality, 5 = severe) scale. Ratings from the SAPS and SANS are divided into three symptom dimensions which include psychoticism, negative symptoms, and disorganization. The psychoticism dimension covers the global ratings of hallucinations and delusions; the negative dimension covers global ratings of affective flattening, alogia, avolition-apathy, and anhedonia-asociality; while the disorganization dimension covers global ratings of bizarre behavior, formal thought disorder, and inappropriate affect. As a research tool, the SAPS is generally utilized less frequently than the SANS.

GENERAL APPLICATIONS

The SAPS is utilized to assess baseline clinical status and change over time in individuals with schizophrenia. It is recommended that it be administered with the SANS.

SELECTED PSYCHOMETRIC PROPERTIES

There is less reliability data for the SAPS compared to the SANS. Interrater reliability for the SAPS is generally good. Weighted kappas for most items have been reported to range from 0.7 to 1.00.

REFERENCES

Andreasen N, "Scale for the Assessment of Positive Symptoms (SAPS)," University of Iowa, Department of Psychiatry, Iowa City, Iowa, 1984.

Andreasen N, "Methods for Assessing Positive and Negative Symptoms," *Schizophrenia: Positive and Negative Symptoms and Syndromes. Modern Problems in Pharmacopsychiatry*, Andreasen N, ed, New York, NY: S. Karger Publisher, Inc, 1990, 73-85.

Miller DD, Arndt S, and Andreasen NC, "Alogia, Attentional Impairment, and Inappropriate Affect: Their Status in the Dimensions of Schizophrenia," *Compr Psychiatry*, 1993, 34(4):221-6.

Moscarelli M, Maffei C, Cesana BM, et al, "An International Perspective on Assessment of Negative and Positive Symptoms in Schizophrenia," *Am J Psychiatry*, 1987, 144(12):1595-8.

COPYRIGHT

N Andreasen
The University of Iowa
Department of Psychiatry
200 Hawkins Drive
Iowa City, Iowa 52242-1057

SCALE GENERALLY DONE BY

Clinicians with training in mental health or a trained rater

TIME TO COMPLETE SCALE

15-20 minutes

REPRESENTATIVE STUDY UTILIZING SCALE

Pallanti S, Quercioli L, Rossi A, et al, "The Emergence of Social Phobia During Clozapine Treatment and Its Response to Fluoxetine Augmentation," *J Clin Psychiatry*, 1999, 60(12):819-23.

G. SCALE FOR ASSESSMENT OF POSITIVE SYMPTOMS (SAPS) *(Continued)*

SAPS

0 = None   1 = Questionable   2 = Mild   3 = Moderate   4 = Marked   5 = Severe

HALLUCINATIONS

1. *Auditory Hallucinations*   0 1 2 3 4 5

   The patient reports voices, noises, or other sounds
   that no one else hears.

2. *Voices Commenting*   0 1 2 3 4 5

   The patient reports a voice which makes a running
   commentary on his behavior or thoughts.

3. *Voices Conversing*   0 1 2 3 4 5

   The patient reports hearing two or more voices
   conversing.

4. *Somatic or Tactile Hallucinations*   0 1 2 3 4 5

   The patient reports experiencing peculiar physical
   sensations in the body.

5. *Olfactory Hallucinations*   0 1 2 3 4 5

   The patient reports experiencing unusual smells which
   no one else notices.

6. *Visual Hallucinations*   0 1 2 3 4 5

   The patient sees shapes or people that are not
   actually present.

7. *Global Rating of Hallucinations*   0 1 2 3 4 5

   This rating should be based on the duration and
   severity of the hallucinations and their effects on the
   patient's life.

DELUSIONS

8. *Persecutory Delusions*   0 1 2 3 4 5

   The patient believes he is being conspired against or
   persecuted in some way.

9. *Delusions of Jealousy*   0 1 2 3 4 5

   The patient believes his spouse is having an affair
   with someone.

SAPS (continued)

0 = None   1 = Questionable   2 = Mild   3 = Moderate   4 = Marked   5 = Severe

DELUSIONS (continued)

10. *Delusions of Guilt or Sin*   0   1   2   3   4   5

The patient believes that he has committed some
terrible sin or done something unforgivable.

11. *Grandiose Delusions*   0   1   2   3   4   5

The patient believes he has special powers or abilities.

12. *Religious Delusions*   0   1   2   3   4   5

The patient is preoccupied with false beliefs of a
religious nature.

13. *Somatic Delusions*   0   1   2   3   4   5

The patient believes that somehow his body is diseased,
abnormal, or changed.

14. *Delusions of Reference*   0   1   2   3   4   5

The patient believes that insignificant remarks or
events refer to him or have some special meaning.

15. *Delusions of Being Controlled*   0   1   2   3   4   5

The patient feels that his feelings or actions are
controlled by some outside force.

16. *Delusions of Mind Reading*   0   1   2   3   4   5

The patient feels that people can read his mind or
know his thoughts.

17. *Thought Broadcasting*   0   1   2   3   4   5

The patient believes that his thoughts are broadcast
so that he himself or others can hear them.

18. *Thought Insertion*   0   1   2   3   4   5

The patient believes that thoughts that are not his
own have been inserted into his mind.

G. SCALE FOR ASSESSMENT OF POSITIVE SYMPTOMS (SAPS) *(Continued)*

SAPS *(continued)*

0 = None   1 = Questionable   2 = Mild   3 = Moderate   4 = Marked   5 = Severe

DELUSIONS *(continued)*

19. *Thought Withdrawal*   0   1   2   3   4   5

The patient believes that thoughts have been taken away from his mind.

20. *Global Rating of Delusions*   0   1   2   3   4   5

This rating should be based on the duration and persistence of the delusions and their effect on the patient's life.

BIZARRE BEHAVIOR

21. *Clothing and Appearance*   0   1   2   3   4   5

The patient dresses in an unusual manner or does other strange things to alter his apperance.

22. *Social and Sexual Behavior*   0   1   2   3   4   5

The patient may do things considered inappropriate according to usual social normal (eg, masturbating in public)

23. *Aggressive and Agitated Behavior*   0   1   2   3   4   5

The patient may behave in an aggressive, agitated manner, often unpredictably.

24. *Repetitive or Stereotyped Behavior*   0   1   2   3   4   5

The patient develops a set of repetitive action or rituals that he must perform over and over.

25. *Global Rating of Bizarre Behavior*   0   1   2   3   4   5

This rating should reflect the type of behavior and the extent to which it deviates from social norms.

POSITIVE FORMAL THOUGHT DISORDER

26. *Derailment*   0   1   2   3   4   5

A pattern or speech in which ideas slip off track onto ideas obliquely related or unrelated.

170

SAPS (*continued*)

0 = None   1 = Questionable   2 = Mild   3 = Moderate   4 = Marked   5 = Severe

POSITIVE FORMAL THOUGHT DISORDER (*continued*)

27. *Tangentiality*   0   1   2   3   4   5

Replying to a question in an oblique or irrelevant manner.

28. *Incoherence*   0   1   2   3   4   5

A pattern of speech which is essentially incomprehensible
at times.

29. *Illogicality*   0   1   2   3   4   5

A pattern of speech in which conclusions are reached
which do not follow logically.

30. *Circumstantiality*   0   1   2   3   4   5

A pattern of speech which is very indirect and
delayed in reaching its goal idea.

31. *Pressure of Speech*   0   1   2   3   4   5

The patient's speech is rapid and difficult to interrupt;
the amount of speech produced is greater than that
considered normal.

32. *Distractible Speech*   0   1   2   3   4   5

The patient is distracted by nearby stimuli which
interrupt his flow of speech.

33. *Clanging*   0   1   2   3   4   5

A pattern of speech in which sounds rather than
meaningful relationships govern word choice.

34. *Global Rating of Positive Formal Thought Disorder* 0   1   2   3   4   5

This rating should reflect the frequency of abnormality
and degree to which it affects the patient's ability to
communicate.

FUNCTIONAL LEVEL / GENERAL SYMPTOM

SCALES

TABLE OF CONTENTS

A. CLINICAL GLOBAL IMPRESSIONS (CGI)

OVERVIEW

The CGI, developed at the National Institute of Mental Health (NIMH), is one of the most widely used brief assessment tools in psychiatry. This is a three-item scale which measures overall illness severity. Repeated, it can evaluate response to treatment. The CGI is rated by the patient's physician or a trained rater who evaluates severity of illness, clinical progress, and therapeutic efficacy. Raters are asked to evaluate the severity of the patient's illness based on the rater's total experience with the specific patient population to which the patient belongs. For example, individuals with depression should be compared to other patients with depression, not to patients with schizophrenia.

The scale includes three items:
- Severity of illness
- Global improvement
- Therapeutic response

Severity of illness is rated on a seven-point spectrum (1 = normal, 7 = among the most severely ill patients). Global improvement is also rated on a seven-point spectrum (1 = very much improved, 7 = very much worse). A zero rating may be assigned for items not assessed. Therapeutic response is rated as a combination of therapeutic effectiveness and adverse effects. In clinical and research situations, only the first two items - severity of illness and global improvement - are often utilized. Each item on the CGI is rated separately and there is no overall score. The CGI is designed to be useful in situations where change over time is to be assessed. The CGI is usually paired with a more specific psychopathology scale, such as the BPRS *on page 130*.

GENERAL APPLICATIONS

The CGI measures overall illness severity and response to treatment in psychiatric patients.

SELECTED PSYCHOMETRIC PROPERTIES

The CGI has high face validity with many other commonly utilized psychopathology scales. Good reliability scores have been reported for severity of illness ratings (0.41 to 0.60), but reliability of global improvement scores appears less good (0.35 to 0.51).

REFERENCES

"Clinical Global Impressions," *ECDEU Assessment Manual for Psychopharmacology*, Guy W, ed, Rockville, MD: U.S. Department of Health, Education, and Welfare, 1976, DHEW Publication No. (ADM) 76-338.

COPYRIGHT

Not applicable

SCALE GENERALLY DONE BY

Clinician or trained rater

TIME TO COMPLETE SCALE

Less than 5 minutes after clinical evaluation.

REPRESENTATIVE STUDY UTILIZING SCALE

Brady K, Pearlstein T, Asnis GM, et al, "Efficacy and Safety of Sertraline Treatment of Post-Traumatic Stress Disorder: A Randomized Controlled Trial," *JAMA*, 2000, 283(14):1837-44.

CLINICAL GLOBAL IMPRESSIONS (CGI)
(ECDEU Version)

1. SEVERITY OF ILLNESS

Considering your total clinical experience with this particular population, how mentally ill is the patient at this time?

0 = Not assessed
1 = Normal, not at all ill
2 = Borderline mentally ill
3 = Mildly ill

4 = Moderately ill
5 = Markedly ill
6 = Severely ill
7 = Among the most extremely ill patients

2. GLOBAL IMPROVEMENT - Rate total improvement whether or not, in your judgment, it is due entirely to drug treatment.

Compared to his condition at admission to the project, how much has he changed?

0 = Not assessed
1 = Very much improved
2 = Much improved
3 = Minimally improved

4 = No change
5 = Minimally worse
6 = Much worse
7 = Very much worse

3. EFFICACY INDEX - Rate this item on the basis of DRUG EFFECT ONLY.

Select the terms which best describe the degrees of therapeutic effect and side effects and record the number in the box where the two items intersect.

EXAMPLE: Therapeutic effect is rated as "Moderate" and side effects are judged "Do not significantly interfere with patient's functioning".

THERAPEUTIC EFFECT	SIDE EFFECTS			
	None	Do not significantly interfere with patient's functioning	Significantly interferes with patient's functioning	Outweighs therapeutic effect
MARKED - Vast improvement. Complete or nearly complete remission of all symptoms	01	02	03	04
MODERATE - Decided improvement. Partial remission of symptoms	05	06	07	08
MINIMAL - Slight improvement which doesn't alter status of care of patient	09	10	11	12
UNCHANGED OR WORSE	13	14	15	16
Not Assessed = 00				

B. GLOBAL ASSESSMENT SCALE (GAS and GAF)

OVERVIEW

These very similar scales, one of which is the fifth axis for the DSM-IV, have their origins in the Health Sickness Rating Scale done by Luborsky in 1962, considered the first effort to evaluate psychological health and illness utilizing a 100-point scale. Later, the scale was divided in groups of 10, called levels, resulting in the Global Assessment Scale (GAS) and in 1987, after some modifications, became the Global Assessment of Functioning Scale (GAF) and Axis V for the DSM III-R and DSM-IV.

The GAS/GAF Scale is used to assess psychiatric patients at the time of admission to an inpatient or outpatient program as part of the multiaxial evaluation recommended by the APA DSM classifications.

The GAF/GAS Scales are both 100-point single-item scales with values ranging from 1 to 100 representing the hypothetically sickest person to the healthiest. The scale is divided into 10 equal 10-point intervals with the 81 to 90 and 91 to 100 intervals for individuals who exhibit superior functioning. The 71 to 80 interval is for persons with minimal psychopathology. Most patients in outpatient settings will receive ratings between 31 and 70, and most inpatients between 1 and 40.

The information needed to assign a numeric value to the health of the patient in question comes from the clinical evaluation done and the information obtained from other sources (family, records, etc). The GAS and GAF are used very widely in both clinical and research settings.

GENERAL APPLICATIONS

The GAS and GAF both measure global functional level of psychiatric patients.

SELECTED PSYCHOMETRIC PROPERTIES

The reliability of the GAF ranges from 0.62 to 0.82. The reliability of the GAS is similar.

REFERENCES

Luborsky L, "Clinicians' Judgment of Mental Health," *Arch Gen Psychiat*, 1962, 7:407-17.

Endicott J, Spitzer RL, Fleiss JL, et al, "The Global Assessment Scale. A Procedure for Measuring Overall Severity of Psychiatric Disturbance," *Arch Gen Psychiat*, 1976, 33(6):766-71.

ECDEU Assessment Manual for Psychopharmacology, Guy W, ed, Washington DC: U.S. Department of Health, Education and Welfare, 1976.

American Psychiatric Association, *Diagnostic and Statistical Manual of Mental Disorders*, 4th ed, Washington, DC: American Psychiatric Association, 1994.

Jones SH, Thornicroft G, Coffey M, et al, "A Brief Mental Health Outcome Scale-Reliability and Validity of the Global Assessment of Functioning (GAF)," *Br J Psychiatry*, 1995, 166(5):654-9.

COPYRIGHT

GAS: Not copyrighted
Copies and details for use may be obtained from:
Jean Endicott, PhD
Chief, Department of Research, Assessment and Training
New York State Psychiatric Institute
1051 Riverside Dr
123 New York, NY 10032

GAF available as part of DSM-IV from:
American Psychiatric Association
Diagnostic and Statistical Manual of Mental Disorders
1400 K. Street NW
Suite 1101
Washington, DC 20005

SCALE GENERALLY DONE BY

A clinical professional (MD, nurse, psychologist, social worker, or other trained mental health professional).

TIME TO COMPLETE SCALE

Once the evaluation of the patient is completed, the assignment of the GAF/GAS scores takes only seconds.

REPRESENTATIVE STUDY UTILIZING SCALE

Segui J, Salvador-Carulla L, Marquez M, et al, "Differential Clinical Features of Late-Onset Panic Disorder," *J Affect Disord*, 2000, 57(1-3):115-24.

B. GLOBAL ASSESSMENT SCALE (GAS and GAF) *(Continued)*

GLOBAL ASSESSMENT SCALE (GAS)

Rate the subject's lowest level of functioning in the last week by selecting the lowest range which describes his functioning on a hypothetical continuum of mental health-illness. For example, a subject whose "behavior is considerably influenced by delusions" (range 21-30), should be given a rating in that range even though he has "major impairment in several areas" (range 31-40). Use intermediary levels when appropriate (eg, 35, 58, 62). Rate actual functioning independent of whether or not subject is receiving and may be helped by medication or some other form of treatment.

Name of Patient_____ ID No._____ Group Code_____

Admission Date_____ Date of Rating_____ Rater_____

GAS Rating:_____

100   Superior functioning in a wide range of activities, life's problems never seem to get out
| of hand, is sought out by others because of his warmth and integrity. No symptoms.
91

90   Good functioning in all areas, many interests, socially effective, generally satisfied with
| life. There may or may not be transient symptoms and "everyday" worries that only
| occasionally get out of hand.
81

80   No more than slight impairment in functioning, varying degrees of "everyday" worries and
| problems that sometimes get out of hand. Minimal symptoms may or may not be
| present.
71

70   Some mild symptoms (eg, depressive mood and mild insomnia) OR some difficulty in
| several areas of functioning, but generally functioning pretty well, has some meaningful
| interpersonal relationships and most untrained people would not consider him "sick".
61

60   Moderate symptoms OR generally functioning with some difficulty (eg, few friends and
| flat affect, depressed mood and pathological self-doubt, euphoric mood and pressure of
51   speech, moderately severe antisocial behavior).

50   Any serious symptomatology or impairment in functioning that most clinicians would think
| obviously requires treatment or attention (eg, suicidal preoccupation or gesture, severe
41   obsessional rituals, frequent anxiety attacks, serious antisocial behavior, compulsive
     drinking, mild but definite manic syndrome).

40   Major impairment in several areas such as work, family relations, judgment, thinking or
| mood (eg, depressed woman avoids friends, neglects family, unable to do housework),
| OR some impairment in reality testing or communication (eg, speech is at time obscure,
| illogical or irrelevant), OR single suicide attempt.
31

30   Unable to function in almost all areas (eg, stays in bed all day) OR behavior is
| considerably influenced by either delusions or hallucinations OR serious impairment in
| communication (eg, sometimes incoherent or unresponsive) or judgment (eg, acts
21   grossly inappropriately).

20   Needs some supervision to prevent hurting self or others, or to maintain minimal
| personal hygiene (eg, repeated suicide attempts, frequently violent, manic excitement,
| smears feces), OR gross impairment in communication (eg, largely incoherent or mute).
11

10   Needs constant supervision for several days to prevent hurting self or others (eg,
| requires an intensive care unit with special observation by staff), makes no attempt to
| maintain minimal personal hygiene, or serious suicide act with clear intent and
1   expectation of death.

The original idea for a single rating scale of 1 to 100 for the health-sickness continuum with defined anchor points is embodied in Luborsky's Health Sickness Rating Scale. The Global Assessment Scale differs from it in the larger number of defined ranges, the avoidance of diagnostic considerations in defining anchoring points, and the use of brief clinical descriptions in the anchoring definitions.

C. SYMPTOM CHECKLIST-90-REVISED (SCL-90-R)

OVERVIEW

The SCL-90-R, developed by LR Derogatis, is a widely-utilized screen for global psychopa-thology and a general symptom measure. The SCL-90-R consists of 90 self-rated items. Each item asks respondents to report how much discomfort he/she experienced over the past week and past day with selected symptoms/psychological states. Responses are scored on a 0 to 4 continuum (O = not at all, 4 = extremely). The SCL-90-R covers nine symptom dimensions: Somatization, obsessive-compulsive symptoms, interpersonal sensitivity, depression, anxiety, hostility, phobic-anxiety, paranoid ideation, and psychoticism. There is also a Global Severity Index, which is the mean of all items. The SCL-90-R is brief to administer and a computerized scoring version of the SCL-90-R is available.

GENERAL APPLICATIONS

The SCL-90-R is a screening instrument for general psychopathology/symptoms.

SELECTED PSYCHOMETRIC PROPERTIES

Reliability of the SCL-90-R is reported by the authors to range from 0.79-0.90 (alpha coeffi-cients). Test-retest stability has been reported to range from 0.78-0.90 at one week, and 0.68-0.80 at 10 weeks.

REFERENCES

Derogatis LR, "SCL-90-R, Brief Symptom Inventory: The Matching Clinical Rating Scales in Psychological Testing," *The Use of Psychological Testing for Treatment Planning and Outcome Assessment,* Maruish ME, ed, Hillsdale, NJ: L. Erlbaum Associates, 1994.

Derogatis LR, Lipman RS, and Covi L, "SCL-90: An Outpatient Psychiatric Rating Scale-Preliminary Report," *Psychopharmacol Bull*, 1973, 9(1):13-28.

COPYRIGHT

Pearson Assessments
5601 Green Valley Drive
Bloomington, MN 55437
Tel: 1-800-627-7271
Website: www.personassessments.com

SCALE GENERALLY DONE BY

Self-rated scale

TIME TO COMPLETE SCALE

15-20 minutes

REPRESENTATIVE STUDY UTILIZING SCALE

Kim JH, Lee BC, Park HJ, et al, "Subjective Emotional Experience and Cognitive Impairment in Drug-Induced Akathisia," *Compr Psychiatry*, 2002, 43(6):456-62.

SOCIAL / FAMILY FUNCTIONING

RATING SCALES

TABLE OF CONTENTS

A. FAMILY ASSESSMENT DEVICE (FAD)

OVERVIEW

The Family Assessment Device (FAD), developed by NB Epstein and colleagues, was designed to measure family functioning along multiple dimensions. The FAD is a 60-item, self-report instrument that evaluates family functioning along six dimensions: Affective involvement, affective responsiveness, behavior control, communication, problem solving, and roles. There is a 12-item General Functioning scale as well. Each item is scored on a 4-point Likert-type format with responses ranging from 1 (strongly agree) to 4 (strongly disagree). Higher scores indicate more severe family dysfunction. While the FAD has been tested in primarily North American settings, there is also research data on the FAD in other cultural settings and the FAD has been translated into 17 languages.

GENERAL APPLICATIONS

The FAD is a multidimensional measure of family functioning.

SELECTED PSYCHOMETRIC PROPERTIES

The authors have reported internal consistency (Cronbach's alpha) ranging from 0.72-0.92, with alpha highest for the General Functioning scale. Test-retest reliability over one week ranges from 0.66-0.76.

REFERENCES

Epstein NB, Baldwin LM, and Bishop DS, "The McMaster Family Assessment Device," *J Marital Fam Ther*, 1983, 9:171-80.

Miller IW, Epstein NB, Bishop DS, et al, "The McMaster Family Assessment Device: Reliability and Validity," *J Marital Fam Ther*, 1985, 11:345-56.

Miller IW, Kabacoff RI, Epstein NB, et al, "The Development of a Clinical Rating Scale for the McMaster Model of Family Functioning," *Fam Process*, 1994, 33(1):53-69.

COPYRIGHT

Dr C Ryan, Director
Brown University Family Research Program
Rhode Island Hospital - Potter 3
593 Eddy Street
Providence, RI 02903
Tel: 401-444-3534
Fax: 401-444-3298
To order scale: e-mail: familyresearch@lifespan.org
For Questions: e-mail: christine_ryan@brown.edu

SCALE GENERALLY DONE BY

Self-rated scale

TIME TO COMPLETE SCALE

15 minutes

REPRESENTATIVE STUDY UTILIZING SCALE

Millikan E, Wamboldt MZ, and Bihun JT, "Perceptions of the Family, Personality Characteristics, and Adolescent Internalizing Symptoms," *J Am Acad Child Adolesc Psychiatry*, 2002, 41(12):1486-94.

FAMILY ASSESSMENT DEVICE

INSTRUCTIONS: The following are statements about families. Please read each statement and indicate whether you strongly agree (SA), agree (A), disagree (D), or strongly disagree (SD) with each by circling the choice corresponding to your response.

STRONGLY AGREE SA	AGREE A	DISAGREE D	STRONGLY DISAGREE SD

1. Planning family activities is difficult because we misunderstand each other. SA A D SD

2. We resolve most everyday problems around the house. SA A D SD

3. When someone is upset, the others know why. SA A D SD

4. When you ask someone to do something, you have to check that they did it. SA A D SD

5. If someone is in trouble, the others become too involved. SA A D SD

6. In times of crisis, we can turn to each other for support. SA A D SD

7. We don't know what to do when an emergency comes up. SA A D SD

8. We sometimes run out of things we need. SA A D SD

9. We are reluctant to show our affection for each other. SA A D SD

10. We make sure members meet their family responsibilities. SA A D SD

11. We cannot talk to each other about the sadness we feel. SA A D SD

12. We usually act on our decisions regarding problems. SA A D SD

13. You only get the interest of others when something is important to them. SA A D SD

14. You can't tell how a person is feeling from what they are saying. SA A D SD

15. Family tasks don't get spread around enough. SA A D SD

16. Individuals are accepted for what they are. SA A D SD

17. You can easily get away with breaking the rules. SA A D SD

18. People come right out and say things instead of hinting at them. SA A D SD

19. Some of us just don't respond emotionally. SA A D SD

20. We know what to do in an emergency. SA A D SD

21. We avoid discussing our fears and concerns. SA A D SD

22. It is difficult to talk to each other about tender feelings. SA A D SD

23. We have trouble meeting our bills. SA A D SD

24. After our family tries to solve a problem, we usually discuss whether it worked or not. SA A D SD

25. We are too self-centered. SA A D SD

26. We can express feelings to each other. SA A D SD

27. We have no clear expectations about personal hygiene. SA A D SD

28. We do not show our love for each other. SA A D SD

29. We talk to people directly rather than through go-betweens. SA A D SD

A. FAMILY ASSESSMENT DEVICE (FAD) *(Continued)*

30.	Each of us has particular duties and responsibilities.	SA	A	D	SD
31.	There are lots of bad feelings in the family.	SA	A	D	SD
32.	We have rules about hitting people.	SA	A	D	SD
33.	We get involved with each other only when something interests us.	SA	A	D	SD
34.	There's little time to explore personal interests.	SA	A	D	SD
35.	We often don't say what we mean.	SA	A	D	SD
36.	We feel accepted for what we are.	SA	A	D	SD
37.	We show interest in each other when we can get something out of it personally.	SA	A	D	SD
38.	We resolve most emotional upsets that come up.	SA	A	D	SD
39.	Tenderness takes second place to other things in our family.	SA	A	D	SD
40.	We discuss who is to do household jobs.	SA	A	D	SD
41.	Making decisions is a problem for our family.	SA	A	D	SD
42.	Our family shows interest in each other only when they can get something out of it.	SA	A	D	SD
43.	We are frank with each other.	SA	A	D	SD
44.	We don't hold to any rules or standards.	SA	A	D	SD
45.	If people are asked to do something, they need reminding.	SA	A	D	SD
46.	We are able to make decisions about how to solve problems.	SA	A	D	SD
47.	If the rules are broken, we don't know what to expect.	SA	A	D	SD
48.	Anything goes in our family.	SA	A	D	SD
49.	We express tenderness.	SA	A	D	SD
50.	We confront problems involving feelings.	SA	A	D	SD
51.	We don't get along well together.	SA	A	D	SD
52.	We don't talk to each other when we are angry.	SA	A	D	SD
53.	We are generally dissatisfied with the family duties assigned to us.	SA	A	D	SD
54.	Even though we mean well, we intrude too much into each others lives.	SA	A	D	SD
55.	There are rules about dangerous situations.	SA	A	D	SD
56.	We confide in each other.	SA	A	D	SD
57.	We cry openly.	SA	A	D	SD
58.	We don't have reasonable transportation.	SA	A	D	SD
59.	When we don't like what someone has done, we tell them.	SA	A	D	SD
60.	We try to think of different ways to solve problems.	SA	A	D	SD

B. MULTIDIMENSIONAL SCALE OF PERCEIVED SOCIAL SUPPORT (MSPSS)

OVERVIEW

The Multidimensional Scale of Perceived Social Support (MSPSS), developed by GD Zimet and colleagues is a 12-item, self-rated measure of social support as perceived by an individual. The MSPSS evaluates social support from family, friends, and significant others and quantifies the degree to which respondents perceive support from each of these three sources. Items 3, 4, 8, and 11 measure family support, items 1, 2, 5, 6, 7, 9, and 12 measure support from friends, and the remaining items measure support from significant others. Scores are derived by summing the individual items and dividing by the number of items. A score can thus be obtained for the total scale, as well as each of the three subscales. Higher scores indicate higher perceived social support. Strengths of the MSPSS include brevity and ease of administration and scoring.

GENERAL APPLICATIONS

The MSPSS measures perceived social support in adults.

SELECTED PSYCHOMETRIC PROPERTIES

The MSPSS has very good internal consistency with reported alpha coefficients of 0.91 for the total score and 0.90 to 0.95 for each of the three subscales.

REFERENCES

Dahlem NW, Zimet GD, and Walker RR, "The Multidimensional Scale of Perceived Social Support: A Confirmation Study," *J Clin Psychol*, 1991, 47(6):756-61.

Zimet GD, Dahlem NW, Zimet SG, et al, "The Multidimensional Scale of Perceived Social Support," *J Pers Assess*, 1988, 52:31-41.

Zimet GD, Powell SS, Farley GK, et al, "Psychometric Characteristics of the Multidimensional Scale of Perceived Social Support," *J Pers Assess*, 1990, 55(3-4):610-7.

COPYRIGHT

Not applicable

For details regarding the scale and its implementation contact:
Dr Gregory D Zimet, PhD
Section of Adolescent Medicine
Indiana University School of Medicine
575 N West Drive, Room 070
Indianapolis, IN 46202
Tel: 317-274-8812
e-mail: gzimet@iupui.edu

B. MULTIDIMENSIONAL SCALE OF PERCEIVED SOCIAL SUPPORT (MSPSS) *(Continued)*

SCALE GENERALLY DONE BY

Self-rated scale

TIME TO COMPLETE SCALE

5-10 minutes

REPRESENTATIVE STUDY UTILIZING SCALE

Zhang J and Norvilitis JM, "Measuring Chinese Psychological Well-Being With Western Developed Instruments," *J Pers Assess*, 2002, 79(3):492-511.

MULTIDIMENSIONAL SCALE OF PERCEIVED SOCIAL SUPPORT

INSTRUCTIONS: We are interested in how you feel about the following statements. Read each statement carefully. Indicate how you feel about each statement.

Circle the "1" if you **Very Strongly Disagree**

Circle the "2" if you **Strongly Disagree**

Circle the "3" if you **Mildly Disagree**

Circle the "4" if you are **Neutral**

Circle the "5" if you **Mildly Agree**

Circle the "6" if you **Strongly Agree**

Circle the "7" if you **Very Strongly Agree**

1.	There is a special person who is around when I am in need.	1	2	3	4	5	6	7
2.	There is a special person with whom I can share joys and sorrows.	1	2	3	4	5	6	7
3.	My family really tries to help me.	1	2	3	4	5	6	7
4.	I get the emotional help and support I need from my family.	1	2	3	4	5	6	7
5.	I have a special person who is a real source of comfort to me.	1	2	3	4	5	6	7
6.	My friends really try to help me.	1	2	3	4	5	6	7
7.	I can count on my friends when things go wrong.	1	2	3	4	5	6	7
8.	I can talk about my problems with my family.	1	2	3	4	5	6	7
9.	I have friends with whom I can share my joys and sorrows.	1	2	3	4	5	6	7
10.	There is a special person in my life who cares about my feelings.	1	2	3	4	5	6	7
11.	My family is willing to help me make decisions.	1	2	3	4	5	6	7
12.	I can talk about my problems with my friends.	1	2	3	4	5	6	7

C. SOCIAL ADJUSTMENT SCALE (SAS, SAS-SR)

OVERVIEW

The Social Adjustment Scale (SAS) is a rating scale for social functioning developed by MM Weissman and S Bothwell. The original SAS is a longer instrument, requiring nearly one hour to administer, while the newer SAS-SR is a shorter, self-rated instrument. Both the SAS and SAS-SR are widely utilized in research and treatment assessment settings. Both scales evaluate multiple dimensions of social functioning including work, social, and leisure activities; relationships with family members; sexual functioning; parental role; and family role. The SAS has 42 questions in 6 areas of role functioning. Each item is rated on a continuum from either 1 (best functioning) to 5 (worst functioning), or 1 (best functioning) to 7 (worst functioning). The SAS evaluates social functioning over a 2-month period, while the SAS-SR evaluates social functioning over a 2-week period. A short version of the SAS-SR, the SAS-S, has also been developed. In addition, there is a version of the SAS for patients with schizophrenia.

GENERAL APPLICATIONS

The SAS measures social functioning in adults.

SELECTED PSYCHOMETRIC PROPERTIES

The SAS-SR shows good internal consistency, with mean Cronbach's alpha of 0.74. The SAS is able to discriminate between social functioning of depressed adults compared to nondepressed adults, with the most robust differences in the work-related domain.

REFERENCES

Edwards DW, Yarvis RM, Mueller DP, et al, "Test-Taking and the Stability of Adjustment Scales: Can We Assess Patient Deterioration?" *Eval Q*, 1978, 2:275-92.

Weissman MM and Bothwell S, "Assessment of Social Adjustment by Patient Self-Report," *Arch Gen Psychiatry*, 1976, 33(9):1111-5.

Weissman MM, Prusoff BA, Thompson WD, et al, "Social Adjustment by Self-Report in a Community Sample and in Psychiatric Outpatients," *J Nerv Ment Dis*, 1978, 166(5):317-26.

COPYRIGHT

SAS:
Myrna M. Weissman, PhD
College of Physicians and Surgeons
Columbia University and School of Public Health Division of Clinical and Genetic Epidemiology
New York State Psychiatric Institute, Unit 24
1051 Riverside Dr
New York, NY 10032
Tel: 212-543-5880
Fax: 212-568-3534
e-mail: mmw@child.cpmc.columbia.edu

SAS-SR and SAS-S:
Multi-Health Systems, Inc
PO Box 950
North Tonawanda, NY 14120-0950
Tel: 800-456-3003
Fax: 888-540-4484
www.mhs.com

SCALE GENERALLY DONE BY

SAS: Trained rater.
SAS-SR: Self-rated, however, it is recommended that a trained rater be available to answer questions and check for response completeness.

TIME TO COMPLETE SCALE

SAS: Up to 60 minutes
SAS-SR: 15 minutes

REPRESENTATIVE STUDY UTILIZING SCALE

Hudson CR, Kirby KC, Firely ML, et al, "Social Adjustment of Family Members and Significant Others (FSOs) of Drug Users," *J Subst Abuse Treat*, 2002, 23(3):171-81.

C. SOCIAL ADJUSTMENT SCALE (SAS, SAS-SR) *(Continued)*

Sample Entries of the
SAS-SR Question Booklet
by Myrna M. Weissman, PhD

We are interested in finding out how you have been doing in the last 2 weeks. We would like you to answer some questions about your work, your spare time, and your family life. There are no right or wrong answers to these questions. Before starting, please fill out the information at the top of the answer form. Answer the questions by circling your response on the answer form.

A. Work for Pay
Do you work 15 hours or more per week for pay?
*If **YES**, please answer question 1. If **NO**, skip to section B. Housework (unpaid).*

1. How many days did you miss from work in the past 2 weeks?
1. I didn't miss any days.
2. I missed one day.
3. I missed about half the time.
4. I missed more than half the time but did work at least one day.
5. I did not work any days.
6. I did not work any days because of scheduled vacation.

Did you work any days in the last 2 weeks?
*If **YES**, please answer questions 2 through 6. If **NO**, skip to section B. Housework (unpaid).*

B. Housework (unpaid)
Is unpaid housework a significant activity in your life?
*If **YES**, please answer question 7. If **NO**, skip to section C. Student.*

7. How often did you do some unpaid housework (eg, cooking, cleaning, laundry, grocery shopping, and errands) in the past 2 weeks?
1. I did the housework every day.
2. I did the housework almost every day.
3. I did the housework about half the time.
4. I did not usually do the housework.
5. I was completely unable to do housework.
6. I was away from home all of the last 2 weeks.

Were you away from home all of the last 2 weeks?
*If **YES**, skip to section C. Student. If **NO**, please answer questions 8 through 12.*

D. Social and Leisure
Everyone please answer questions 19 through 27.

19. How many friends have you seen or been in contact with (eg, on the telephone, via e-mail, etc) in the last 2 weeks?
1. Nine or more friends.
2. Five to eight friends.
3. Two to four friends.
4. One friend.
5. No friends.

E. Family Outside the Home

Answer questions 30-37 about your parents, brothers, sisters, in-laws, and children not living at home.

Have you been in contact with any of them in the last 2 weeks?
*If **YES**, please answer questions 30-37. If **NO**, skip to question 36.*

36. During the last 2 weeks, have you been thinking that you have let any of your relatives down or been unfair to them at any time?

1. I did not feel that I let them down at all.
2. I usually did not feel that I let them down.
3. About half the time I felt that I let them down.
4. Most of the time I felt that I let them down.
5. I always felt that I let them down.

F. Primary Relationship

Are you living with your spouse or have you been living with a partner in an intimate relationship?
*If **YES**, please answer questions 38 through 46. If **NO**, skip to section G. Parental.*

39. How often have you been able to talk about your feelings and problems with your partner during the last 2 weeks?

1. I could always talk freely about my feelings.
2. I could usually talk about my feelings.
3. About half the time I felt able to talk about my feelings.
4. I was not usually able to talk about my feelings.
5. I was never able to talk about my feelings.

H. Family Unit

Have you ever been married, ever lived with a partner in an intimate relationship, or ever had children?
*If **YES**, please answer questions 51 through 53. If **NO**, skip to question 54.*

54. Have you had enough money to take care of your own and your immediate family's financial needs during the last 2 weeks?

1. I had enough money for needs.
2. I usually had enough money with minor problems.
3. About half the time I did not have enough money but did not have to borrow money.
4. I usually did not have enough money and had to borrow from others.
5. I had great financial difficulty.

THANK YOU FOR YOUR PARTICIPATION.

GENERAL HEALTH
ASSESSMENT SCALES

TABLE OF CONTENTS

A. THE COOP CHARTS FOR ADULT PRIMARY CARE PRACTICE

OVERVIEW

The COOP, developed by E Nelson and colleagues in 1987, provides a rapid, visual way to assess the health and functioning of patients in primary care and can provide a rapid view of the health of a patient from a clinical point of view.

This instrument was developed as part of the Dartmouth Primary Care Cooperative Information Project (COOP) in New Hampshire for measuring health status in physician's offices and consists of 9 charts depicting cartoons and a 5-point system of scoring. The charts are designed to measure physical fitness, feelings, daily activities, social activities, pain, change in health, overall health, social support, and quality of life. Initially, it was recommended that the charts be presented by a trained staff member, but the COOP can be completed by the patient in the office waiting room. The COOP charts are considered as separate dimensions of functioning and there is no overall score.

The COOP Charts have been utilized in different countries with a good deal of success due in great part to the illustrations utilized. These illustrations represent an alternative way to do these evaluations and are adaptable to a variety of cultural and clinical settings.

The COOP Charts have been utilized in different countries with a good deal of success due in great part to the illustrations utilized. These illustrations represent an alternative way to do these evaluations and are adaptable to a variety of cultural and clinical settings.

GENERAL APPLICATIONS

The COOP measures health and functioning of adolescents and adults in a primary care clinic.

SELECTED PSYCHOMETRIC PROPERTIES

Interrater agreement measured by the intraclass correlation has been reported to average 0.77. Retest reliability is 0.67.

In terms of validity, the COOP Charts have been used in a wide variety of studies and it has been found that the charts are well understood by patients and enjoyed by them.

REFERENCES

Larson CO, Hays RD, and Nelson EC, "Do the Pictures Influence Scores on the Dartmouth COOP Charts?" *Qual Life Res*, 1992, 1(4):247-9.

Meyboom-de Jong B and Smith Rja, "Studies With the Dartmouth COOP Charts in General Practice: Comparison With the Nottingham Health Profile and the General Health Questionnaire," *Functional Status Measurement in Primary Care*, New York, NY: Springer-Verlag, 1990, 132-49.

Nelson E, Wasson J, Kirk J, et al, "Assessment of Function in Routine Clinical Practice: Description of the COOP Chart Method and Preliminary Findings," *J Chronic Dis*, 1987, 40(Suppl 1):55S-63S.

COPYRIGHT

John Wasson, MD
Dartmouth Medical School
Hanover, NH 03755
Tel: 603-650-1823

SCALE GENERALLY DONE BY

Self-report instrument

TIME TO COMPLETE SCALE

5-10 minutes

REPRESENTATIVE STUDY UTILIZING SCALE

Lam CL and Lauder IJ, "The Impact of Chronic Diseases on the Health-Related Quality of Life (HRQOL) of Chinese Patients in Primary Care," *Fam Pract*, 2000, 17(2):159-66.

A. THE COOP CHARTS FOR ADULT PRIMARY CARE PRACTICE
(Continued)

The following graphics have been used with permission from John Wasson, MD, Dartmouth Medical School, Hanover, NH 03755

QUALITY OF LIFE

How have things been going for you during the past 4 weeks?

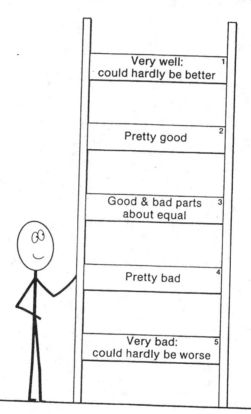

Very well: could hardly be better — 1

Pretty good — 2

Good & bad parts about equal — 3

Pretty bad — 4

Very bad: could hardly be worse — 5

PHYSICAL FITNESS

During the past 4 weeks . . .
What was the hardest physical activity
you could do for at least 2 minutes ?

Very heavy, (for example)
- Run, fast pace
- Carry a heavy load
  upstairs or uphill
  (25 lbs/10 kgs)

1

Heavy, (for example)
- Jog, slow pace
- Climb stairs or a hill
  moderate pace

2

Moderate, (for example)
- Walk, medium pace
- Carry a heavy load
  level ground
  (25 lbs/10 kgs)

3

Light, (for example)
- Walk, medium pace
- Carry light load
  on level ground
  (10 lbs/5kgs)

4

Very light, (for example)
- Walk, slow pace
- Wash dishes

5

A. THE COOP CHARTS FOR ADULT PRIMARY CARE PRACTICE
(Continued)

FEELINGS

During the past 4 weeks . . .
    How much have you been bothered by
    emotional problems such as feeling anxious,
    depressed, irritable or downhearted and blue ?

Not at all		1
Slightly		2
Moderately		3
Quite a bit		4
Extremely		5

DAILY ACTIVITIES

During the past 4 weeks . . .
How much difficulty have you had doing your usual
activities or task, both inside and outside the house
because of your physical and emotional health ?

No difficulty at all		1
A little bit of difficulty		2
Some difficulty		3
Much difficulty		4
Could not do		5

A. THE COOP CHARTS FOR ADULT PRIMARY CARE PRACTICE
(Continued)

SOCIAL ACTIVITIES

During the past 4 weeks . . .
 Has your physical and emotional health limited
 your social activities with family, friends,
 neighbors or groups ?

Not at all		1
Slightly		2
Moderately		3
Quite a bit		4
Extremely		5

PAIN

During the past 4 weeks . . .
How much bodily pain have you
generally had ?

No pain		1
Very mild pain		2
Mild pain		3
Moderate pain		4
Severe pain		5

A. THE COOP CHARTS FOR ADULT PRIMARY CARE PRACTICE
(Continued)

CHANGE IN HEALTH

How would you rate your overall health
now compared to 4 weeks ago ?

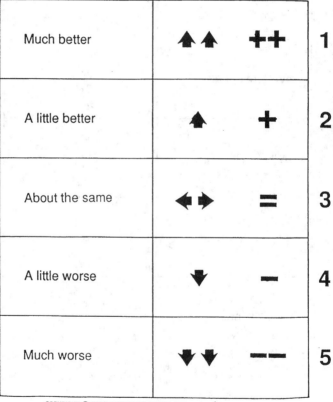

Much better	⬆⬆ ++	1
About the same	⬆ +	2
About the same	⬅➡ =	3
A little worse	⬇ —	4
Much worse	⬇⬇ ——	5

OVERALL HEALTH

During the past 4 weeks . . .
How would you rate your health in general ?

Excellent		**1**
Very good		**2**
Good		**3**
Fair		**4**
Poor		**5**

A. THE COOP CHARTS FOR ADULT PRIMARY CARE PRACTICE
(Continued)

SOCIAL SUPPORT

During the past 4 weeks . . .

Was someone available to help you if you
needed and wanted help? For example if you

— felt very nervous, lonely, or blue
— got sick and had to stay in bed
— needed someone to talk to
— needed help with daily chores
— needed help just taking care of yourself

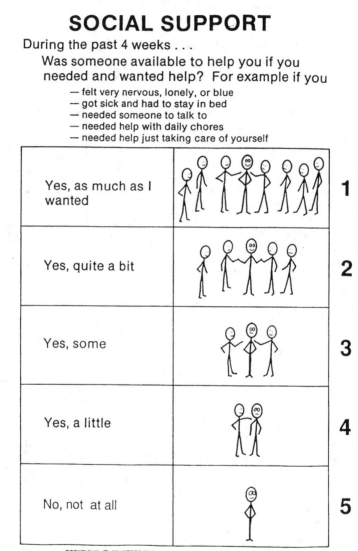

Yes, as much as I wanted		1
Yes, quite a bit		2
Yes, some		3
Yes, a little		4
No, not at all		5

B. THE DUKE HEALTH PROFILE (DUKE)

OVERVIEW

The Duke Health Profile (DUKE), developed by G Parkerson, is derived from the Duke-UNC Health Profile, a 63-item measure designed to evaluate outcomes in primary care settings. This lengthy instrument was modified to become a 17-item generic health status profile intended to be used as a brief and practical instrument in primary care settings.

The DUKE includes all the elements recommended by the World Health Organization (WHO), physical, mental, and social health, plus issues related to self-esteem and self-perception of health. There are also dysfunction scores covered by anxiety, depression, pain, and disability. All the items are self-scored.

The profile has raw scores for each one of the responses on a scale from 0 to 2. Scores for each measure are calculated by adding the raw scores for the items on that measure, dividing by the maximum raw score and then multiplying by 100. The resulting scores may run from 0 to 100 with the high scores indicating good health in opposition to the dysfunction measures where the high scores indicate poor health.

GENERAL APPLICATIONS

The DUKE is a general health status measure for adults.

SELECTED PSYCHOMETRIC PROPERTIES

The correlation between items has been reported by the authors to be somewhat low (0.37 to 0.45) but alpha reliabilities and intraclass coefficients have been reported to be approximately 0.5. In terms of validity, the DUKE has been compared with a series of other instruments showing a good correlation.

REFERENCES

Beaton DE, Bombardier C, and Hogg-Johnson S, "Choose Your Tool: A Comparison of the Psychometric Properties of Five Generic Health Instruments in Workers With Soft Tissue Injuries," *Qual Life Res*, 1994, 3:50-6.

Parkerson GR Jr, Broadhead WE, and Tse CK, "The Duke Health Profile. A 17-Item Measure of Health and Dysfunction," *Med Care*, 1990, 28(11):1056-72.

COPYRIGHT

George R Parkerson
Duke University
Department of Community and Family Medicine
348 Hanes House
Box 3886 Medical Center
Durham NC, 27710
Tel: (919) 681-3043

SCALE GENERALLY DONE BY

Self rated, or may be administered by trained interviewer

TIME TO COMPLETE SCALE

Less than 5 minutes

REPRESENTATIVE STUDY UTILIZING SCALE

Seelert KR, Hill RD, Rigdon MA, et al, "Measuring Patient Distress in Primary Care," *Fam Med*, 1999, 31(7):483-7.

B. THE DUKE HEALTH PROFILE (DUKE) *(Continued)*

DUKE HEALTH PROFILE (Duke)

INSTRUCTIONS: Here are some questions about your health and feelings. Please read each question carefully and check your best answer. You should answer the questions in your own way. There are no right or wrong answers. (Please ignore the small scoring numbers next to each blank.)

	Yes, describes me exactly	Somewhat describes me	No, doesn't describe me at all
1. I like who I am	12	11	10
2. I am not an easy person to get along with	20	21	22
3. I am basically a healthy person	32	31	30
4. I give up too easily	40	41	42
5. I have difficulty concentrating	50	51	52
6. I am happy with my family relationships	62	61	60
7. I am comfortable being around people	72	71	70

TODAY would you have any physical trouble or difficulty:

	None	Some	A Lot
8. Walking up a flight of stairs	82	81	80
9. Running the length of a football field	92	91	90

DURING THE PAST WEEK: How much trouble have you had with:

	None	Some	A Lot
10. Sleeping	102	101	100
11. Hurting or aching in any part of your body	112	111	110
12. Getting tired easily	122	121	120
13. Feeling depressed or sad	132	131	130
14. Nervousness	142	141	140

DURING THE PAST WEEK: How often did you:

	None	Some	A Lot
15. Socialize with other people (talk or visit with friends or relatives)	150	151	152
16. Take part in social, religious, or recreation activities (meetings, church, movies, sports, parties)	160	161	162

DURING THE PAST WEEK: How often did you:

	None	1-4 Days	5-7 Days
17. Stay in your home, a nursing home, or hospital because of sickness, injury, or other health problem	172	171	170

MANUAL SCORING FOR THE DUKE HEALTH PROFILE

To calculate the scores in this column, the raw scores must be revised as follows:

If 0, change to 2; if 2, change to 0; if 1, no change

Item	Raw Score*		PHYSICAL HEALTH SCORE
8	= _____		
9	= _____		
10	= _____		
11	= _____		
12	= _____		
Sum	= _____	x 10 =	

Item	Raw Score*		MENTAL HEALTH SCORE
1	= _____		
4	= _____		
5	= _____		
13	= _____		
14	= _____		
Sum	= _____	x 10 =	

Item	Raw Score*		SOCIAL HEALTH SCORE
2	= _____		
6	= _____		
7	= _____		
15	= _____		
16	= _____		
Sum	= _____	x 10 =	

ANXIETY SCORE

Item	Raw Score*	Revised
2	= _____	– _____
5	= _____	– _____
7	= _____	– _____
10	= _____	– _____
12	= _____	– _____
14	= _____	= _____
	Sum = _____	x 8.333 =

DEPRESSION SCORE

Item	Raw Score*	Revised
4	= _____	– _____
5	= _____	– _____
10	= _____	– _____
12	= _____	– _____
13	= _____	– _____
	Sum = _____	x 10 =

GENERAL HEALTH SCORE

Physical Health score = _____

Mental Health score = _____

Social Health score = _____

Sum = _____ + 3 =

ANXIETY-DEPRESSION (DUKE-AD) SCORE

Item	Raw Score*	Revised
4	= _____	– _____
5	= _____	– _____
7	= _____	– _____
10	= _____	– _____
12	= _____	– _____
13	= _____	– _____
14	= _____	– _____
	Sum = _____	x 7.143 =

PERCEIVED HEALTH SCORE

Item	Raw Score*	
3	= _____	x 50 =

PAIN SCORE

Item	Raw Score*	Revised	
11	= _____	– _____	x 50 =

SELF-ESTEEM SCORE

Item	Raw Score*	
1	= _____	
2	= _____	
4	= _____	
6	= _____	
7	= _____	
Sum	= _____	x 10 =

DISABILITY SCORE

Item	Raw Score*	Revised	
17	= _____	– _____	x 50 =

*Raw Score = last digit of the numeral adjacent to the blank checked by the respondent for each item. For example, if the second blank is checked for item 10 (blank numeral = 101), then the raw score is "1", because 1 is the last digit of 101.

Final Score is calculated from the raw scores as shown and entered into the box for each scale. For physical health, mental health, social health, general health, self-esteem, and perceived health, 100 indicates the best health status, and 0 indicates the worse health status. For anxiety, depression, anxiety-depression, pain, and disability, 100 indicates the worst health status and 0 indicates the best health status.

Missing Values: If one or more responses are missing within one of the eleven scales, a score cannot be calculated for that particular scale.

C. THE SHORT FORM 36 HEALTH SURVEY (SF-36)

OVERVIEW

This widely-used scale was designed as a general indicator of health status and is utilized to evaluate functional health, well-being, and general health perceptions in population surveys, evaluative studies of health policies, and clinical trials. In 1992, a million forms had been administered.

The SF-36 is derived from work done by the Rand Corporation of Santa Monica, which has developed a series of outcome measures over the last three decades. Initially, a 20-item scale called the SF-20, was developed to evaluate chronic medical and psychiatric conditions. This was later revised to become the SF-36.

The SF-36, as a generic instrument, was designed to be applicable to a wide range of types and severities of conditions. Ware, one of its creators, maintained that the SF-36 should cover both physical and mental concepts including behavioral functioning, perceived well-being, social and role disability, and personal evaluations of health in general. The SF-36 includes questions about work, self-care, mobility, as well as feeling states.

The items of the SF-36 were drawn from the original Medical Outcomes Study questionnaire and the Psychological General Well Being Schedule by Dupuy (see PGWB *on page 271*) and are organized in the following eight dimensions:

- Physical functioning (ten items)
- Role limitations due to physical health problems (four items)
- Bodily pain
- Social functioning
- General mental health, covering psychological distress and well being (five items)
- Role limitations due to emotional problems
- Vitality, energy, or fatigue
- General health perceptions

The SF-36 has two types of scoring which are somewhat different. The first, developed by the Rand group, records the answers to the questions as a 0 to 100 score with the higher scores representing the most favorable scores. The second format, developed by the Health Institute, gives different weights to some responses. The former is analyzed by an optical scanner which reads the forms and prints a graphical display of the results. An acute version of the SF-36 also exists which focuses on health status over the last week. A copy of this version may be obtained from the copyright holder.

GENERAL APPLICATIONS

The SF-36 is a general indicator of health status in adults.

SELECTED PSYCHOMETRIC PROPERTIES

The reliability and validity of the SF-36 has been demonstrated in multiple studies which have surveyed more than 3000 patients with various medical and psychiatric conditions. In general, the median alpha reliability for all scales exceeds 0.80 and the two weeks test-retest correlations exceeds 0.8, with the test-retest correlation after a delay of six months ranging between 0.6 and 0.9.

The manual for the SF-36 has the criterion validity information for all the scales, suggesting a significant and consistent association with the validation criteria. Several studies have demonstrated good correlation with other scales such as the Sickness Impact Profile (see SIP *on page 284*), the Quality of Well-Being Scale, and the EuroQol Quality of Life.

REFERENCES

Medical Outcomes Trust, *How to Score the SF-36 Short Form Health Survey*, Boston, MA: The Medical Outcomes Trust, 1992.

Ware JE Jr and Sherbourne CD, "The MOS 36-Item Short-Form Health Survey (SF-36). I. Conceptual Framework and Item Selection," *Med Care*, 1992, 30(6):473-83.

Ware JE, Kosinski M, and Keller SD, *SF-36 Physical and Mental Health Summary Scores: A User's Manual*, Boston, MA: The Health Institute, New England Medical Center, 1994.

Ware JE, Snow KK, Kosinski M, et al, *SF-36 Health Survey: Manual and Interpretation Guide*, Boston, MA: The Health Institute, New England Medical Center, 1993.

Hays RD, Wells KB, Sherbourne CD, et al, "Functioning and Well-Being Outcomes of Patients With Depression Compared to Chronic Medical Illnesses," *Arch Gen Psychiat*, 1994, 52(1):11-9.

COPYRIGHT

The Medical Outcomes Trust
The Health Institute
New England Medical Center
198 Tremont St, PMB #503
Boston, MA 02116
Tel: 617-426-4046
Website: www.outcomestrust.org

Computerized Scoring System
Response Technologies, Inc
3399 South County Trail
East Greenwich, RI

Technical information:
SF-36 Health Survey
The Health Institute
New England Medical Center Hospitals
Box 345
750 Washington Street
Boston, MA 02111

SCALE GENERALLY DONE BY

The SF-36 may be self administered or used in personal or telephone interviews; machine-readable forms and instruction sheets for each version are available from The Health Institute.

TIME TO COMPLETE SCALE

10 minutes

REPRESENTATIVE STUDY UTILIZING SCALE

Mundinger MO, Kane RL, Lenz ER, et al, "Primary Care Outcomes in Patients Treated by Nurse Practitioners or Physicians: A Randomized Trial," *JAMA*, 2000, 283(1):59-68.

C. THE SHORT FORM 36 HEALTH SURVEY
(SF-36) *(Continued)*

SF-36 HEALTH SURVEY (Standard US Version)

INSTRUCTIONS: This survey asks for your views about your health. This information will help keep track of how you feel and how well you are able to do your usual activities.

Answer every question by marking the answer as indicated. If you are unsure about how to answer a question, please give the best answer you can.

1. In general, would you say your health is:

(circle one)

Excellent 1
Very good 2
Good 3
Fair 4
Poor 5

2. Compared to one year ago, how would you rate your health in general <u>now</u>?

(circle one)

Much better now than one year ago 1
Somewhat better now than one year ago 2
About the same as one year ago 3
Somewhat worse now than one year ago 4
Much worse now than one year ago 5

3. The following items are about activities you might do during a typical day. Does <u>your health now limit you</u> in these activities? If so, how much?

(circle one number on each line)

ACTIVITIES	Yes, Limited a Lot	Yes, Limited a Little	No, Not Limited at All
a. Vigorous activities, such as running, lifting heavy objects, participating in strenuous sports	1	2	3
b. Moderate activities, such as moving a table, pushing a vacuum cleaner, bowling, or playing golf	1	2	3
c. Lifting or carrying groceries	1	2	3
d. Climbing several flights of stairs	1	2	3
e. Climbing one flight of stairs	1	2	3
f. Bending, kneeling, or stooping	1	2	3
g. Walking more than a mile	1	2	3
h. Walking several blocks	1	2	3
i. Walking one block	1	2	3
j. Bathing or dressing yourself	1	2	3

4. During the past 4 weeks, have you had any of the following problems with your work or other regular daily activities as a result of your physical health?

(circle one number on each line)

	YES	NO
a. Cut down on the amount of time you spent on work or other activities	1	2
b. Accomplished less than you would like	1	2
c. Were limited in the kind of work or other activities	1	2
d. Had difficulty performing the work or other activities (for example, it took extra effort)	1	2

5. During the past 4 weeks, have you had any of the following problems with your work or other regular daily activities as a result of any emotional problems (such as feeling depressed or anxious)?

(circle one number on each line)

	YES	NO
a. Cut down on the amount of time you spent on work or other activities	1	2
b. Accomplished less than you would like	1	2
c. Didn't do work or other activities as carefully as usual	1	2

6. During the past 4 weeks, to what extent has your physical health or emotional problems interfered with your normal social activities with family, friends, neighbors, or groups?

(circle one)

Not at all 1
Slightly 2
Moderately 3
Quite a bit 4
Extremely 5

7. How much bodily pain have you had during the past 4 weeks?

(circle one)

None 1
Very mild 2
Mild 3
Moderate 4
Severe 5
Very severe 6

8. During the past 4 weeks, how much did pain interfere with your normal work (including both work outside the home and housework)?

(circle one)

Not at all 1
A little bit 2
Moderately 3
Quite a bit 4
Extremely 5

C. THE SHORT FORM 36 HEALTH SURVEY
(SF-36) (Continued)

9. These questions are about how you feel and how things have been with you <u>during the past 4 weeks</u>. For each question, please give the one answer that comes closest to the way you have been feeling. How much of the time during the <u>past 4 weeks</u>.....

(circle one number on each line)

	All of the Time	Most of the Time	A Good Bit of the Time	Some of the Time	A Little of the Time	None of the Time
a. Did you feel full of pep?	1	2	3	4	5	6
b. Have you been a very nervous person?	1	2	3	4	5	6
c. Have you felt so down in the dumps that nothing could cheer you up?	1	2	3	4	5	6
d. Have you felt calm and peaceful?	1	2	3	4	5	6
e. Did you have a lot of energy?	1	2	3	4	5	6
f. Have you felt downhearted and blue?	1	2	3	4	5	6
g. Did you feel worn out?	1	2	3	4	5	6
h. Have you been a happy person?	1	2	3	4	5	6
i. Did you feel tired?	1	2	3	4	5	6

10. During the <u>past 4 weeks</u>, how much of the time has your physical health or emotional problems interfered with your social activities (like visiting with friends, relatives, etc)?

(circle one)

All of the time 1
Most of the time 2
Some of the time 3
A little of the time 4
None of the time 5

11. How TRUE or FALSE is <u>each</u> of the following statements for you?

(circle one number on each line)

	Definitely True	Mostly True	Don't Know	Mostly False	Definitely False
a. I seem to get sick a little easier than other people	1	2	3	4	5
b. I am as healthy as anybody I know	1	2	3	4	5
c. I expect my health to get worse	1	2	3	4	5
d. My health is excellent	1	2	3	4	5

INSIGHT ASSESSMENT

RATING SCALES

TABLE OF CONTENTS

A. INSIGHT AND TREATMENT ATTITUDE QUESTIONNAIRE (ITAQ)

OVERVIEW

The ITAQ, developed by JP McEvoy and colleagues, is an 11-item rating scale to evaluate patient recognition of illness and need for treatment in psychiatric illness, particularly schizophrenia. Each item is scored on a 0 to 2 scale (0 = no insight, 2 = good insight). The ITAQ has been well-researched and is easy to administer. Although the scale is good for assessing patient acceptance of a diagnosis and need for treatment, it is limited in its evaluation of other dimensions of insight, such as awareness of the consequences of a mental illness.

GENERAL APPLICATIONS

The ITAQ is used to assess insight into psychiatric illness, particularly psychotic illness.

SELECTED PSYCHOMETRIC PROPERTIES

The authors have reported a high interrater reliability (r = 0.82, p <.001). Construct validity, checked by correlating scores with an open interview and medication compliance was also good (r = 0.85, p <.001).

REFERENCES

McEvoy JP, Apperson LJ, Applebaum PS, et al, "Insight in Schizophrenia: Its Relationship to Acute Psychopathology," *J Nerv Ment Dis*, 1989, 177(1):43-7.

McEvoy JP, Applebaum PS, Apperson LJ, et al, "Why Must Some Schizophrenic Patients Be Involuntarily Committed? The Role of Insight," *Comp Psychiatry*, 1989, 30(1):13-7.

COPYRIGHT

Joseph McEvoy
John Umstead Hospital
103 12th Street
Butner, NC 27509
Tel: 919-575-7213

SCALE GENERALLY DONE BY

Clinician or trained rater

TIME TO COMPLETE SCALE

10 minutes

REPRESENTATIVE STUDY UTILIZING SCALE

Carroll A, Fattah S, Clyde Z, et al, "Correlates of Insight and Insight Change in Schizophrenia," *Schizophr Res*, 1999, 35(3):247-53.

INSIGHT AND TREATMENT ATTITUDES QUESTIONNAIRE (ITAQ)

INFORMATION NOT OBTAINED ☐

Check or tick (√) one answer for each of the questions below.

1. Have you *at any time* had mental ("nerve," "worry") problems that were different from most other people's?

   ☐ 2 The patient acknowledges the presence of delusional beliefs, hallucinatory experiences or disorganized thoughts, and views these as serious problems which required substantial intervention.

   ☐ 1 The patient acknowledges only anxiety, sleep disturbances, arguing, or being upset, and believes the treatment may not have been necessary; or states that he went along with treatment because important others (eg, family or physician) felt he was ill and should be treated.

   ☐ 0 The patient states that no problems existed and that treatment was completely unnecessary, or gives nonsensical answer (eg, "I came for coffee.")

2. Have you *at any time* needed treatment (hospitalization or outpatient care) for mental ("nerve," "worry") problems?

   ☐ 2 The patient acknowledges the presence of delusional beliefs, hallucinatory experiences or disorganized thoughts, and views these as serious problems which required substantial intervention.

   ☐ 1 The patient acknowledges only anxiety, sleep disturbances, arguing, or being upset, and believes the treatment may not have been necessary; or states that he went along with treatment because important others (eg, family or physician) felt he was ill and should be treated.

   ☐ 0 The patient states that no problems existed and that treatment was completely unnecessary, or gives nonsensical answer (eg, "I came for coffee.")

3. Do you *now* have mental ("nerve," "worry") problems?

   ☐ 2 The patient acknowledges that some psychopathology is still present, or if symptoms have cleared, that the illness has been controlled but not completely cured. He or she views recovery as the happy result of successful treatment.

   ☐ 1 The patient states that all problems which had been present are now completely gone, and that there is no more need for concern. He or she is unclear as to why treatment is continuing but willing to go along if told to do so by his family or physician.

   ☐ 0 The patient believes there never were any problems, there are no problems now, and there is certainly no need for treatment.

215

A. INSIGHT AND TREATMENT ATTITUDE QUESTIONNAIRE (ITAQ)
(Continued)

INSIGHT AND TREATMENT ATTITUDES QUESTIONNAIRE (ITAQ)

4. Do you *now* need treatment (hospitalization or outpatient care) for mental ("nerve," "worry") problems?

☐ 2 The patient acknowledges that some psychopathology is still present, or if symptoms have cleared, that the illness has been controlled but not completely cured. He or she views recovery as the happy result of successful treatment.

☐ 1 The patient states that all problems which had been present are now completely gone, and that there is no more need for concern. He or she is unclear as to why treatment is continuing but wiling to go along if told to do so by his family or physician.

☐ 0 The patient believes there never were any problems, there are no problems now, and there is certainly no need for treatment.

5. Is it possible that *in the future* you may have mental ("nerve," "worry") problems?

☐ 2 The patient is aware that schizophrenia is a chronic illness, like diabetes or hypertension, and that maintenance treatment, including attendance at outpatient follow-up appointments, is required to prevent relapse.

☐ 1 The patient is unsure about the possibility of relapse or the need for maintenance treatment, but will participate if told to do so by his family or physician.

☐ 0 The patient assures us that there will be no mental problems in his future, and that maintenance treatment is completely unnecessary.

6. Will you *in the future* need continued treatment (outpatient care or, possibly, hospitalization) for mental ("nerve," "worry") problems?

☐ 2 The patient is aware that schizophrenia is a chronic illness, like diabetes or hypertension, and that maintenance treatment, including attendance at outpatient follow-up appointments, is required to prevent relapse.

☐ 1 The patient is unsure about the possibility of relapse or the need for maintenance treatment, but will participate if told to do so by his family or physician.

☐ 0 The patient assures us that there will be no mental problems in his future, and that maintenance treatment is completely unnecessary.

INSIGHT AND TREATMENT ATTITUDES QUESTIONNAIRE (ITAQ)

7. Have you *at any time* needed to take medications for mental problems ("nerves," "worry")?

☐₂ The patient views antipsychotic medications as having favorable therapeutic effects in alleviating delusions, hallucinations, or disorganized thoughts, and states that continued treatment will be required to prevent a recurrence of these symptoms.

☐₁ The patient states that medications were helpful in relieving anxieties, improving sleep, or diminishing irritability. He is unsure as to whether medications will be required on a regular basis in the future but will take them if told to do so by his family or physician.

☐₀ The patient believes that medications have not been indicated, and certainly are not required in the future.

8. Do you *now* need to take medications for mental problems ("nerves," "worry")?

☐₂ The patient views antipsychotic medications as having favorable therapeutic effects in alleviating delusions, hallucinations, or disorganized thoughts, and states that continued treatment will be required to prevent a recurrence of these symptoms.

☐₁ The patient states that medications were helpful in relieving anxieties, improving sleep, or diminishing irritability. He is unsure as to whether medications will be required on a regular basis in the future but will take them if told to do so by his family or physician.

☐₀ The patient believes that medications have not been indicated, and certainly are not required in the future.

9. Will you *in the future* need to take medications for mental problems ("nerves", "worry")?

☐₂ The patient views antipsychotic medications as having favorable therapeutic effects in alleviating delusions, hallucinations, or disorganized thoughts, and states that continued treatment will be required to prevent a recurrence of these symptoms.

☐₁ The patient states that medications were helpful in relieving anxieties, improving sleep, or diminishing irritability. He is unsure as to whether medications will be required on a regular basis in the future but will take them if told to do so by his family or physician.

☐₀ The patient believes that medications have not been indicated, and certainly are not required in the future.

A. INSIGHT AND TREATMENT ATTITUDE QUESTIONNAIRE (ITAQ)
(Continued)

INSIGHT AND TREATMENT ATTITUDES QUESTIONNAIRE (ITAQ)

10. Will you take the medications?

☐$_2$ The patient states that he will take medications because he has a chronic psychiatric illness which the medications control (prevent relapse).

☐$_1$ The patient states that he probably will take medications because they help him to sleep or because his family or physician tell him to.

☐$_0$ The patient states that the medications are unnecessary and do no good, and that he will not take them.

11. Do the medications do you any good?

☐$_2$ The patient states that he will take medications because he has a chronic psychiatric illness which the medications control (prevent relapse).

☐$_1$ The patient states that he probably will take medications because they help him to sleep, or because his family or physician tell him to.

☐$_0$ The patient states that the medications are unnecessary and do no good, and that he will not take them.

B. SCALE TO ASSESS UNAWARENESS OF MENTAL DISORDER (SUMD)

OVERVIEW

The SUMD, developed by XF Amador and DH Strauss, is a 74-item scale used to evaluate awareness of illness or insight in patients with psychiatric disorder, particularly psychotic illness. The authors have categorized insight as multidimensional with two main components: Awareness of illness and attribution regarding illness. Information for rating is obtained via a semistructured interview. The scale requires that the patient have a mental disorder with one or more symptoms listed on a symptom checklist. Severity of unawareness of illness is rated on a 0 to 5 scale with 5 being poorest insight (zero score = not applicable). The SUMD can be used to evaluate either current or past illness. It may provide information on patient acceptance of a diagnosis or understanding of effects of medication. Strengths of the scale include its wide use in insight evaluation and evaluation over a wide range of signs and symptoms. A limitation of the scale includes no assessment of the patient's beliefs regarding need for treatment. The authors (Amador, 1994) have also published an abridged version of the scale with nine items.

GENERAL APPLICATIONS

The SUMD is used to assess insight in psychiatric disorders, particularly schizophrenia.

SELECTED PSYCHOMETRIC PROPERTIES

Examination of the SUMD across training sites showed generally strong intraclass correlation coefficients ranging from 0.52 to 0.99 (median: 0.64) for scores on awareness and attribution of current illness. Test-retest intraclass correlation coefficients have been reported to range from 0.36 to 0.80 (median: 0.51).

REFERENCES

Amador XF, Flaum M, Andreasen NC, et al, "Awareness of Illness in Schizophrenia and Schizoaffective and Mood Disorders," *Arch Gen Psychiat*, 1994, 51(10):826-36.

Amador XF, Strauss DH, Yale SA, et al, "Awareness of Illness in Schizophrenia," *Schizophr Bull*, 1991, 17(1):113-32.

COPYRIGHT

Xavier F Amador, PhD
New York State Psychiatric Institute
722 West 168th St, Unit 2
New York, NY 10032

SCALE GENERALLY DONE BY

Clinician or trained rater

TIME TO COMPLETE SCALE

Full version: Up to 40 minutes; abridged version: 10-20 minutes

REPRESENTATIVE STUDY UTILIZING SCALE

Arango C, Adami H, Sherr JD, et al, "Relationship of Awareness of Dyskinesia in Schizophrenia to Insight Into Mental Illness," *Am J Psychiatry*, 1999, 156(7):1097-9.

B. SCALE TO ASSESS UNAWARENESS OF MENTAL DISORDER (SUMD) *(Continued)*

SAMPLE ENTRIES OF THE

SCALE TO ASSESS UNAWARENESS OF MENTAL DISORDERS (SUMD)

Directions:

This scale requires that the subject has a mental disorder with one of the symptoms listed below. For each symptom-item on the scale, it must first be ascertained that the subject has exhibited the particular symptom during the period under investigation. The severity of the symptom is not relevant, only that it is clearly present. The symptom checklist must be completed prior to filling out the scale in order to determine which symptom-items are relevant. The three nonsymptom "summary" items (1, 2, and 3) are usually relevant and should be completed if this is the case.

In the **current** column "C", rate the highest level of awareness obtained at the time of the interview for "current" psychopathology.

In the **past** column "P", rate the present level of awareness for each item occurring during the period of time preceding the current period of investigation. In other words, when questioned about a particular episode in the past, would the subject currently say s/he was delusional, thought disordered, asocial, mentally ill, etc at that time.

Longer or shorter time periods may be used to assess current and retrospective awareness and attributions depending on the goals of the investigation.

Following each symptom item (4-20), you are asked to rate the subject's understanding of the cause of the symptom (ie, attribution). **NOTE:** For any symptom, attribution items are rated only if the subject received a score between 1 and 3 on the awareness item.

Symptom Checklist:

Circle either "c" for current, or "p" for past, next to the item number to denote which symptom-items and time periods are to be rated.

Item			Symptom
4.	c	p	Hallucinations
5.	c	p	Delusion(s)
6.	c	p	Thought disorder
7.	c	p	Inappropriate affect
8.	c	p	Unusual dress or appearance
9.	c	p	Stereotypic or ritualistic behavior
10.	c	p	Poor social judgment
11.	c	p	Poor control of aggressive impulses
12.	c	p	Poor control of sexual impulses
13.	c	p	Alogia
14.	c	p	Flat or blunt affect
15.	c	p	Avolition-Apathy
16.	c	p	Anhedonia-Asociality
17.	c	p	Poor attention
18.	c	p	Confusion-Disorientation
19.	c	p	Unusual eye contact
20.	c	p	Poor social relationships

1. Awareness of mental disorder.

In the most general terms, does the subject believe that s/he has a mental disorder, psychiatric problem, emotional difficulty, etc?

C	P	
0	0	Cannot be assessed
1	1	Aware: Subject clearly believes that s/he has a mental disorder
2	2	
3	3	Somewhat: Is unsure about whether s/he has a mental disorder, but can entertain the idea that s/he might
4	4	
5	5	Unaware: Believes s/he does not have a mental disorder

2. Awareness of the achieved effects of medication.

What is the subject's belief regarding the effects of medication? Does the subject believe that medications have lessened the intensity or frequency of his/her symptoms (ie, if applicable)?

C	P	
0	0	Cannot be assessed or item not relevant
1	1	Aware: Subject clearly believes medications have lessened the intensity or frequency of his/her symptoms
2	2	
3	3	Somewhat: Is unsure about whether medications have lessened the intensity or frequency of his/her symptoms, but can entertain the idea
4	4	
5	5	Unaware: Believes that medications have not lessened the intensity or frequency of his/her symptoms

3. Awareness of the social consequences of mental disorder.

What is the subject's belief regarding the reason s/he has been admitted to the hospital, involuntarily hospitalized, arrested, evicted, fired, injured, etc?

C	P	
0	0	Cannot be assessed or item not relevant
1	1	Aware: Subject clearly believes that the relevant social consequences are related to having a mental disorder
2	2	
3	3	Somewhat: Is unsure about whether the relevant social consequences are related to having a mental disorder
4	4	
5	5	Unaware: Believes that the relevant social consequences have nothing to do with having a mental disorder

C. SCHEDULE FOR ASSESSMENT OF INSIGHT (SAI)

OVERVIEW

The SAI, developed by A David, is a three-item rating scale used to evaluate insight in psychotic illness. The SAI evaluates insight in three dimensions: 1. the recognition of mental illness, 2. the ability to recognize abnormal mental events (eg, hallucinations) as pathological, 3. treatment compliance. Responses are scored on a 0 to 2 scale (0 = never, 2 = often). The SAI has the advantage of brevity and ease of administration; however, like the ITAQ, its evaluation of insight is fairly narrow. An expanded version of the SAI (Kemp, 1997) has been published which incorporates awareness of change into the evaluation.

GENERAL APPLICATIONS

The SAI is used to rate insight in psychotic illness.

SELECTED PSYCHOMETRIC PROPERTIES

The SAI has been reported to have a correlation of 0.527 with the BPRS total and 0.525 with the Beck total.

REFERENCES

David AS, "Insight and Psychosis," *Br J Psychiatry*, 1990, 156:798-808.

David A and Kemp R, "Five Perspectives on the Phenomenon of Insight in Psychosis," *Psychiatric Annals*, 27(12):791-7.

Kemp R and David A, "Insight and Compliance," *Compliance and the Treatment of Alliance in Serious Mental Illness*, Blackwell B, ed, Neward, NJ: Gordon and Breach Publishing Group, 1997, 61-84.

COPYRIGHT

Anthony David, Professor
Department of Psychological Medicine
King's College School of Medicine and Dentistry and the Institute of Psychiatry
103 Denmark Hill
London SE5 8AZ, England

SCALE GENERALLY DONE BY

Clinician or trained rater

TIME TO COMPLETE SCALE

Under 10 minutes

REPRESENTATIVE STUDY UTILIZING SCALE

MacPherson R, Jerrom B, and Hughes A, "Relationship Between Insight, Educational Background, and Cognition in Schizophrenia," *Br J Psychiatry*, 1996, 168(6):718-22.

SCHEDULE FOR ASSESSMENT OF INSIGHT (SAI)

1a. Does patient accept (includes passive acceptance) treatment (medication and/or admission and/or other physical and psychological therapies)?

  Often = 2 (may rarely question need for treatment)

  Sometimes = 1 (may occasionally question need for treatment)

  Never = 0 (ask why)

  If 1 or 2, proceed to 1b.

1b. Does patient ask for treatment unprompted?

  Often = 2 (excludes inappropriate requests for medication, etc)

  Sometimes = 1 (rate here if forgetfulness/disorganization leads to occasional requests only)

  Never = 0 (accepts treatment after prompting)

2a. Ask patient: "Do you think you have an illness?" or "Do you think there is something wrong with you?" (mental physical, unspecified)

  Often = 2 (thought present most of the day, most days)

  Sometimes = 1 (thought present occasionally)

  Never = 0 (ask why doctors/others think he/she does)

  If 1 or 2, proceed to 2b.

2b. Ask patient: "Do you think you have a mental/psychiatric illness?"

  Often = 2 (thought present most of the day, most days)

  Sometimes = 1 (thought present occasionally, minimum once per day)

  Never = 0

  If 1 or 2 proceed to 2c.

2c. Ask patient: "How do you explain your illness?"

  Reasonable account given based on plausible mechanisms (appropriate given patient's social, cultural, and educational background, eg, excess stress, chemical imbalance, family history, etc) = 2

  Confused account given, repetition of overheard explanation without adequate understanding or "don't know" = 1

  Delusional explanation = 0

3a. Ask patient: "Do you think the belief that.... (insert specific delusion) is not really true/ happening?" or "Do you think that ..... (insert specific hallucination) is not really there/ happening?"

  Often = 2 (thought present most of the day, most days)

  Sometimes = 1 (thought present occasionally, minimum once per day)

  Never = 0

  If 1 or 2 present, proceed to 3b.

3b. Ask patient: "How do you explain these phenomena (the belief that .... hearing that voice/ seeing that image, etc)?"

  Part of my illness = 2

  Reaction to outside event/s (eg, tiredness, stress, etc) = 1

  Attributed to outside forces (may be delusional) = 0

Maximum score = 14.

INVOLUNTARY MOVEMENTS

ASSESSMENT SCALES

TABLE OF CONTENTS

A. ABNORMAL INVOLUNTARY MOVEMENT SCALE (AIMS)

OVERVIEW

The AIMS is a 12-item instrument developed at the National Institute of Mental Health (NIMH) and utilized to provide a numeric measure to the observed abnormal movements in different parts of the body. These abnormal movements can be produced by a number of conditions including exposure to psychotropic medication such as may occur with tardive dyskinesia. For this reason, the AIMS is heavily used in the clinical trials evaluating new antipsychotic medications.

The AIMS information is collected after a brief neurological examination, which if done systematically, can provide very accurate information. This information is scored in a five-point scale (0 = none, 4 = severe) which evaluates abnormal movements in three main anatomic areas (orofacial area, extremities, and trunk). The AIMS has a global rating of severity, a rating of the incapacitation due to the abnormal movements, and an assessment of the patient awareness of the abnormal movements.

The scale can be utilized to measure abnormal movements in different kinds of patients, including adults, children, and adolescents. The original developers did not produce guidelines for the scoring of the AIMS and throughout the years it has been scored by clinicians following their clinical judgment for severity. Some investigators have proposed guidelines which include factors such as amplitude of movements and frequency or diagnosis, but none of the guidelines have been universally accepted or implemented.

The AIMS does not make the diagnosis of the disorder causing the movement abnormality unless some criteria have been established *a priori* to facilitate the diagnostic process.

GENERAL APPLICATIONS

The AIMS is used to assess abnormal involuntary movements of the body in adults, children, and adolescents.

SELECTED PSYCHOMETRIC PROPERTIES

A number of authors have demonstrated satisfactory levels of interrater reliability for the AIMS. Experienced raters obtain higher levels of agreement compared to those who are less well-versed in using the scale. Test-retest reliability at 6-8 weeks ranges from 0.40-0.82 for individual items and is 0.71 for overall severity.

REFERENCES

ECDEU Assessment Manual for Psychopharmacology, Guy W, ed, Washington DC: U.S. Department of Health, Education and Welfare, 1976 (Reprinted 1991).

Lane RD, Glazer WM, Hansen TE, et al, "Assessment of Tardive Dyskinesia Using the Abnormal Involuntary Movement Scales," *J Nerv Ment Dis*, 1985, 173:353-7.

Munetz MR and Benjamin S, "How to Examine Patients Using the Abnormal Involuntary Movement Scale," *Hosp Community Psychiatry*, 1988, 39:1171-7.

COPYRIGHT

Not applicable

SCALE GENERALLY DONE BY

The scale can be done as part of a physical-neurological examination by a trained clinician.

TIME TO COMPLETE SCALE

10-15 minutes

REPRESENTATIVE STUDY UTILIZING SCALE

Sajatovic M, Bingham CR, Garver D, et al, "An Assessment of Clinical Practice of Clozapine Therapy for Veterans," *Psychiatric Services*, 2000, 51(5):669-71.

A. ABNORMAL INVOLUNTARY MOVEMENT SCALE (AIMS) *(Continued)*

ABNORMAL INVOLUNTARY MOVEMENT SCALE (AIMS)

(ECDEU Version)

INSTRUCTIONS: Movement Ratings: Rate highest severity observed. Rate movements that occur upon activation one <u>less</u> than those observed spontaneously.

Code: 0 = None
1 = Minimal, may be extreme normal
2 = Mild
3 = Moderate
4 = Severe

				Circle One		
FACIAL AND ORAL MOVEMENTS	1. Muscles of Facial Expression (eg, movements of forehead, eyebrows, periorbital area, cheeks; include frowning, blinking, smiling, grimacing)	0	1	2	3	4
	2. Lips and Perioral Area (eg, puckering, pouting, smacking)	0	1	2	3	4
	3. Jaw (eg, biting, clenching, chewing, mouth opening, lateral movement)	0	1	2	3	4
	4. Tongue Rate only increase in movement both in and out of mouth, NOT inability to sustain movement	0	1	2	3	4
EXTREMITY MOVEMENTS	5. Upper (arms, wrists, hands, fingers) Include choreic movements (ie, rapid, objectively purposeless, irregular, spontaneous), athetoid movements (ie, slow, irregular, complex serpentine). Do NOT include tremor (ie, repetitive, regular, rhythmic)	0	1	2	3	4
	6. Lower (legs, knees, ankles, toes) (eg, lateral knee movement, foot tapping, heel dropping, foot squirming, inversion and eversion of foot)	0	1	2	3	4
TRUNK MOVEMENTS	7. Neck, shoulders, hips (eg, rocking, twisting, squirming, pelvic gyrations)	0	1	2	3	4
GLOBAL JUDGMENTS	8. Severity of abnormal movements	None, normal Minimal Mild Moderate Severe				0 1 2 3 4
	9. Incapacitation due to abnormal movements	None, normal Minimal Mild Moderate Severe				0 1 2 3 4
	10. Patient's awareness of abnormal movements Rate only patient's report	No awareness Aware, no distress Aware, mild distress Aware, moderate distress Aware, severe distress				0 1 2 3 4
DENTAL STATUS	11. Current problems with teeth and/or dentures	No Yes				0 1
	12. Does patient usually wear dentures?	No Yes				0 1

B. BARNES AKATHISIA SCALE (BAS, BARS)

OVERVIEW

The BAS, developed by T Barnes in 1989, has a global approach to the evaluation of akathisia associated with the use of antipsychotic medications, including an objective and a subjective component plus a global impression rating for the overall disorder. These components are rated on a scale of 0 to 3 for the objective and subjective items, and 0 to 5 for the global clinical assessment. The manual for the scale has good instructions for the administration; excellent definition for the items and for the severity points; plus definitions for mild, moderate, and severe akathisia. In the global clinical assessment a rating of 2 or more is diagnostic of the condition.

GENERAL APPLICATIONS

The BAS is used to evaluate drug-induced akathisia in adults, children, and adolescents.

SELECTED PSYCHOMETRIC PROPERTIES

The interrater reliability is good (reported as weighted Cohen's kappa ranging from 0.736 to 0.955 with highest figure for the global item) as well as its validity, which is derived from its basis in signs and symptoms identified in multiple studies involving patients being treated with psychotropic medications in various clinical situations.

REFERENCES

Barnes TRE, "A Rating Scale for Drug-Induced Akathisia," *Br J Psychiatry*, 1989, 154:672-6.

Barnes TRE, "Clinical Assessment of the Extrapyramidal Side Effects of Antipsychotic Drugs," *J Psychopharm*, 1992, 6:214-21.

COPYRIGHT

Thomas RE Barnes
The Royal College of Psychiatrists
The British Journal of Psychiatry
17 Belgrave Square, SW1X 8PG

SCALE GENERALLY DONE BY

The scale can be done as part of a general physical-neurological examination done by a trained clinician.

TIME TO COMPLETE SCALE

10-15 minutes

REPRESENTATIVE STUDY UTILIZING SCALE

Sajatovic M, Perez D, Brescan D, et al, "Olanzapine Therapy in Elderly Patients With Schizophrenia," *Psychopharmacol Bull*, 1998, 34(4):819-23.

B. BARNES AKATHISIA SCALE (BAS, BARS) *(Continued)*

RATING SCALE FOR DRUG-INDUCED AKATHISIA
(BAS, BARS SCALE)

Patient should be observed while seated, then standing while engaged in neutral conversation. Symptoms observed in other situations (eg, in activity on the ward) may also be rated. Subsequently, the subjective phenomena should be elicited by direct questioning.

1. OBJECTIVE

0 = Normal, occasional fidgety movements of limbs

1 = Presence of characteristic restless movements; shuffling, tramping, swinging of one leg while sitting, rocking from foot to foot, or "walking on the spot" when standing, present for less than half the time observed

2 = Observed phenomena, present for at least half the observation period

3 = Constantly engaged in characteristic restless movements, has inability to remain seated or standing without walking or pacing, during time observed

2. SUBJECTIVE (Awareness of Restlessness)

0 = Absence of inner restlessness

1 = Nonspecific sense of inner restlessness

2 = Aware of an inability to keep legs still, complaints of inner restlessness aggravated by being required to stand still

3 = Awareness of intense compulsion to move most of the time and/or reports strong desire to walk or pace most of the time

DISTRESS RELATED TO RESTLESSNESS

0 = No distress

1 = Mild

2 = Moderate

3 = Severe

3. GLOBAL CLINICAL ASSESSMENT OF AKATHISIA

0 = Absent - no evidence of awareness of restlessness, observation of characteristic movements of akathisia in the absence of a subjective report of inner restlessness or compulsive desire to move legs should be classified as pseudoakathisia

1 = Questionable - nonspecific inner tension and fidgety movements

2 = Mild akathisia - awareness of restlessness in legs, and/or inner restlessness worse when required to stand still, fidgety movements present, but characteristic restless movements of akathisia not necessarily observed, causes little or no distress

3 = Moderate akathisia - awareness of restlessness as described for mild akathisia above, combined with characteristic restless movements, such as rocking from foot to foot when standing, patient finds condition distressing

4 = Marked akathisia - subjective experience of restlessness, compulsive desire to walk or pace; however, patient is able to remain seated for at least 5 minutes, condition obviously distressing

5 = Severe akathisia - patient reports strong compulsion to pace up and down most of the time, unable to sit or lie for more than a few minutes, constant restlessness associated with intense distress and insomnia

C. EXTRAPYRAMIDAL SYMPTOM RATING SCALE (ESRS)

OVERVIEW

The ESRS, developed by G Chouinard and collaborators, includes 12 questionnaire items to identify subjective symptomatology. Eight items are devoted to parkinsonian signs, under which is included akathisia.

Each item is rated on a seven-point scale. This scale has a novel approach to resolve the problem of how to judge severity by recommending the rating in two modalities: Frequency and amplitude. The ESRS has become a very widely utilized instrument in clinical trials to assess side effects of antipsychotic medications.

GENERAL APPLICATIONS

The ESRS measures extrapyramidal symptoms in children, adolescents, and adults.

SELECTED PSYCHOMETRIC PROPERTIES

The ESRS is considered comprehensive and its statistical properties appear good.

REFERENCES

Chouinard G, Ross-Chouinard A, Annable L, et al, "Extrapyramidal Rating Scale," *Can J Neurolog Sci*, 1980, 7:233.

Chouinard G, Annable L, Mercier P, et al, "A Five-Year Follow-Up Study of Tardive Dyskinesia," *Psychopharm Bull*, 1986, 22:259-63.

COPYRIGHT

Guy Chouinard, MD
Centre de Recherche Fernand-Seguin
Hospital Louis-H. Lafontaine
7401 Rue Hochelaga
Montreal (Quebec) Canada H1N 3M5
Tel: 514-251-4000

SCALE GENERALLY DONE BY

The scale can be done as part of a physical-neurological examination by a trained clinician.

TIME TO COMPLETE SCALE

15-20 minutes

REPRESENTATIVE STUDY UTILIZING SCALE

Madhussodanon S, Brenner R, Suresh P, et al, "Efficacy and Tolerability of Olanzapine in Elderly Patients with Psychotic Disorders: A Prospective Study," *Ann Clin Psychiatr*, 2000, 12(1):11-8.

C. EXTRAPYRAMIDAL SYMPTOM RATING SCALE (ESRS) *(Continued)*

EXTRAPYRAMIDAL SYMPTOM RATING SCALE

1) Period _____
                          1   2   3

2) Subject number _____
                          4   5   6

3) Sex (M=1, F=2) _____
                                    7

4) Evaluator _____
                          8   9

5) Project _____
                     10   11   12   13

I. PARKINSONISM, DYSTONIA AND DYSKINESIA: QUESTIONNAIRE

Inquire into the status of each symptom as reported by the patient and rate accordingly.

	Absent	Mild	Moderate	Severe
1. Impression of slowness or weakness, difficulty in carrying out routine tasks	0	1	2	3
2. Difficulty walking or with balance	0	1	2	3
3. Difficulty swallowing or talking	0	1	2	3
4. Stiffness, stiff posture	0	1	2	3
5. Cramps or pains in limbs, back or neck	0	1	2	3
6. Restless, nervous, unable to keep still	0	1	2	3
7. Tremors, shaking	0	1	2	3
8. Oculogyric crisis or abnormal sustained posture	0	1	2	3
9. Increased salivation	0	1	2	3
10. Abnormal involuntary movements (dyskinesia) of extremities or trunk	0	1	2	3
11. Abnormal involuntary movements (dyskinesia) of tongue, jaw, lips or face	0	1	2	3
12. Dizziness when standing up (especially in the morning)	0	1	2	3

II. PARKINSONISM: EXAMINATION

1. Expressive automatic movements
(facial mask/speech)

0: normal
1: very mild decrease in facial expressiveness
2: mild decrease in facial expressiveness
3: rare spontaneous smile, decreased blinking, voice slightly monotonous
4: no spontaneous smile, staring gaze, low monotonous speech, mumbling
5: marked facial mask, unable to frown, slurred speech
6: extremely severe facial mask with unintelligible speech

|__|__|
   14

2. Bradykinesia

0: absent
1: global impression of slowness in movements
2: definite slowness in movements
3: very mild difficulty in initiating movements
4: mild to moderate difficulty in initiating movements
5: difficulty in starting or stopping any movement, or freezing on initiating voluntary act
6: rare voluntary movement, almost completely immobile

|__|__|
   15

3. Rigidity   Total _____
   right upper limb _____
   left upper limb _____
   right lower limb _____
   left lower limb _____

0: normal muscle tone
1: very mild, barely perceptible
2: mild, (some resistance to passive movements)
3: moderate (definite resistance to passive movements)
4: moderately severe (moderate resistance but still easy to move limb)
5: severe (marked resistance with definite difficulty to move the limb)
6: extremely severe (limb nearly frozen)

|__|__|
   16

4. Gait & posture

0: normal
1: mild decrease of pendular arm movement
2: moderate decrease of pendular arm movement, normal steps
3: no pendular arm movement, head flexed, steps more or less normal
4: still posture (neck, back), small steps (shuffling gait)
5: more marked, festination or freezing on turning
6: triple flexion, barely able to walk

|__|__|
   17

5. Tremor   Total _____
   right upper limb _____ head _____
   left upper limb _____ jaw/chin _____
   right lower limb _____ tongue _____
   left lower limb _____ lips _____

			FREQUENT	CONSTANT OR ALMOST SO
none	0			
borderline	1			
small amplitude		2	3	4
moderate amplitude		3	4	5
large amplitude		4	5	6

OCCASIONAL   FREQUENT

|__|__|
   18

6. Akathisia

0: absent
1: looks restless, nervous, impatient, uncomfortable
2: needs to move at least one extremity
3: often needs to move one extremity or to change position
4: moves one extremity almost constantly if sitting, or stamps feet while standing
5: unable to sit down for more than a short period of time
6: moves or walks constantly

|__|__|
   19

EXTRAPYRAMIDAL SYMPTOM RATING SCALE *(continued)*

7. Sialorrhea

0: absent
1: very mild
2: mild
3: moderate: impairs speech
4: moderately severe
5: severe
6: extremely severe: drooling

| | 20 |

8. Postural stability

0: normal
1: hesitation when pushed but no retropulsion
2: retropulsion but recovers unaided
3: exaggerated retropulsion without falling
4: absence of postural response, would fall if not caught by examiner
5: unstable while standing, even without pushing
6: unable to stand without assistance

| | 21 |

III. DYSTONIA: EXAMINATION

1. Acute torsion dystonia   Total _____

right upper limb _____   head _____
left upper limb _____   jaw _____
right lower limb _____   tongue _____
left lower limb _____   lips _____   trunk _____
   eyes _____   other _____

0: absent
1: very mild
2: mild
3: moderate
4: moderately severe
5: severe
6: extremely severe

| | 22 |

1. Nonacute or chronic or tardive dystonia   Total _____

right upper limb _____   head _____
left upper limb _____   jaw _____
right lower limb _____   tongue _____
left lower limb _____   lips _____   trunk _____
   face _____   other _____

0: absent
1: very mild
2: mild
3: moderate
4: moderately severe
5: severe
6: extremely severe

| | 23 |

IV. DYSKINETIC MOVEMENTS: EXAMINATION

1. Lingual movements (slow lateral or torsion movement of tongue)

	OCCASIONAL*	FREQUENT**	CONSTANT OR ALMOST SO	
none	0			
borderline	1			
clearly present, within oral cavity	2	3	4	24
with occasional partial protrusion	3	4	5	
with complete protrusion	4	5	6	

2. Jaw movements (lateral movement, chewing, biting, clenching)

none	0			
borderline	1			
clearly present, small amplitude	2	3	4	25
moderate amplitude, but without mouth opening	3	4	5	
large amplitude, with mouth opening	4	5	6	

3. Bucco-labial movements (puckering, pouting, smacking, etc)

none	0			
borderline	1			
clearly present, small amplitude	2	3	4	26
moderate amplitude, forward movement of lips	3	4	5	
large amplitude; marked, noisy smacking of lips	4	5	6	

4. Truncal movements (rocking, twisting, pelvic gyrations)

none	0			
borderline	1			
clearly present, small amplitude	2	3	4	27
moderate amplitude	3	4	5	
greater amplitude	4	5	6	

5. Upper extremities (choreoathetoid movements only: Arms, wrists, hands, fingers)

none	0			
borderline	1			
clearly present, small amplitude, movement of one limb	2	3	4	28
moderate amplitude, movement of one limb or				
movement of small amplitude involving two limbs	3	4	5	
greater amplitude, movement involving two limbs	4	5	6	

C. EXTRAPYRAMIDAL SYMPTOM RATING SCALE (ESRS) *(Continued)*

EXTRAPYRAMIDAL SYMPTOM RATING SCALE *(continued)*

		OCCASIONAL*	FREQUENT**	CONSTANT OR ALMOST SO	
6. Lower extremities (choreoathetoid movements only: Legs, knees, ankles, toes)					
none	0				
borderline	1				
clearly present, small amplitude, movement of one limb		2	3	4	29
moderate amplitude, movement of one limb or					
movement of small amplitude involving two limbs		3	4	5	
greater amplitude movement involving two limbs		4	5	6	

		OCCASIONAL*	FREQUENT**	CONSTANT OR ALMOST SO	
7. Other involuntary movements (swallowing, irregular respiration, frowning, blinking, grimacing, sighing, etc)					
none	0				
borderline	1				
clearly present, small amplitude		2	3	4	30
moderate amplitude		3	4	5	
greater amplitude		4	5	6	

SPECIFY _____

* when activated or rarely spontaneous
** frequently spontaneous and present when activated

Examiner signature _____ Date _____

EXTRAPYRAMIDAL SYMPTOM RATING SCALE MANUAL

1) Period _____

                                  1   2   3

2) Subject number _____

                                  4   5   6

3) Sex (M=1, F=2) _____

                                      7

4) Evaluator _____

                               8   9

5) Project _____

                        10 11 12 13

Global
0 = Absent
1 = Borderline
2 = Very mild
3 = Mild
4 = Moderate
5 = Moderately severe
6 = Marked
7 = Severe
8 = Extremely severe

Global Items

V. Clinical Global Impression of Severity of Parkinsonism

Considering your clinical experience, how severe is the Parkinsonism at this time?

      |___|
       14

VI. Clinical Global Impression of Severity of Dystonia

Considering your clinical experience, how severe is the dystonia at this time?

      |___|
       15

VII. Clinical Global Impression of Severity of Dyskinesia

Considering your clinical experience, how severe is the dyskinesia at this time?

      |___|
       16

VIII. Clinical Global Impression of Severity of Akathisia

Considering your clinical experience, how severe is the akathisia (subjective and objective components) at this time?

      |___|
       17

Stage of Parkinsonism

IX. Stage of Parkinsonism |___|
(Hoehn & Yahr)   18

0 = Normal
1 = Unilateral involvement only, minimal or no functional impairment (stage 1)
2 = Bilateral or midline involvement, without impairment of balance (stage 2)
3 = Mildly to moderately disabling: First signs of impaired righting or postural reflex (unsteadiness as the patient turns or when he is pushed from standing equilibrium with the feet together and eyes closed), patient is physically capable of leading independent life (stage 3)
4 = Severely disabling: patient is still able to walk and stand unassisted but is markedly incapacitated (stage 4)
5 = Confinement to bed or wheelchair (stage 5)

Examiner signature _____   Date _____

D. SIMPSON ANGUS SCALE (SAS)

OVERVIEW

The Simpson Angus Scale, known also as the Extrapyramidal Side Effects Rating Scale, is a 10-item instrument developed by GM Simpson and JW Angus and utilized to measure the symptoms of parkinsonism or parkinsonian side effects related to the use of antipsychotic medications. The scale has items that measure the parkinsonian symptoms of rigidity, tremor, akinesia, and salivation. Multiple versions of the scale are in existence.

The 10 items are rated on a five-point scale (0 = complete absence of the condition, 4 = presence of the condition on extreme form). A majority, 7 of the 10 items, measure rigidity in different parts of the body with only one item (gait) looking at the symptom of akinesia, a common side effect associated with the use of antipsychotic medication. The items are easily scored after a simple neurological examination and observation of the patient's gait. The global score is the sum of all scores divided by the total number of items. Final scores of up to 0.3 are considered within the normal range. The SAS is very widely used in clinical trials for evaluating the side effects of antipsychotic medications.

GENERAL APPLICATIONS

The SAS is used to measure drug-induced parkinsonism in adults, adolescents, and children.

SELECTED PSYCHOMETRIC PROPERTIES

The authors have reported that mean correlation coefficients for the SAS range from 0.87 for glabellar tap to 0.52 for gait. Correlations between two raters on the total scales ranged from 0.71 to 0.96 in the original study.

REFERENCES

Simpson GM and Angus JW, "A Rating Scale for Extrapyramidal Side Effects," *Acta Psychiatr Scand*, 1970, 212(Suppl 44):11-9.

COPYRIGHT

Acta Psychiatrica Scandinavica
Munksgaard
35 Norre Sogade
Postbox 173, DK-1005
Copenhagen K
Denmark
e-mail: direct@munksgaarddirect.dk

SCALE GENERALLY DONE BY

The scale can be done as part of a physical-neurological examination.

TIME TO COMPLETE SCALE

10-15 minutes

REPRESENTATIVE STUDY UTILIZING SCALE

Friedman JH and Factor SA, "Atypical Antipsychotics in the Treatment of Drug-Induced Psychosis in Parkinson's Disease," *Movement Disorder*, 2000, 15(2):201-11.

SIMPSON ANGUS SCALE (SAS)

1. GAIT

The patient is examined as he walks into the examining room; his gait, the swing of his arms, his general posture, all form the basis for an overall score for this item. This is rated as follows:

0 = Normal

1 = Diminution in swing while the patient is walking

2 = Marked diminution in swing with obvious rigidity in the arm

3 = Stiff gait with arms held rigidly before the abdomen

4 = Stooped shuffling gait with propulsion and retropulsion

2. ARM DROPPING

The patient and the examiner both raise their arms to shoulder height and let them fall to their sides. In a normal subject a stout slap is heard as the arms hit the sides. In the patient with extreme Parkinson's syndrome, the arms fall very slowly.

0 = Normal, free fall with loud slap and rebound

1 = Fall slowed slightly with less audible contact and little rebound

2 = Fall slowed, no rebound

3 = Marked slowing, no slap at all

4 = Arms fall as though against resistance; as though through glue

3. SHOULDER SHAKING

The subject's arms are bent at a right angle at the elbow and taken one at a time by the examiner who grabs one hand and also clasps the other around the patient's elbow. The subject's upper arm is pushed to and from and the humerus is externally rotated. The degree of resistance from normal to extreme rigidity is scored as follows:

0 = Normal

1 = Slight stiffness and resistance

2 = Moderate stiffness and resistance

3 = Marked rigidity with difficulty in passive movement

4 = Extreme stiffness and rigidity with almost a frozen shoulder

4. ELBOW RIGIDITY

The elbow joints are separately bent at right angles and are passively extended and flexed, with the subject's biceps observed and simultaneously palpated. The resistance to the procedure is rated. (The presence of cogwheel rigidity is noted separately.)

0 = Normal

1 = Slight stiffness and resistance

2 = Moderate stiffness and resistance

3 = Marked rigidity with difficulty in passive movement

4 = Extreme stiffness and rigidity with almost a frozen shoulder

D. SIMPSON ANGUS SCALE (SAS) *(Continued)*

5. FIXATION OF POSITION OR WRIST RIGIDITY

The wrist is held in one hand and then the fingers held by the examiner's other hand with the wrist moved to extension, and both ulnar and radial deviation. The resistance to this procedure is rated:

0 = Normal

1 = Slight stiffness and resistance

2 = Moderate stiffness and resistance

3 = Marked rigidity with difficulty in passive movement

4 = Extreme stiffness and rigidity with almost a frozen shoulder

6. LEG PENDULOUSNESS

The patient sits on a table with his legs hanging down and swinging free. The ankle is grasped by the examiner and raised until the knee is partially extended. It is then allowed to fall. The resistance to falling and the lack of swinging form the basis for the score on this item.

0 = The legs swing freely

1 = Slight diminution in the swing of the legs

2 = Moderate resistance to swing

3 = Marked resistance to damping of swing

4 = Complete absence of swing

7. HEAD DROPPING

The patient lies on a well-padded examining table and his head is raised by the examiner's hand. The hand is then withdrawn and the head allowed to drop. In the normal subject, the head will drop upon the table. The movement is delayed in extrapyramidal system disorder, and in extreme parkinsonism, it is absent. The neck muscles are rigid and the head does not reach the examining table. Score is as follows:

0 = The head falls completely with a good thump as it hits the table

1 = Slight slowing in fall, mainly noted by lack of slap as head meets the table

2 = Moderate slowing in the fall quite noticeable to the eye

3 = Head falls stiffly and slowly

4 = Head does not reach examining table

8. GLABELLA TAP

Subject is told to open his eyes and not blink. The glabella region is tapped at a steady, rapid speed. The number of times patient blinks in succession is noted:

0 = 0-5 blinks

1 = 6-10 blinks

2 = 11-15 blinks

3 = 16-20 blinks

4 = 21 and more blinks

9. TREMOR

Patient is observed walking into examining room and then is examined for this item:

0 = Normal

1 = Mild finger tremor, obvious to sight and touch

2 = Tremor of hand or arm occurring spasmodically

3 = Persistent tremor of one or more limbs

4 = Whole body tremor

10. SALIVATION

Patient is observed while talking and then asked to open his mouth and elevate his tongue. The following ratings are given:

0 = Normal

1 = Excess salivation to the extent that pooling takes place if the mouth is open and the tongue raised

2 = When excess salivation is present and might occasionally result in difficulty in speaking

3 = Speaking with difficulty because of excess salivation

4 = Frank drooling

E. UDVALG FOR KLINISKE UNDERSOGELSER (UKU) SIDE EFFECT RATING SCALE

OVERVIEW

The UKU was developed to collect information about the side effects of psychotropic medication in a systematized and comprehensive way following 48 well-defined and operationalized items. The scale has three components with the first one having 48 items, the second component is a global assessment of the interference of the side effects with the functioning of the individual, and the third one is to record the action taken to resolve the problem.

The 48 single items which are scored in a 4-point scale (0 = none, 1 = present to a mild degree, 2 = present to a moderate degree, and 3 = present to a severe degree) are very well defined in an accompanying manual which also provides detailed definitions of the anchor points. These items are organized in four categories:

1. The psychic subscale has 9 items, some of which may be related to the illness. Here it is important to make the judgment if the information recorded has or has not an association with the medication under consideration.

2. The neurological subscale has items from the Simpson Angus Scale *on page 236* plus items for paresthesia and seizures.

3. The autonomic scale has 11 items covering anticholinergic effects, polydipsia, and polyuria.

4. The other scale has 19 miscellaneous items covering dermatological, sexual, and other side effects.

It is important to keep in mind that each item is scored based on the presence of the symptom, whether this effect is considered a side effect or not. The time frame for scoring is the present but sometimes a window of 3-4 days is utilized. As with most other scales, all available information can be utilized to score the item, and when there is a discrepancy, the judgment of the clinician prevails.

Once all the items have been scored, the rater has to make a judgment about the presence or absence of a causal relationship between the symptom and the medication being studied. The terms utilized are impossible, possible, or probable.

GENERAL APPLICATIONS

The UKU evaluates sides effects in patients receiving psychotropic medication on a clinical or research basis.

SELECTED PSYCHOMETRIC PROPERTIES

Studies done in the Nordic European countries show a very good score for intraclass correlations with reported reliability ranging from 0.3 to 0.9. Also, several studies have shown good face, content, and concurrent validity.

REFERENCES

Lingjaerde O, Ahlfors UG, Bech P, et al, "The UKU Side Effect Rating Scale. A New Comprehensive Rating Scale for Psychotropic Drugs and a Cross-Sectional Study of Side Effects in Neuroleptic-Treated Patients," *Acta Psychiatr Scand Suppl*, 1987, 334:1-100.

COPYRIGHT

Not applicable

SCALE GENERALLY DONE BY

Physician, nurse, or rater trained to administer the scale

TIME TO COMPLETE SCALE

10-30 minutes

REPRESENTATIVE STUDY UTILIZING SCALE

Marder SR and Meibach RC, "Risperidone in the Treatment of Schizophrenia," *Am J Psychiatry*, 1994, 151:825-35.

E. UDVALG FOR KLINISKE UNDERSOGELSER (UKU) SIDE EFFECT RATING SCALE *(Continued)*

ATTACHMENT XIII - UKU SIDE EFFECT RATING SCALE

ITEM   ASSESSMENT

1   MENORRHAGIA (Hypermenorrhoea, polymenorrhoea, or metrorrhagia during the last 3 months)

   0   No or doubtful increase in frequency or intensity of menstrual flow.
   1   Hypermenorrhoea, ie, the menstrual flow is more intense than usual, the intervals between are normal.
   2   Polymenorrhoea, ie, the menstrual flow occurs more frequently and is more intense than normal.
   3   Metrorrhagia, ie, irregular intervals and intensity, the blood loss being more frequent and intense compared with the usual pattern.

2   AMENORRHOEA (Hypermenorrhoea, oligomenorrhoea, or amenorrhoea, during the past 3 months)

   0   No or doubtful reduction in frequency or intensity of menstrual flow.
   1   Hypomenorrhoea, ie, uterine bleeding of less than the normal amount, but occurring at normal intervals.
   2   Oligomenorrhoea, ie, prolonged intervals compared with the usual condition; the intensity may also be lower than usual.
   3   Amenorrhoea, ie, menstruation has been absent for more than 3 months.

3   GALACTORRHOEA (Increased secretion of milk outside periods of breast feeding)

   0   No galactorrhoea.
   1   Galactorrhoea present, but to a very slight degree.
   2   Galactorrhoea is present to a moderate degree and is felt to be somewhat disturbing.
   3   Galactorrhoea is very pronounced and clearly disturbing.

4   GYNAECOMASTIA (Excessive development of the male mammary gland)

   0   No gynecomastia.
   1   Gynaecomastia present to a very slight degree compared with the usual state.
   2   Gynaecomastia clearly present; however, only hampering when the patient is undressed.
   3   Gynaecomastia present to such a severe degree that it affects the patient cosmetically, as it can be observed even if he is dressed.

5   INCREASED SEXUAL DESIRE (Increase desire for sexual activity)

   0   No or doubtful.
   1   Slight increase, which is, however, still felt as natural by the partner.
   2   Clear increase that has given rise to comments and discussions with the partner.
   3   When the usual desire has increased to such a severe extent that the patient's life with his partner is considerably disturbed.

ITEM   ASSESSMENT

6   DIMINISHED SEXUAL DESIRE (Reduced desire for sexual activity)

    0   No or doubtful.

    1   The desire for sexual activity is slightly diminished, but without hampering the patient.

    2   A distinct reduction of the patient's desire for and interest in sexual activities so that it becomes a problem for the patient.

    3   Desire and interest have diminished to such an extent that sexual intercourse occurs extremely seldom or has stopped.

7   ERECTILE DYSFUNCTION (Difficulty in attaining or maintaining an erection)

    0   No or doubtful.

    1   Slightly diminished ability to attain or maintain an erection.

    2   A distinct change in the patient's ability to attain or maintain an erection.

    3   The patient only rarely (or never) can attain or maintain an erection.

8   EJACULATORY DYSFUNCTION (Dysfunction of the patient's ability to control ejaculation. Includes a) premature or b) delayed ejaculation. On the scoring sheet it should be indicated whether a) or b) is present.)

    0   No or doubtful.

    1   It is somewhat more difficult than usual for the patient to control ejaculation, but it does not trouble him.

    2   A distinct change in the patient's ability to control ejaculation, so that it becomes a problem for him.

    3   The patient's ability to control ejaculation is influenced to such an extent that it has become a dominating problem in his sexual intercourse and, thus, to a great extent, influences his experience of orgasm.

9   ORGASTIC DYSFUNCTION (Difficulty in obtaining and experiencing satisfactory orgasm)

    0   No or doubtful.

    1   It is more difficult for the patient than usual to obtain orgasm and/or the experience of orgasm is slightly influenced.

    2   The patient states that there is a clear change in the ability to obtain orgasm and/or in the experience of orgasm. This change has reached such a degree that it troubles the patient.

    3   When the patient rarely or never can obtain orgasm and/or the experience of orgasm is markedly reduced.

10   DRY VAGINA (Dryness of vagina with sexual stimulation)

    0   No or doubtful.

    1   Slight dryness of vagina with sexual stimulation.

    2   Moderately disturbing dryness of vagina with sexual stimulation.

    3   Severely disturbing, marked dryness of vagina making coitus difficult (or necessitating the use of lubricants).

PATIENT SATISFACTION / ATTITUDE TOWARDS TREATMENT

SCALES

TABLE OF CONTENTS

A. DRUG ATTITUDE INVENTORY (DAI)

OVERVIEW

The Drug Attitude Inventory (DAI-30), developed by AG Awad, is a 30-item, self-report inventory that focuses on the subjective effect of neuroleptic medications in patients with schizophrenia. The DAI also addresses insight into illness.

The initial pool of scale items was largely derived from clinical practice, according to the authors. Data was obtained from individuals with schizophrenia regarding their medication treatments. One hundred items were selected by the ability of each item to distinguish between patients who took the medication from those who were not compliant. These items were given to a sample of outpatients and 30 of the items were found to discriminate significantly between the two groups. Subjective responses are scored on a euphoric-dysphoric continuum, with scores ranging from -44 (maximum dysphoric response) to +44 (maximum euphoric response).

There is a 10-item scale called the DAI-10 which was derived from stepwise discriminate analyses of responses of 150 schizophrenic patients to the DAI-30. In this case, six of the items are scored as True and four are scored as False. A correct answer to these items is scored as plus one. An incorrect response is scored as minus one. The final score is the sum of the total pluses and minuses. A positive total score means a positive subjective response (compliant). A negative total score means a negative subjective response (noncompliant).

GENERAL APPLICATIONS

The DAI evaluates subjective response to neuroleptic medication in individuals with schizophrenia.

SELECTED PSYCHOMETRIC PROPERTIES

The reliability of the 30-item scale was found to be 0.93, as determined by the developers using the Kuder-Richardson formula. The scale also shows a high discriminative validity.

REFERENCES

Awad AG, "Subjective Response to Neuroleptics in Schizophrenia," *Schizophr Bull*, 1993, 19(3):609-18.

COPYRIGHT

A George Awad
Clarke Institute of Psychiatry
250 College Street
Toronto, Ontario, MST 1R8 Canada
Tel: 416-979-6865

SCALE GENERALLY DONE BY

Self-report scale; may also be administered by clinician or trained rater

TIME TO COMPLETE SCALE

15-30 minutes for 30-item version; approximately 10 minutes for 10-item version

REPRESENTATIVE STUDY UTILIZING SCALE

Cabeza IG, Amador MS, Lopez CA, et al, "Subjective Response to Antipsychotics in Schizophrenic Patients: Clinical Implications and Related Factors," *Schizophr Res*, 2000, 41(2):349-55.

B. PATIENT SATISFACTION QUESTIONNAIRE (PSQ)

OVERVIEW

The Patient Satisfaction Questionnaire (PSQ), developed by JE Ware and colleagues, is a self-rated scale to measure patient satisfaction with medical care. Two current versions of the PSQ are the PSQ-II (Ware, 1984) and the PSQ-III (Marshall, 1993). The PSQ-II contains 55 items with an additional 46-item short form. The PSQ-III contains 50 items. The PSQ evaluates general satisfaction with health care and includes a variety of subscales, which differ slightly depending on the version of the scale. Strengths of the PSQ include its brevity and ease of use. The PSQ is designed to measure satisfaction with medical care in general and, thus, may be less useful for assessment of satisfaction with specific services.

GENERAL APPLICATIONS

The PSQ is a measure of patient satisfaction with medical care in general.

SELECTED PSYCHOMETRIC PROPERTIES

For the PSQ-II: Internal consistency has been reported based upon four large samples. For the 18 subscales, 68 out of 72 coefficients (using Cronbach's alpha) were above a recommended standard of 0.5. Only one was below 0.46. For the PSQ-III: Internal consistency of the seven subscales has been reported to range from 0.82 to 0.88 (Cronbach's alpha).

For the PSQ-III: Internal consistency of the seven subscales has been reported to range from 0.82 to 0.88 (Cronbach's alpha).

REFERENCES

Marshal GN, Hays RD, Sherbourne CD, et al, "The Structure of Patient Satisfaction With Outpatient Medical Care," *Psychol Assess*, 1993, 5:477-83.

Ware JE, Snyder MK, Wright WR, et al, "Defining and Measuring Patient Satisfaction With Medical Care," *Eval Program Plann*, 1984, 6:247-63.

Ware JE, Snyder MK, and Wright WR, "Development and Validation of Scales to Measure Patient Satisfaction With Health Care Services," *Review of Literature, Overview of Methods, and Results Regarding Construction of Scales,* Springfield, VA: National Technical Information Service, 1976, Vol 1 of a final report, Pt A, 288-329.

Ware JE, Snyder MK, and Wright WR, "Development and Validation of Scales to Measure Patient Satisfaction With Health Care Services," *Results Regarding Scales Constructed From the Patient Satisfaction Questionnaire and Measures of Other Health Care Perceptions,* Springfield, VA: National Technical Information Service, 1976, Vol 1 of a final report, Pt B, 288-329.

COPYRIGHT

PSQ-II:
    John E Ware, Jr
    Boston University
    Sargent College of Health and Rehabilitation Sciences
    635 Commonwealth Avenue
    Boston, MA 02215-1605

B. PATIENT SATISFACTION QUESTIONNAIRE (PSQ) *(Continued)*

PSQ-III:
Psychological Assessment
American Psychological Association
750 First St NE
Washington, DC 20002-4242
Tel: 202-336-5541
Fax: 202-336-5633

SCALE GENERALLY DONE BY

Self-rated scale

TIME TO COMPLETE SCALE

15 minutes

REPRESENTATIVE STUDY UTILIZING SCALE

Millar M, "Patient Satisfaction With General Practice in Ireland," *Ir Med J*, 2001, 94(4):106, 108-9.

C. THE CLIENT SATISFACTION QUESTIONNAIRE (CSQ)

OVERVIEW

Patient satisfaction with treatment has become an important factor to evaluate in the measurement of health and outcomes research. There are many scales which measure patient satisfaction as a component of quality improvement. The University of California, San Francisco (UCSF) has developed two scales designed to measure patient and service satisfaction: The Client Satisfaction Questionnaire (CSQ) and the Service Satisfaction Scale (SSS-30) *on page 251.*

The CSQ questionnaire, developed by C Attkisson et al, is intended to measure satisfaction with healthcare services received by an individual. Questions cover nine conceptual domains of patient satisfaction: Physical surroundings; procedures; support staff; kind or type of service; treatment staff; quality of service; amount, length or quantity of service; outcome of service; and general satisfaction.

GENERAL APPLICATIONS

The CSQ measures patient satisfaction with healthcare services.

SELECTED PSYCHOMETRIC PROPERTIES

The scale has high levels of internal consistency, with alphas ranging from 0.86 to 0.94, and excellent acceptability by patients. It is utilized in conjunction with the Service Satisfaction Scale (SSS-30), having a good correlation with this scale. The scoring involves the unweighted summation of the direction-corrected response values and calculation of measures such as mean, standard deviation, etc.

REFERENCES

Attkisson CC and Greenfield TK, "The Client Satisfaction Questionnaire-8 and the Service Satisfaction Questionaire-30," *The Use of Psychological Testing for Treatment Planning and Outcome Assessment*, Maruish ME, ed, Hillsdale, NJ: Erlbaum Associates, 1994.

Attkisson CC and Pascoe GC, eds, "Patient Satisfaction in Health and Mental Health Services," *Eval Prog Planning*, 1983, 6(Suppl 3 and 4):185-418.

Larsen DL, Attkisson CC, Hargreaves WA, et al, "Assessment of Client/Patient Satisfaction: Development of a General Scale," *Eval Program Plann*, 1979, 2(3):197-207.

Rosenblatt A and Attkisson CC, "Assessing Outcomes for Sufferers of Severe Mental Disorder: A Conceptual Framework and Review," *Eval Prog Planning*, 1993, 16:347-63.

COPYRIGHT

C Clifford Attkisson, PhD
Professor of Medical Psychology
Department of Psychiatry
Box 33-C, University of California
San Francisco, CA 94143
Fax: 415-476-9690

C. THE CLIENT SATISFACTION QUESTIONNAIRE (CSQ) *(Continued)*

SCALE GENERALLY DONE BY

The CSQ scale is self-reported, but the information can be obtained by a clinician doing a regular interview.

TIME TO COMPLETE SCALE

5-10 minutes

REPRESENTATIVE STUDY UTILIZING SCALE

Greenwood N, Key A, Burns T, et al, "Satisfaction With In-Patient Psychiatric Services. Relationship to Patient and Treatment Factors," *Br J Psychiatry*, 1999, 174:159-63.

D. THE SERVICE SATISFACTION SCALE (SSS-30)

OVERVIEW

The SSS-30, like its companion the CSQ *on page 249*, is a direct measure of service satisfaction designed to be used with a wide variety of patient groups and settings and is intended to assess multiple factors of service. These factors were identified as the most common or important by consumers of various human services. The SSS-30 was developed by TK Greenfield and CC Attkisson. In comparison with the CSQ, the SSS-30 uses more items which are less global and more specific. Analyses of the scale in different settings have shown two types of subscales: Practitioner Manner and Skills (nine items) and Perceived Outcome (eight items). Other potential subscales are Office Procedures and Accessibility.

GENERAL APPLICATIONS

The SSS-30 measures health service satisfaction of adults in mental health centers, primary care health clinics, and health maintenance organizations. Derivative versions are available for clients with serious mental disorders in residential settings or care management.

SELECTED PSYCHOMETRIC PROPERTIES

According to the developers, the SSS-30 total score can serve as a composite satisfaction measure with high internal consistency. The Cronbach's values have ranged from 0.93 to 0.96 with the subscales having very good internal reliability. The correlation between the SSS-30 and the CSQ-8 is very good. As with its companion, the CSQ-8, scoring involves the unweighted summation of the response values and the calculation of measures such as the mean, standard deviation, etc.

REFERENCES

Greenfield TK and Attkisson CC, "The UCSF Client Satisfaction Scales: II The Service Satisfaction Scale-30," *The Use of Psychological Testing for Treatment Planning and Outcomes Assessment*, 2nd ed, Maruish ME, ed, Mahwah, NJ: Lawrence Erlbaum Associates, 1999, 1347-67.

COPYRIGHT

Dr Thomas K Greenfield
Public Health Institute
2000 Hearst Ave, Suite 300
Berkeley, CA 94709-2176

Copies can be obtained from the author at:
e-mail: tgreenfield@arg.org
Fax: 510-642-7175

C Clifford Attkisson, PhD
Professor of Medical Psychology
Department of Psychiatry
Box 33-C, University of California
San Francisco, CA 94143
Fax: 415-476-9690

D. THE SERVICE SATISFACTION SCALE
(SSS-30) *(Continued)*

SCALE GENERALLY DONE BY

Self-report scale

TIME TO COMPLETE SCALE

15-20 minutes

REPRESENTATIVE STUDY UTILIZING SCALE

Greenfield TK, "Consumer Satisfaction With the Delaware Drinking Driver Program in 1993," Berkley, CA, Public Health Institute, 1994.

Greenfield TK and Attkisson CC, "Progress Toward a Multifactorial Satisfaction Scale for Primary Care and Mental Health Services," *Evaluation and Program Planning*, 1989, 12:271-8.

SERVICES EVALUATION (SSS-30 Practitioner Version)

CONFIDENTIAL

SUBSCALE KEY

Please read the following statements carefully. Indicate the answer that best describes your feeling about each aspect of the services you have received. We are interested in your *overall experience* based on all visits or contacts you have had *during the last year*. By "practitioner" we mean the one or more doctors, psychologists, counselors, clinicians, etc, who have worked with you.

What is your overall feeling about the …

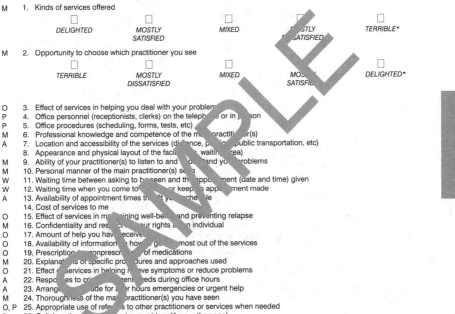

M 1. Kinds of services offered

    ☐ DELIGHTED   ☐ MOSTLY SATISFIED   ☐ MIXED   ☐ MOSTLY DISSATISFIED   ☐ TERRIBLE*

M 2. Opportunity to choose which practitioner you see

    ☐ TERRIBLE   ☐ MOSTLY DISSATISFIED   ☐ MIXED   ☐ MOSTLY SATISFIED   ☐ DELIGHTED*

O 3. Effect of services in helping you deal with your problems
P 4. Office personnel (receptionists, clerks) on the telephone or in person
P 5. Office procedures (scheduling, forms, tests, etc)
M 6. Professional knowledge and competence of the main practitioner(s)
A 7. Location and accessibility of the services (distance, parking, public transportation, etc)
   8. Appearance and physical layout of the facility (waiting area)
M 9. Ability of your practitioner(s) to listen to and understand your problems
M 10. Personal manner of the main practitioner(s) seen
W 11. Waiting time between asking to be seen and the appointment (date and time) given
W 12. Waiting time when you come to office or keep an appointment made
A 13. Availability of appointment times that fit your schedule
   14. Cost of services to me
O 15. Effect of services in maintaining well-being and preventing relapse
M 16. Confidentiality and respect for your rights as an individual
O 17. Amount of help you have received
O 18. Availability of information on how to get the most out of the services
O 19. Prescription or nonprescription of medications
M 20. Explanations of specific procedures and approaches used
O 21. Effect of services in helping relieve symptoms or reduce problems
A 22. Responses to crisis or emergent needs during office hours
A 23. Arrangements made for after hours emergencies or urgent help
M 24. Thoroughness of the main practitioner(s) you have seen
O, P 25. Appropriate use of referrals to other practitioners or services when needed
P 26. Collaboration among service providers (if more than one)
   27. Publicity or information about programs and services offered
P 28. Handling and accuracy of your records (as best you can tell)
O 29. Contribution of services to achievement of your life goals
M 30. In an overall general sense, how satisfied are you with the service you have received?
   31. (If applicable) Support of the group as a whole, helpfulness and caring of its members

SUBSCALE KEY

M = Manner and Skill (9-items; average α = .88)
O = Perceived Outcome (8-items; average α = .83)
P = Procedures (5-items; average α = .74)
A = Accessibility (4-items; average α = .67)
W = Waiting (2 items, may optionally be combined with Access)

*Example Item scale. Note that individual item scale anchors alternate direction throughout the instrument; scoring reverses every other item, allowing validity check for role responding.

D. THE SERVICE SATISFACTION SCALE
(SSS-30) *(Continued)*

SERVICES EVALUATION (SSS-30 Practitioner Version), *continued*

It is important to know something about our clients as a whole, so we request some demographic information. Only grouped data will be used, and you will never be identified. However, if you prefer not to answer any or all questions, you may freely do so.

32. About how many miles (one way) from the facility do you live?

☐ 5 or Less   ☐ 6-10   ☐ 11-15   ☐ 16-20   ☐ 20-25   ☐ 26 or more

33. Approximately how many *weeks* have you been involved with this program?

☐ Less than 1   ☐ 1-2   ☐ 3-4   ☐ 5-6   ☐ 7-12   ☐ More than 12

34. Including today's, approximately how many sessions have you had in this program?

☐ 0   ☐ 1   ☐ 2   ☐ 3   ☐ 4   ☐ 5   ☐ 6-10   ☐ 11-2   ☐ -30   ☐ 31-50   ☐ 51+

35. Your Sex: MALE ☐   FEMALE ☐

36. Your Age: ☐ Under 20   ☐ 21-25   ☐ 26-35   ☐ 36-45   ☐ 4   ☐ 56-6   ☐ 66-75   ☐ 76-85   ☐ 86+

37. Yearly Family Income:

Under $10,000 ☐ $10,000 - ,000 ☐
$20,001 - $40,000 ☐ $,001 - $ ☐
$60,001 - $80,000 ☐   1 - $100 ☐
                        $,0 or more ☐

38. Your Education:

Grade 8 or less ☐   Some igh sc. ☐
High school grad ☐   ome lege ☐
College grad ☐   ou. grad ☐
Masters ☐   PhD, M c ☐

39. Ethnic Background:

Caucasian/White ☐   Asian/Pacific American ☐
Native American/Indian ☐   Hispanic/Latino ☐
Afric an/Black ☐   Other (Specify) ☐
Pre not to answer ☐   _____

40. In genera. ese , how you feel about your life as a whole?

☐ TERRIBLE   ☐ UNHAPP   ☐ MOSTLY DISSATISFIED   ☐ MIXED   ☐ MOSTLY SATISFIED   ☐ PLEASED   ☐ DELIGHTED

41. In general these days, how do you feel about your health?

☐ TERRIBLE   ☐ UNHAPPY   ☐ MOSTLY DISSATISFIED   ☐ MIXED   ☐ MOSTLY SATISFIED   ☐ PLEASED   ☐ DELIGHTED

THANK YOU VERY MUCH FOR YOUR HELP WITH THIS SURVEY. WE WOULD APPRECIATE ANY ADDITIONAL COMMENTS ABOUT THIS SERVICE YOU WOULD CARE TO ADD. YOU MAY WRITE THEM BELOW.

42. The thing I have liked best about my experience here is:

43. What I liked least was:

44. If I could change one thing about this service it would be:

QUALITY OF LIFE

SCALES

TABLE OF CONTENTS

A. LEHMAN QUALITY OF LIFE INTERVIEW (QOLI)

OVERVIEW

This scale, by A Lehman, initially developed in 1983 for use in a survey of severely ill patients living in board and care homes in Los Angeles, has been applied in many studies with chronically mentally ill persons, including the national evaluation of the Robert Wood Johnson Program on Chronic Mental Illness and the Evaluation of Assertive Community Treatment (ACT) Programs in Baltimore, Maryland. The QOLI is a widely-used and well-validated scale. A limitation for use is the relatively long administration time (approximately 45 minutes) required for completion of the entire scale. This is a limitation of many of the current Quality of Life assessment instruments.

The QOLI is a structured self-report interview administered by a lay interviewer. It consists of 153 items. Its purpose is to assess the quality of life of persons with severe mental disorders from two perspectives: 1) Their personal experience of what they do and experience (objective quality of life) and 2) The feelings associated with these experiences (subjective quality of life).

The scale, originally developed to be utilized in populations of patients with severe mental disorders and living in institutions, has been utilized in a number of situations. This includes both inpatient and outpatient studies, the evaluation of drug studies, and use for individuals with chronic physical disorders.

The scale is administered by a face-to-face interview with scoring based on patient self-reports and involving a variety of areas including:

- Living situation
- Family relations
- Social relations
- Leisure activities
- Finances
- Safety and legal problems
- Work and school
- Health
- Religion
- Neighborhood

A shorter version of the scale, the Quality of Life Interview, Brief Version (QOLI-Brief Version), was developed in 1994 as a response to many requests for an abbreviated version. This scale has 74 items requiring less time for the interview without losing its reliability and/or validity.

GENERAL APPLICATIONS

The QOLI is used to assess quality of life in the severely mentally ill.

SELECTED PSYCHOMETRIC PROPERTIES

According to the author, the scale shows a very good internal consistency reliability with median scores of 0.85 for the life satisfaction scales and 0.68 for the objective quality of life scales. The test-retest reliabilities (one week) are very good. The construct and predictive validity have been assessed in multiple studies, and the scale is capable of differentiating patients living in hospitals and supervised community residential programs. There are also several papers published on the relationship between quality of life, clinical symptoms, gender, and housing type.

REFERENCES

Lehman AF, "The Well-Being of Chronic Mental Patients," *Arch Gen Psychiatry*, 1983, 40(4):369-73.

Lehman AF, "A Quality of Life Interview for the Chronically Mentally Ill," *Evaluation and Program Planning*, 1988, Vol 11, 51-62.

Lehman AF, et al, "Quality of Life Experiences of the Chronic Mentally Ill: Gender and Stages of Life Effects," *Evaluation and Program Planning*, 1992, Vol 15, 7-12.

COPYRIGHT

Anthony Lehman
University of Maryland
Department of Psychiatry
645 West Redwood St
Baltimore, MD 21201
Tel: 410-706-2490

SCALE GENERALLY DONE BY

Trained lay interviewers

TIME TO COMPLETE SCALE

45 minutes

REPRESENTATIVE STUDY UTILIZING SCALE

Traver T, Duckmanton RA, and Chiu E, "A Study of Quality of Life of the Severely Mentally Ill," *Int J Soc Psych*, 1998, 44(2):79-91.

A. LEHMAN QUALITY OF LIFE INTERVIEW (QOLI) *(Continued)*

QUALITY OF LIFE INTERVIEW

Full Version

SECTION A: DEMOGRAPHICS

Time Began (military time): _____ : _____

First, I'm going to ask you a few background questions.

1. SEX OF RESPONDENT (Code by observation)	Male	1
	Female	2
2. What is your date of birth?	_____ / _____ / _____	
3. How old are you?	Age	____
	Missing	99
4. What is your marital status?	Married	1
	Separated	2
	Divorced	3
	Widowed	4
	Never married	5
	Co-habitating	6
	Missing	9
5. A. How many children do you have?	No. of children	____
	None	00
	Missing	99
B. How many of your children are under 18 years of age?	No. of children	____
6. What is the highest grade in school or year of college you have completed?		
	Grade	____
	None	00
	Missing	99

IF Q6 CODED 12 OR MORE, GO TO Q8

7. Did you pass a high school equivalency test?	No	0
	Yes	1
	Missing	9
8. Do you have a college degree?	No (go to Q10)	0
	Yes	1
	Missing	9
9. What degree is that?	Associate	1
	Bachelors	2
	Masters	3
	Doctorate	4
	Other (specify)	5

SPECIFY: _____

258

10. Do you have any other training?	No (go to Q12)	0
	Yes	1
	Missing	9

11. What kind of training?

_____

12. Which of the following best describes your race?	Caucasian (not Hispanic)	1
	African-American (not Hispanic)	2
	Hispanic	3
	American Indian ...	4
	Asian	5
	Other (specify)	6
	Missing	9

SPECIFY: _____

13. Did you ever serve in the Armed Forces of the United States?	No (go to next section)	0
	Yes	1
	Missing	9

14. What branch of the Armed Forces?	Army	1
	Navy	2
	Marines	3

15. What type of discharge did you receive when you left the Armed Forces?		
	Honorable	1
	General	2
	Undesirable	3
	Bad conduct	4
	Dishonorable or dismissal	5
	Other	6

SECTION B: GENERAL LIFE SATISFACTION

Please look at this card (hand subject the delighted-terrible scale). This is called the Delighted-Terrible Scale (D/T Scale).

The scale goes from terrible, which is the lowest ranking of 1, to delighted, which is the highest ranking of 7. There are also points 2 through 6 with descriptions below them. (Read points on the scale.)

During the interview we'll be using this scale from time to time to help you tell me how you feel about different things in your life. All you have to do is tell me what on the scale best describes how you feel. For example, if I ask "how do you feel about chocolate ice cream" and you are someone who loves chocolate ice cream, you might point to "delighted." On the other hand, if you hate chocolate ice cream, you might point to "terrible." If you feel equally satisfied and dissatisfied with chocolate ice cream, then you would point to the middle of the scale.

Do you have any questions about the scale? Please show me how you feel about chocolate ice cream. Let's begin.

A. LEHMAN QUALITY OF LIFE INTERVIEW (QOLI) *(Continued)*

The first question is a very general one.

1. How do you feel about your life in general?
   D-T SCALE: _____

   Missing   9

Now, set the scale aside. I'll let you know when we need it again.

SECTION C: LIVING SITUATION

Now I am going to ask you some questions about your living situation.

1. What is your *current* living situation? _____

(If respondent is currently in the hospital, and this hospitalization has lasted less than 3 months, living situation = living situation just prior to the hospitalization. If the hospitalization has been for 3 months or more, code "HOSPITAL".)

   01   Hospital
   02   Skilled nursing facility - 24-hour nursing service
   03   Intermediate care facility - less than 24-hour nursing facility
   04   Supervised group living (generally long term)
   05   Transitional group home (halfway or quarterway house)
   06   Family foster care
   07   Cooperative apartment, supervised (staff on premises)
   08   Cooperative apartment, unsupervised (staff not on premises)
   09   Board and care home (private proprietary home for adults, with program and supervision)
   10   Boarding house (includes meals, no program or supervision)
   11   Rooming or boarding house or hotel (includes single room occupancy, no meals are provided, cooking facilities may be available)
   12   Private house or apartment
   13   Shelter
   14   Jail
   15   No current residence (including the streets, bus stations, missions, etc)
   16   Other _____
   99   No information

2. Have you lived any place else during the past <year>? (including hospital)

   No (go to Q5)   0
   Yes (go to Q3)   1
   Missing (go to Q5) . . .   9

3. List in order the places you have lived during the past <year>, including hospitalizations, beginning with your *current* living situation (use codes in Q1 above).

	CODE		DESCRIPTION
a.	_____	_____	_____
b.	_____	_____	_____
c.	_____	_____	_____
d.	_____	_____	_____
e.	_____	_____	_____
f.	_____	_____	_____
g.	_____	_____	_____
h.	_____	_____	_____

Total number of different, nonhospital residences, during past <year>? _____

4. Which of these was your usual residence during the past   _____
    <year>? (use codes in Q1 above)

5. During the past <year> did you sleep in any of the following locations?

LOCATION	NO	YES	MISSING
a. Outside without shelter	0	1	9
b. Inside an empty building	0	1	9
c. In a public shelter	0	1	9
d. In a church/mission	0	1	9

6. Do you *currently* have a regular place to live where you spend at least 5 out of 7 nights
    on the average?

    No 0
    Yes 1
    Missing 9

7. NOW LOOK AT THE D-T SCALE AGAIN AND ANSWER THE FOLLOWING (Hand
    respondent the D-T scale. If respondent is currently in the hospital for less than 3 months,
    use most recent residence prior to hospitalization. If respondent is in the hospital 3
    months or more, use hospital as the residence. Skip if homeless).

    How do you feel about:

    A. The living arrangements where you live?   _____
    B. The food there?   _____
    C. The rules there?   _____
    D. The privacy you have there?   _____
    E. The amount of freedom you have?   _____
    F. The prospect of staying on where you currently live for a long period of   _____
        time?

8. STILL USING THE D-T SCALE, ANSWER THE FOLLOWING: (If respondent is in the
    hospital for less than 3 months, use most recent residence prior to hospitalization. If
    respondent is in the hospital 3 months or more, use hospital as the residence. Skip if
    homeless).

    How do you feel about:

    A. The people who live in the houses and apartments near yours?   _____
    B. People who live in this community?   _____
    C. The outdoor space there is for you to use outside your home?   _____
    D. The particular neighborhood as a place to live?   _____
    E. This community as a place to live?   _____
    F. How safe do you feel in this neighborhood?   _____

A. LEHMAN QUALITY OF LIFE INTERVIEW (QOLI) *(Continued)*

SECTION D: DAILY ACTIVITIES AND FUNCTIONING

1. Now let's talk about some of the things you did with your time in the *past week*. I'm going to read you a list of things people may do with their free time. For each of these, please tell me if you did it during the past week. Did you......? (Read options A-P)

		NO	YES	MISS
A.	Go for a walk?	0	1	9
B.	Go to a movie or play?	0	1	9
C.	Watch television?	0	1	9
D.	Go shopping?	0	1	9
E.	Go to a restaurant or coffee shop?	0	1	9
F.	Go to a bar?	0	1	9
G.	Read a book, magazine, or newspaper?	0	1	9
H.	Listen to a radio?	0	1	9
I.	Play cards?	0	1	9
J.	Go for a ride in a bus or car?	0	1	9
K.	Prepare a meal?	0	1	9
L.	Work on a hobby?	0	1	9
M.	Play a sport?	0	1	9
N.	Go to a meeting of some organization or social group? (Include program-related meetings)	0	1	9
O.	Go to a park?	0	1	9
P.	Go to a library?	0	1	9

2. Overall, how would you rate your functioning in home, social, school, and work settings at the present time? Would you say your functioning in these areas is excellent, good, fair, or poor?

Excellent	1
Good	2
Fair	3
Poor	4
Missing	9

3. NOW PLEASE LOOK AT THE D-T SCALE AGAIN.

    How do you feel about... ? (Read options A-F)

    A. The way you spend your spare time? _____

    B. The amount of time you have to do the things you want to do? _____

    C. The chance you have to enjoy pleasant or beautiful things? _____

    D. The amount of fun you have? _____

    E. The amount of relaxation in your life? _____

    F. The pleasure you get from the television or radio? _____

SECTION E: FAMILY

The next few questions are about your relationship with your family including any relatives with whom you live.

1. In the past <year>, how often did you talk to a member of your family on the telephone? Would you say at least once a day, at least once a week, at least once a month, less than once a month but at least once during the year, or not at all?

At least once a day	5
At least once a week	4
At least once a month	3
Less than once a month ...	2
Not at all	1
No family (go to Section F)	0
Missing	9

2. In the past <year>, how often did you get together with a member of your family - at least once a day, at least once a week, at least once a month, less than once a month but at least once during the year, or not at all?

At least once a day	5
At least once a week	4
At least once a month	3
Less than once a month ...	2
Not at all	1
No family (go to Section F)	0
Missing	9

3. PLEASE LOOK AT THE D-T SCALE AGAIN.

    How do you feel about.....? (Read options A-D)

    A. Your family in general? _____

    B. How often you have contact with your family? _____

    C. The way you and your family act toward each other? _____

    D. The way things are in general between you and your family? _____

SECTION F: SOCIAL RELATIONS

Now I'd like to know about other people in your life, that is, people who are not in your family.

1. About how often do you do the following? Would you say at least once a day, once a week, once a month, less than once a month, or not at all?

At least once a day	5
At least once a week	4
At least once a month	3
Less than once a month ...	2
Not at all	1
Missing	9

    A. Do things with a close friend? _____

    B. Visit with someone who does not live with you? _____

263

A. LEHMAN QUALITY OF LIFE INTERVIEW (QOLI) *(Continued)*

    C. Telephone someone who does not live with you? _____

    D. Write a letter to someone? _____

    E. Do something with another person that you planned ahead of time? _____

    F. Spend time with someone you consider more than a friend, like a spouse, boyfriend, or girlfriend? _____

2. PLEASE LOOK AT THE D-T SCALE AGAIN.

   How do you feel about:

   A. The things you do with other people? _____
   B. The amount of time you spend with other people? _____
   C. The people you see socially? _____
   D. How you get along with other people in general? _____
   E. The chance you have to know people with whom you really feel comfortable? _____
   F. The amount of friendship in your life? _____

SECTION G: FINANCES

A few questions about money.

1. In the past <year>, have you had any financial support from the following sources?

	YES	NO	MISS
A. Earned income	1	0	9
B. Social Security Benefits (SSA)	1	0	9
C. Social Security Disability Income (SSDI)	1	0	9
D. Supplemental Security Income (SSI)	1	0	9
E. Armed Service connected disability payments	1	0	9
F. Other Social Welfare benefits - state or county (general welfare, Aid to Families with Dependent Children (AFDC))	1	0	9
G. Vocational program (Comprehensive Employment and Training Act (CETA)), vocational rehabilitation, sheltered workshop	1	0	9
H. Unemployment compensation	1	0	9
I. Retirement, investment, or savings income	1	0	9
J. Rent supplements (including HUD, Section 8 certificates, living programs receiving public assistance support)	1	0	9
K. Alimony and child support	1	0	9
L. Food stamps	1	0	9
M. Family and/or spouse contribution	1	0	9
N. Other source(s) (SPECIFY):	1	0	9

2. How much money did you receive during the *past month* from all these sources?

    $_____

    Missing   9999

2A. Was this a usual *month* in terms of the amount of money you received?

Yes (go to Q3)	1
No (go to Q2B)	0
Missing (go to Q2B)	9

2B. Would you say that the amount of money you received during the *past month* was more than or less than usual?

More than usual	1
Less than usual	2
Missing	9

2C. How much would you say that you have usually received *per month* during the past year?

$ _____

Missing	9999

3. On the average, how much money did you have to spend on yourself in the *past month*, not counting money for room and meals?

$ _____

Missing	9999

INTERVIEWER RATING:

HOW RELIABLE DO YOU THINK R'S RESPONSES WERE TO Q1:

VERY RELIABLE	4
GENERALLY RELIABLE . . .	3
GENERALLY UNRELIABLE	2
VERY UNRELIABLE	1

4. Is there anyone who handles your money for you?

No (go to Q5)	0
Yes	1

A. Are your checks mailed directly to this person?

No	0
Yes	1

5. During the past <year>, did you generally have enough money each month to cover.....? (Read options A-F)

	YES	NO	MISS
A. Food?	0	1	9
B. Clothing?	0	1	9
C. Housing?	0	1	9
D. Medical care?	0	1	9
E. Traveling around the city for things like shopping, medical appointments, or visiting friends and relatives?	0	1	9
F. Social activities like movies or eating in restaurants?	0	1	9

A. LEHMAN QUALITY OF LIFE INTERVIEW (QOLI) *(Continued)*

6. NOW, I'D LIKE YOU TO USE THE D-T SCALE AGAIN. In general, how do you feel about......? (Read options A-D)

    A. The amount of money you get?   _____

    B. The amount of money you have to cover basic necessities such as food,   _____
        housing, and clothes?

    C. How comfortable and well-off are you financially?   _____

    D. The amount of money you have available to spend for fun?   _____

SECTION H: WORK AND SCHOOL

1. During a usual week, what do you do *most of the time*?

Work at a job for pay (go to Q3) ...	1
Go to a structured day program ...	2
Go to school	3
Do volunteer work	4
Keep house	5
Nothing much (eg, drink coffee, smoke cigarettes, watch TV)	6
Something else (specify)	7
Missing	9

    SPECIFY: _____

2. Are you currently working in a job for pay?

No (go to Q11)	0
Yes	1
Missing	9

3. I'd like to know about the job you have now. What kind of business or industry do you work in? (If more than one job, use the job at which the person earns the higher weekly salary)

    Describe _____

    A. What kind of work do you do?

    Specify: _____

    B. What are your most important activities or duties?

    Specify: _____

4. How long have you been working at this job?

# of months	_____
Less than one month	995
Less than one week	996
Missing	999

5. Is this a job in a sheltered workshop?

No	0
Yes	1
Missing	9

6. Do you have a special supervisor or a job coach?

No	0
Yes	1
Missing	9

7. Is this a job you can keep as long as you wish?

No	0
Yes (go to Q9)	1
Missing	9

8. Is this a job that ends after a certain period of time when you are expected to find another job at another place of work?

No	0
Yes	1
Missing	9

9. How many hours a week do you usually work?

# of hours	____
Missing	999

10. How much do you earn per hour/week at this job? (Choose one)

$ per hour	____
$ per week	____

SKIP TO Q17

11. Have you ever worked in the past <year>?

No	0
Yes	1
Missing	9

12. How long has it been since you had a job for pay?

# of years	____
Less than a year	01
Missing	99

13. What do you think is the main reason that you don't have a steady job right now?

Psychiatric reasons . .	1
Physical problems . . .	2
Laid off	3
Looking/can't find a job	4
Other reason	5
Missing	9

14. Are you looking for work right now?

No (go to Q18)	0
Yes, full-time	1
Yes, part-time	2
Yes, casual	3
Missing (go to Q18)	9

A. LEHMAN QUALITY OF LIFE INTERVIEW (QOLI) *(Continued)*

15. How long have you been looking?

<1 month	0
1-3 months	1
4-6 months	2
7-12 months	3
1-5 years	4
5-10 years	5
>10 years	6
Missing (go to Q18)	9

16. During the past <year> have you either:

   A. Filled out an application for a job?

No	0
Yes	1
Missing	9

   B. Interviewed for a job?

No	0
Yes	1
Missing	9

SKIP TO Q18

17. JOB SATISFACTION (USE D-T SCALE) (Skip if unemployed)
    How do you feel about.....?

   A. Your job? _____

   B. The people you work with? _____

   C. What it is like where you work (the physical surroundings)? _____

   D. The number of hours you work? _____

   E. The amount you get paid? _____

18. Have you been a student during the past <year>?

No (go to next section) . . .	0
Yes	1
Missing (go to next section)	9

19. At what level was the schooling?

High school (grades 9-12, including GED)	1
Adult Education	2
College (undergraduate) . .	3
Graduate school	4
Vocational/technical school	5
Job training	6
Other (specify) _____	7

20. Did you carry a full-time load of studies?

No	0
Yes	1
Missing	9

21. Are you attending now?

No	0
Yes	1
Missing	9

268

22. Using the D-T Scale again, how do you feel about......?

    A. Being a student?   _____

    B. Your school?   _____

    C. The other students at your school?   _____

SECTION I: LEGAL AND SAFETY ISSUES

1. In the past <year>, were you a victim of:
   A. Any violent crimes, such as assault, rape, mugging, or robbery?

No	0
Yes	1
Missing	9

   B. Any nonviolent crimes, such as burglary, theft of your property or money, or being cheated?

No	0
Yes	1
Missing	9

2. Have you been arrested or picked up for any crimes in the past <year>?
                                      # ARRESTS .... ____

3. Have you spent any nights in jail in the past <year>?
                                      # NIGHTS .... ____

4. PLEASE LOOK AT THE D-T SCALE AGAIN.
   How do you feel about.....? (Read options A-E)

       A. Your personal safety?   _____

       B. How safe you are on the streets in your neighborhood?   _____

       C. How safe you are where you live?   _____

       D. The protection you have against being robbed or attacked?   _____

       E. Your chance of finding a policeman if you need one?   _____

SECTION J: HEALTH

NOW I'D LIKE TO ASK YOU ABOUT YOUR HEALTH.

1. In general, would you say your health is:

Excellent	1
Very good	2
Good	3
Fair	4
Poor	5
Missing	9

A. LEHMAN QUALITY OF LIFE INTERVIEW (QOLI) *(Continued)*

2. *Compared to six months ago*, how would you rate your health in general *now*?

Much better now than 6 months ago	1
Somewhat better now than 6 months ago	2
About the same	3
Somewhat worse now than 6 months ago	4
Much worse now than 6 months ago	5
Missing	9

3. How do you feel about.....? (Use the D-T scale)

   A. Your health in general? _____

   B. The medical care available to you if you need it? _____

   C. How often you see a doctor? _____

   D. The chance you have to talk with a therapist? _____

   E. Your physical condition? _____

   F. Your emotional well-being? _____

SECTION K: GLOBAL RATING

1. And a very general question again. USING THE D-T SCALE AGAIN, how do you feel about your life in general?

   _____

Time ended (military time): _____ : _____

CARD I: DELIGHTED - TERRIBLE SCALE

1	2	3	4	5	6	7
Terrible	Unhappy	Mostly Dissatisfied	Mixed (About equally satisfied and dissatisfied)	Mostly satisfied	Pleased	Delighted

B. PSYCHOLOGICAL GENERAL WELL BEING SCHEDULE (PGWB)

OVERVIEW

The PGWB scale was developed in 1970 for the National Center for Health Statistics by HJ Dupuy who wrote the conceptual description of the scale in an unpublished paper. According to Dupuy, the scale assesses how the individual feels about his "inner personal state" rather than about external conditions such as income, work environment, or home environment.

The scale has 22 items that are aggregated to provide scores in six subscales:

- Anxiety
- Depressed mood
- Positive well-being
- Self-control
- General health
- Vitality

The scale, a self-administered questionnaire, includes both positive and negative questions with a time-frame and a six-point response representing intensity or frequency for the first 14 questions. The last four questions use a 0 to 10 rating.

GENERAL APPLICATIONS

The PGWB scale evaluates how an individual rates his/her "inner personal state."

SELECTED PSYCHOMETRIC PROPERTIES

The test-retest reliability coefficients after three months are between 0.68 to 0.85 with an internal consistency of 0.95.

The correlational validity of the scale is very high. The scale has been compared with several other scales, particularly with various mood disorder scales, and has been reported to have values between 0.65 and 0.90. Several psychometric studies have shown that the overall score is fairly stable over time but is sensitive to change in patient status.

REFERENCES

Dupuy HJ, "Self-Representations of General Psychological Well-Being of American Adults," Paper Presented at American Public Health Association Meeting, Los Angeles, October 1978.

Dupuy HJ, "The Psychological General Well-Being Index," *Assessment of Quality of Life in Clinical Trials of Cardiovascular Therapies*, Wenger NK, Mattson ME, Furberg CD, Elinson J, eds, New York, NY: LeJacq, 1984, 170-83.

Himmelfarb S and Murrell SA, "Reliability and Validity of Five Mental Health Scales in Older Persons," *J Gerontol*, 1983, 38(3):333-9.

Stephens T, "Physical Activity and Mental Health in the United States and Canada: Evidence From Four Population Surveys," *Prev Med*, 1988, 17(1):35-47.

B. PSYCHOLOGICAL GENERAL WELL BEING SCHEDULE (PGWB)
(Continued)

COPYRIGHT

Not applicable
Copies available from author:
Harold J Dupuy, PhD
263 Alto Road
Vesuvius, VA 24483-9410

SCALE GENERALLY DONE BY

Self-administered

TIME TO COMPLETE SCALE

10-15 minutes

REPRESENTATIVE STUDY UTILIZING SCALE

Herlitz J, Wiklund I, Sjoland H, et al, "Impact of Age on Improvement in Health-Related Quality of Life 5 Years After Coronary Artery Bypass Grafting," *Scand J Rehav Med*, 2000, 32(1):41-8.

THE PSYCHOLOGICAL GENERAL WELL-BEING SCHEDULE*

NAME:_____SEX: M: [ ] F: [ ]
Last   First   Middle

AGE:_____

READ: This section of the examination contains questions about how you feel and how things have been going with you. For each question check [✓] the answer which best applies to you.

1. How have you been feeling in general? (DURING THE PAST MONTH)

5 [ ] In excellent spirits
4 [ ] In very good spirits
3 [ ] In good spirits mostly
2 [ ] I have been up and down in spirits a lot
1 [ ] In low spirits mostly
0 [ ] In very low spirits

2. How often were you bothered by any illness, bodily disorder, aches or pains? (DURING THE PAST MONTH)

0 [ ] Every day
1 [ ] Almost every day
2 [ ] About half of the time
3 [ ] Now and then, but less than half the time
4 [ ] Rarely
5 [ ] None of the time

3. Did you feel depressed? (DURING THE PAST MONTH)

0 [ ] Yes—to the point that I felt like taking my life
1 [ ] Yes—to the point that I did not care about anything
2 [ ] Yes—very depressed almost every day
3 [ ] Yes—quite depressed several times
4 [ ] Yes—a little depressed now and then
5 [ ] No—never felt depressed at all

4. Have you been in firm control of your behavior, thoughts, emotions, or feelings? (DURING THE PAST MONTH)

5 [ ] Yes, definitely so
4 [ ] Yes, for the most part
3 [ ] Generally so
2 [ ] Not too well
1 [ ] No, and I am somewhat disturbed
0 [ ] No, and I am very disturbed

*A longer research version of the schedule is available from the author, Harold Dupuy, PhD.

B. PSYCHOLOGICAL GENERAL WELL BEING SCHEDULE (PGWB)
(Continued)

5. Have you been bothered by nervousness or your "nerves"? (DURING THE PAST MONTH)
   - 0 [ ] Extremely so—to the point where I could not work or take care of things
   - 1 [ ] Very much so
   - 2 [ ] Quite a bit
   - 3 [ ] Some—enough to bother me
   - 4 [ ] A little
   - 5 [ ] Not at all

6. How much energy, pep, or vitality did you have or feel? (DURING THE PAST MONTH)
   - 5 [ ] Very full of energy—lots of pep
   - 4 [ ] Fairly energetic most of the time
   - 3 [ ] My energy level varied quite a bit
   - 2 [ ] Generally low in energy or pep
   - 1 [ ] Very low in energy or pep most of the time
   - 0 [ ] No energy or pep at all—I felt drained, sapped

7. I felt downhearted and blue DURING THE PAST MONTH.
   - 5 [ ] None of the time
   - 4 [ ] A little of the time
   - 3 [ ] Some of the time
   - 2 [ ] A good bit of the time
   - 1 [ ] Most of the time
   - 0 [ ] All of the time

8. Were you generally tense or did you feel any tension? (DURING THE PAST MONTH)
   - 0 [ ] Yes—extremely tense, most or all of the time
   - 1 [ ] Yes—very tense most of the time
   - 2 [ ] Not generally tense, but did feel fairly tense several times
   - 3 [ ] I felt a little tense a few times
   - 4 [ ] My general tension level was quite low
   - 5 [ ] I never felt tense or any tension at all

9. How happy, satisfied, or pleased have you been with your personal life? (DURING THE PAST MONTH)
   - 5 [ ] Extremely happy—could not have been more satisfied or pleased
   - 4 [ ] Very happy most of the time
   - 3 [ ] Generally satisfied—pleased
   - 2 [ ] Sometimes fairly happy, sometimes fairly unhappy
   - 1 [ ] Generally dissatisfied, unhappy
   - 0 [ ] Very dissatisfied or unhappy most or all the time

10. Did you feel healthy enough to carry out the things you like to do or had to do? (DURING THE PAST MONTH)
    - 5 [ ] Yes—definitely so
    - 4 [ ] For the most part
    - 3 [ ] Health problems limited me in some important ways
    - 2 [ ] I was only healthy enough to take care of myself
    - 1 [ ] I needed some help in taking care of myself
    - 0 [ ] I needed someone to help me with most or all of the things I had to do

11. Have you felt so sad, discouraged, hopeless, or had so many problems that you wondered if anything was worthwhile? (DURING THE PAST MONTH)

    0 [ ] Extremely so—to the point that I have just about given up
    1 [ ] Very much so
    2 [ ] Quite a bit
    3 [ ] Some—enough to bother me
    4 [ ] A little bit
    5 [ ] Not at all

12. I woke up feeling fresh and rested DURING THE PAST MONTH.

    0 [ ] None of the time
    1 [ ] A little of the time
    2 [ ] Some of the time
    3 [ ] A good bit of the time
    4 [ ] Most of the time
    5 [ ] All of the time

13. Have you been concerned, worried, or had any fears about your health? (DURING THE PAST MONTH)

    0 [ ] Extremely so
    1 [ ] Very much so
    2 [ ] Quite a bit
    3 [ ] Some, but not a lot
    4 [ ] Practically never
    5 [ ] Not at all

14. Have you had any reason to wonder if you were losing your mind, or losing control over the way you act, talk, think, feel or of your memory? (DURING THE PAST MONTH)

    5 [ ] Not at all
    4 [ ] Only a little
    3 [ ] Some—but not enough to be concerned or worried about
    2 [ ] Some and I have been a little concerned
    1 [ ] Some and I am quite concerned
    0 [ ] Yes, very much so and I am very concerned

15. My daily life was full of things that were interesting to me DURING THE PAST MONTH.

    0 [ ] None of the time
    1 [ ] A little of the time
    2 [ ] Some of the time
    3 [ ] A good bit of the time
    4 [ ] Most of the time
    5 [ ] All of the time

16. Did you feel active, vigorous, or dull, sluggish? (DURING THE PAST MONTH)

    5 [ ] Very active, vigorous every day
    4 [ ] Mostly active, vigorous—never really dull, sluggish
    3 [ ] Fairly active, vigorous—seldom dull, sluggish
    2 [ ] Fairly dull, sluggish—seldom active, vigorous
    1 [ ] Mostly dull, sluggish—never really active, vigorous
    0 [ ] Very dull, sluggish every day

17. Have you been anxious, worried, or upset? (DURING THE PAST MONTH)

    0 [ ] Extremely so—to the point of being sick or almost sick
    1 [ ] Very much so
    2 [ ] Quite a bit
    3 [ ] Some—enough to bother me
    4 [ ] A little bit
    5 [ ] Not at all

18. I was emotionally stable and sure of myself DURING THE PAST MONTH.

    0 [ ] None of the time
    1 [ ] A little of the time
    2 [ ] Some of the time
    3 [ ] A good bit of the time
    4 [ ] Most of the time
    5 [ ] All of the time

B. PSYCHOLOGICAL GENERAL WELL BEING SCHEDULE (PGWB)
(Continued)

19. Did you feel relaxed, at ease *or* high strung, tight, or keyed-up? DURING THE PAST MONTH)

    5 [ ] Felt relaxed and at ease the whole month
    4 [ ] Felt relaxed and at ease most of the time
    3 [ ] Generally felt relaxed but at times felt fairly high strung
    2 [ ] Generally felt high strung but at times felt fairly relaxed
    1 [ ] Felt high strung, tight, or keyed-up most of the time
    0 [ ] Felt high strung, tight, or keyed up the whole month

20. I felt cheerful, lighthearted DURING THE PAST MONTH.

    0 [ ] None of the time
    1 [ ] A little of the time
    2 [ ] Some of the time
    3 [ ] A good bit of the time
    4 [ ] Most of the time
    5 [ ] All of the time

21. I felt tired, worn out, used up, or exhausted DURING THE PAST MONTH.

    5 [ ] None of the time
    4 [ ] A little of the time
    3 [ ] Some of the time
    2 [ ] A good bit of the time
    1 [ ] Most of the time
    0 [ ] All of the time

22. Have you been under or felt you were under any strain, stress, or pressure? (DURING THE PAST MONTH)

    0 [ ] Yes—almost more than I could bear or stand
    1 [ ] Yes—quite a bit of pressure
    2 [ ] Yes, some—more than usual
    3 [ ] Yes, some—but about usual
    4 [ ] Yes—a little
    5 [ ] Not at all

C. QUALITY OF LIFE SCALE

OVERVIEW

The Quality of Life Scale by DW Heinrichs and WT Carpenter was developed at the Maryland Psychiatric Research Center in Baltimore. It is a 21-item scale which is not a pure quality of life scale, but is a scale which also evaluates negative/deficit symptoms of schizophrenia utilizing a semistructured interview. The scale has been widely used in the evaluation of different treatments in patients with schizophrenia, and despite the fact that it was originally designed for outpatient utilization, it has been used in a variety of studies with hospitalized patients. The items are organized in four categories that cover physical functioning, occupational role, interpersonal relationships, and psychological functioning. These four categories are:

- Intrapsychic foundations
- Interpersonal relations
- Instrumental role
- Common objects and activities

Each item is rated on a 7-point scale which requires a clinical judgment from the interviewer.

GENERAL APPLICATIONS

The Quality of Life Scale assesses quality of life in individuals with schizophrenia.

SELECTED PSYCHOMETRIC PROPERTIES

The authors have reported very good interrater reliability with excellent intraclass correlations. Although data on validity is limited, there appears to be a good correlation with the Quality of Life Interview developed by Lehman (see QOLI *on page 256*).

REFERENCES

Heinrichs DW, Hanlon TE, and Carpenter WT Jr, "The Quality of Life Scale: An Instrument for Rating the Schizophrenic Deficit Syndrome," *Schizophrenia Bull*, 1984, 10(3):338-98.

COPYRIGHT

William T Carpenter, PhD
Maryland Psychiatric Research Center
PO Box 21247
Catonsville, MD 21228

SCALE GENERALLY DONE BY

Trained clinical personnel

TIME TO COMPLETE SCALE

30-45 minutes

REPRESENTATIVE STUDY UTILIZING SCALE

Bow-Thomas CC, Velligan DI, Miller AL, et al, "Predicting Quality of Life From Symptomatology in Schizophrenia at Exacerbation and Stabilization," *Psychiatry Res*, 1999, 86(2):131-42.

C. QUALITY OF LIFE SCALE *(Continued)*

QUALITY OF LIFE SCALES

Delighted - Terrible Scales

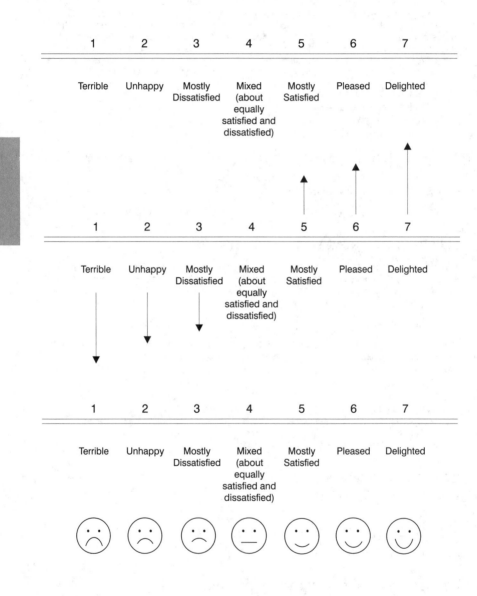

Adapted from the "Delighted - Terrible Scale," Maryland Psychiatric Research Center, Baltimore, Maryland.

D. THE NOTTINGHAM HEALTH PROFILE (NHP)

OVERVIEW

The Nottingham Health Profile (NHP), developed by S McKenna et al, is a generic quality of life questionnaire designed to give a brief indication of perceived physical, social, and emotional health problems. The NHP is a fairly well utilized instrument, especially in Europe, because of its simplicity and its broad coverage. Limitations of the NHP is that it does not include items indicating positive well-being and that in many instances the responders do not record problems in the NHP. This 38-item scale was developed through surveys of 768 patients with acute and chronic illnesses. Section I contains the following items, organized in 6 sections:

- Energy
- Pain
- Emotional reactions
- Sleep
- Social isolation
- Physical mobility

Section II is optional and contains 7 items that record the effects of health problems on occupation, tasks around the home, social, home, and sex life, plus hobbies and holidays. The NHP has been found to be sensitive to differences in perceived distress with a number of disease states in various different studies and research protocols. The instrument has also been utilized in different cultural settings with favorable results.

GENERAL APPLICATIONS

The NHP is used to assess general quality of life.

SELECTED PSYCHOMETRIC PROPERTIES

The test-retest reliability for the scale has ranged from 0.75 to 0.88 and the content validity is very high. The NHP has been shown to discriminate between different types of patients and has shown correlation with other questionnaires, in particular the McGill Pain Questionnaire and the General Health Questionnaire.

REFERENCES

Alonso J, Anto JM, and Moreno C, "Spanish Version of the Nottingham Health Profile: Translation and Preliminary Validity," *Am J Public Health*, 1990, 80(6):704-8.

Ebrahim S, Barer D, and Nouri F, "Use of the Nottingham Health Profile With Patients After a Stroke," *J Epidemiol Community Health*, 1986, 40(2):166-9.

Hunt SM, McEwen J, and McKenna SP, "Measuring Health Status: A New Tool for Clinicians and Epidemiologists," *J R Coll Gen Pract*, 1985, 35(273):185-8.

COPYRIGHT

D. THE NOTTINGHAM HEALTH PROFILE (NHP) *(Continued)*

SCALE GENERALLY DONE BY

Self-rated

TIME TO COMPLETE SCALE

10-15 minutes

REPRESENTATIVE STUDY UTILIZING SCALE

Herlitz J, Wiklund I, Sjoland H, et al, "Impact of Age on Improvement in Health-Related Quality of Life 5 Years After Coronary Artery Bypass Grafting," *Scand J Rehav Med*, 2000, 32(1):41-8.

E. THE QUALITY OF WELL BEING SCALE (QWB)

OVERVIEW

This scale has been renamed twice in order to focus on the quality of life issues. Originally called the Health Status Index when developed by JW Bush and colleagues in 1970, the scale was renamed the Index of Well-Being in 1976, and later, the Quality of Well Being Scale in 1982 by Kaplan and collaborators.

This is a scale that has adapted to the changes in the evaluation of healthcare and is, at the moment, one of the most utilized instruments to calculate the quality-adjusted life years which "integrate mortality and morbidity to express health status in terms of equivalents of well-years of life" according to Kaplan, one of the developers of the instrument. Kaplan has described the QWB scale on a three-component model of health. The assessment of health begins with an objective appraisal of current functional status, based on performance. Second, a value reflecting the utility (relative desirability) is associated to each functional level which is anchored at zero, representing death. The third is the prognostic component.

The QWB exists in two forms: An interviewer-administered version and a self-administered version.

> For the rater-administered version, a structured interview is used to record the symptoms and medical problems experienced on each of the previous eight days at the same time that a classification of the respondent's level of function is ascertained. The questions cover three dimensions of functioning: Mobility and confinement, physical activity, and social activity. The interview also records the presence of 27 problem complexes (CPX).
>
> The self-administered form is currently the most widely used. It contains 58 symptoms and problems.

All the items have weights which reflect judgments that members of society associate with each function level. The overall QWB score ranges from 1 (complete well-being) to 0 (death) and the scoring of each one of the items is a somewhat complicated procedure explained in the manual obtained from the developers.

GENERAL APPLICATIONS

The QWB measures quality of life adjusted for health status.

SELECTED PSYCHOMETRIC PROPERTIES

The reliability coefficient for functional level is 0.90. Kaplan and Bush have reported that in applying the scale to 50,000 person-days, the classification accuracy exceeded 96%. In terms of validity, this has been a widely-used instrument which has correlated well with other instruments and has shown to be useful in the evaluation of change produced by treatment. It is also considered the most important scale in the calculation of Quality adjusted life-years (QALYs) at the present time. The self-administerd QWB has been reported to work well with older adults, as well as younger populations.

REFERENCES

Fanshel S and Bush JW, "A Health-Status Index and Its Application to Health-Services Outcomes," *Operations Res*, 1970, 18:1021-65.

Kaplan RI and Atkins CJ, "The Well-Year of Life as a Basis for Patient Decision-Making," *Patient Educ Couns*, 1989, 13(3):281-95.

Kaplan RM and Bush JW, "Health Related Quality of Life Measurement for Evaluation, Research and Policy Analysis," *Health Psychol*, 1982, 1:61-80.

Kaplan RM, Anderson JP, Wu AW, et al, "The Quality of Well-Being Scale: Applications in AIDS, Cystic Fibrosis, and Arthritis," *Med Care*, 1989, 27(Suppl 3):27S-43S.

Andresen EM, Rothenberg BM, and Kaplan RM, "Performance of a Self-Administered Mailed Version of the Quality of Well Being (QWB-SA) Questionnaire Among Older Adults," *Medical Care*, 1998, 36(9):1349-60.

E. THE QUALITY OF WELL BEING SCALE (QWB) *(Continued)*

COPYRIGHT

Robert M Kaplan, PhD
Professor and Chair
Department of Family and Preventative Medicine
Mail Code 0628
School of Medicine
University of California, San Diego
La Jolla, California 92093-0628

SCALE GENERALLY DONE BY

Trained interviewer or self-rated, depending on version

TIME TO COMPLETE SCALE

Interviewer administered: 15-30 minutes
Self-administered: 7-10 minutes

REPRESENTATIVE STUDY UTILIZING SCALE

Chang JA, Curtis JR, Patrick DL, et al, "Assessment of Health-Related Quality of Life in Patients With Interstitial Lung Disease," *Chest*, 1999, 116(5):1175-82.

SAMPLE ENTRIES OF THE
QUALITY OF WELL-BEING SCALE

Self-Administered QWB-SA, V1.04

Part V - Usual Activity

8. *Over the last 3 days ... (Please fill in all days that apply)*

a. because of any physical or emotional health reasons, on which days did you avoid, need help with, or were limited in doing some of your usual activities, such as work, school or housekeeping?

○ No Days ○ Yesterday ○ 2 days ago ○ 3 days ago

b. because of any physical or emotional health reasons, on which days did you avoid or feel limited in doing some of your usual activities, such as visiting family or friends, hobbies, shopping, recreational, or religious activities?

○ No Days ○ Yesterday ○ 2 days ago ○ 3 days ago

c. on which days did you have to change any of your plans or activities because of your health? (Consider only activities that you did not report in the last 2 questions.)

○ No Days ○ Yesterday ○ 2 days ago ○ 3 days ago

If limited, please describe:

F. THE SICKNESS IMPACT PROFILE (SIP)

OVERVIEW

The Sickness Impact Profile (SIP), developed by M Bergner, evaluates the changes in a person's behavior caused by the presence of an illness. This is a health-related quality of life instrument. In this scale, what is important is the evaluation of the impact of a "sickness" on the individual and its impact on daily activities, feelings, attitudes, and beliefs plus the effects of treatment in the same areas.

The SIP measures health status by assessing the way sickness changes daily activities and behavior utilizing statements such as "I sit during most of the day", "I sometimes behave as if I were confused or disoriented in place or time", or, "I have difficulty reasoning and solving problems". There are 136 statements in 12 categories. Respondents check only the items that describe them on a given day and which are related to their health. The items have different weights, which indicate the relative severity of compromise reflected by each statement. The profile can be administered by an individual or it can be self-scored.

GENERAL APPLICATIONS

The SIP measures health-related quality of life in adults.

SELECTED PSYCHOMETRIC PROPERTIES

The test-retest reliability is high (0.88 to 0.92). Internal consistency has been reported to be good and the interrater reliability is good (0.92) with a kappa of 0.87. The validity scores comparing the SIP with other subjective ratings has been reported as good, with the SIP being compared to other established health indices. A limitation is that the SIP may not be sensitive to small changes on a daily basis. Despite some limitations, the SIP has been used extensively and is considered well established and appropriate when the research is looking for a comprehensive health-related quality of life assessment.

REFERENCES

Bergner M, Bobbitt RA, Kressel S, et al, "The Sickness Impact Profile: Conceptual Formulation and Methodology for the Development of a Health Status Measure," *Int J Health Serv*, 1976, 6(3):393-415.

Bergner M, Bobbitt RA, Pollard WE, et al, The Sickness Impact Profile: Validation of a Health Status Measure," *Med Care*, 1976, 14(1):57-67.

Brooks WB, Jordan JS, Divine GW, et al, "The Impact of Psychologic Factors on Measurement of Functional Status: Assessment of the Sickness Impact Profile," *Med Care*, 1990, 28(9):793-804.

Read JL, Quinn RJ, and Hoefer MA, "Measuring Overall Health: An Evaluation of Three Important Approaches," *J Chronic Dis*, 1987, 40(Suppl 1):7S-21S.

COPYRIGHT

Johns Hopkins University
Medical Outcomes Trust PMB 503
198 Tremont St
Boston, MA 021160-4705
Tel: 617-426-4040
Fax: 617-587-4232

SCALE GENERALLY DONE BY

The scale can be applied by an individual or can be self-scored.

TIME TO COMPLETE SCALE

20 minutes

REPRESENTATIVE STUDY UTILIZING SCALE

Raaymakers TW, "Functional Outcome and Quality of Life After Angiography and Operation for Unruptured Intracranial Aneurysms," *J Neurol Neurosurg Psychiatry*, 2000, 68(5):571-6.

SUBSTANCE ABUSE

RATING SCALES

TABLE OF CONTENTS

A. ADDICTION SEVERITY INDEX (ASI)

OVERVIEW

The ASI, developed by AT McLellan et al, is a very widely used scale to provide information about the areas of an individual's life that may contribute to his or her substance abuse disorder. The ASI evaluates seven functional life areas including medical status, employment and support, drug use, alcohol use, legal status, family/social status, and psychiatric status. Each area is examined separately to identify problem symptoms. The ASI provides a 10-point interviewer-determined severity rating of lifetime problems and a multiple item total score for problem severity over the last 30 days. There are 142 items which include general demographics plus a common format for each of the seven problem areas.

GENERAL APPLICATIONS

The ASI is used to assess the severity and nature of life problems/symptoms experienced as a result of substance abuse.

SELECTED PSYCHOMETRIC PROPERTIES

Validity of the ASI has been demonstrated in multiple treatment settings. The ASI problem severity scores have been reported to correlate with various independent variables (eg, total number of substance use convictions), with correlations ranging from 0.43 to 0.72.

REFERENCES

McLellan AT, Luborsky L, Woody GE, et al, "An Improved Diagnostic Instrument for Substance Abuse Patients. The Addiction Severity Index," *J Nerv Ment Dis*, 1980, 168(1):26-33.

McLellan AT, Luborsky L, Cacciola J, et al, "New Data From the Addiction Severity Index. Reliability and Validity in Three Centers," *J Nerv Ment Dis*, 1985, 173(7):412-23.

COPYRIGHT

The ASI is in the public domain and there is no charge for use. Training and support information may be obtained from:

ASI Information Service
c/o Treatment Research Institute
2005 Market Street, Suite 1020
Philadelphia, PA 19103-7220
Tel: 1-800-238-2433

SCALE GENERALLY DONE BY

Clinician or trained rater

TIME TO COMPLETE SCALE

Approximately 60 minutes. Follow-up interviews: 15-20 minutes

REPRESENTATIVE STUDY UTILIZING SCALE

Petry NM and Bickel WK, "Gender Differences in Hostility of Opioid-Dependent Outpatients: Role in Early Treatment Termination," *Drug Alcohol Depend*, 2000, 1; 58(1-2):27-33.

ADDICTION SEVERITY INDEX 5th Edition

Remember: This is an interview, not a test.

Item numbers circled are to be asked at follow-up.

Items with an asterisk are cumulative and should be rephrased at follow-up.

INTRODUCING THE ASI:

Introduce and explain the seven potential problem areas: Medical, Employment/Support Status, Alcohol, Drug, Legal, Family/Social, and Psychiatric. All clients receive this same standard interview. All information gathered is confidential; explain what that means in your facility; who has access to the information and the process for the release of information.

There are two time periods we will discuss:

1. The past 30 days
2. Lifetime

Patient Rating Scale: Patient input is important. For each area, I will ask you to use this scale to let me know how bothered you have been by any problems in each section. I will also ask you how important treatment is for you for the area being discussed.

The scale is:

0 = Not at all
1 = Slightly
2 = Moderately
3 = Considerably
4 = Extremely

Inform the client that he/she has the right to refuse to answer any question. If the client is uncomfortable or feels it is too personal or painful to give an answer, instruct the client not to answer. Explain the benefits and advantages of answering as many questions as possible in terms of developing a comprehensive and effective treatment plan to help them.

Please try not to give inaccurate information!

INTERVIEWER INSTRUCTIONS:

1. Leave no blanks.
2. Make plenty of comments (if another person reads this ASI, they should have a relatively complete picture of the client's perceptions of his/her problems).
3. X = Question not answered
   N = Question not applicable
4. Terminate interview if client misrepresents two or more sections.
5. When noting comments, please write the question number.
6. Tutorial/clarification notes are preceded with "•".

HALF TIME RULE:

If a question asks the number of months, round up periods of 14 days or more to 1 month. Round up 6 months or more to 1 year.

CONFIDENCE RATINGS:

Last two items in each section.

Do not overinterpret.

Denial does not necessarily warrant misrepresentation.

Misrepresentation = overt contradiction in information.

Probe, cross-check, and make plenty of comments!

A. ADDICTION SEVERITY INDEX (ASI) *(Continued)*

HOLLINGSHEAD CATEGORIES:

1. Higher execs, major professionals, owners of large businesses.
2. Business managers if medium-sized businesses, lesser professions (ie, nurses, opticians, pharmacists, social workers, teachers).
3. Administrative personnel, managers, minor professionals, owners/proprietors of small businesses (ie, bakery, car dealership, engraving business, plumbing business, florist, decorator, actor, reporter, travel agent).
4. Clerical and sales, technicians, small businesses (bank teller, bookkeeper, clerk, drafts-person, timekeeper, secretary).
5. Skilled manual - usually having had training (baker, barber, brakeperson, chef, electrician, fireman, machinist, mechanic, paperhanger, painter, repair person, tailor, welder, police, plumber).
6. Semi-skilled (hospital aide, painter, bartender, bus driver, cutter, cook, drill press, garage guard, checker, waiter, spot welder, machine operator).
7. Unskilled (attendant, janitor, construction helper, unspecified labor, porter, *including unemployed*).
8. Homemaker
9. Student, disabled, no occupation

LIST OF COMMONLY USED DRUGS:

Alcohol:	Beer, wine, liquor
Methadone:	Dolophine, LAAM
Opiates:	Pain killers = morphine, Dilaudid, Demerol, Percocet, Darvon, Talwin, codeine, Tylenol 2,3,4, Robitussin, fentanyl
Barbiturates:	Nembutal, Seconal, Tuinal, Amytal, pentobarbital, secobarbital, phenobarbital, Fiorinal
Sed/Hyp/Tranq:	Benzodiazepines = Valium, Librium, Ativan, Serax, Tranxene, Xanax, Miltown Other = Chloral hydrate (Nortex), quaaludes, Dalmane, Halcion
Cocaine:	Cocaine crystal, free-base cocaine or "crack", and "Rock Cocaine"
Amphetamines:	Monster, Crank, Benzedrine, Dexedrine, Ritalin, Preludin, methamphetamine, Speed, Ice, Crystal
Cannabis:	Marijuana, hashish
Hallucinogens:	LSD (Acid), mescaline, mushrooms (psilocybin), peyote, green, PCP (phencyclidine), Angel Dust, Ecstasy
Inhalants:	Nitrous oxide, amyl nitrate (Whippits, Poppers), glue, solvents, gasoline, toluene, etc
Just note if these are used:	Antidepressants; ulcer meds = Zantac, Tagamet; asthma meds = Ventolin inhaler, Theodur; other meds = antipsychotics, lithium

---

ALCOHOL/DRUG USE INSTRUCTIONS:

The following questions refer to two time periods: The past 30 days and lifetime. Lifetime refers to the time prior to the last 30 days.

- 30 day questions only require the number of days used.
- Lifetime use is asked to determine extended periods of use.
- Regular use = 3 or more times per week, binges, or problematic irregular use in which normal activities are compromised.
- Alcohol to intoxication does not necessarily mean "drunk", use the words "to feel or felt the effects", "got a buzz", "high", etc, instead of intoxication. As a rule, 3 or more drinks in one sitting, or 5 or more drinks in one day defines "intoxication."
- How to ask these questions:
  - "How many days in the past 30 have you used....?"
  - "How many years in your life have you regularly used....?"

GENERAL INFORMATION

G1. ID No.: ☐☐☐☐☐☐☐☐☐☐☐

G2. SS No. ☐☐☐ - ☐☐ - ☐☐☐☐

G4. Date of Admission ☐☐ / ☐☐ / ☐☐

G5. Date of Interview ☐☐ / ☐☐ / ☐☐

G6. Time Begun (Hr:Min) ☐☐ : ☐☐

G7. Time Ended (Hr:Min) ☐☐ : ☐☐

G8. Class: 1. Intake   2. Follow-up ☐

G9. Contact Code: 1. In person
                  2. Telephone (intake ASI
                     must be in person) ☐

G10. Gender: 1. Male   2. Female

G11. Interviewer Code No./Initials ☐☐☐

_____
Name

_____
Address 1

_____
Address 2
                              ( )
City   State   Zip Code   Telephone Number

G14. How long have you lived
     at this address? ☐☐ / ☐☐
                      Yrs.   Mos.

G15. Is this residence owned
     by you or your family? 0-No 1-Yes ☐

G16. Date of birth:
     (Month/Day/Year) ☐☐ / ☐☐ / ☐☐

G17. Of what race do you consider yourself?
     1. White (not Hisp)   5. Asian/Pacific
     2. Black (not Hisp)   6. Hispanic-Mexican   ☐
     3. American Indian   7. Hispanic-Puerto Rican
     4. Alaskan Native   8. Hispanic-Cuban
                           9. Other Hispanic

G18. Do you have a religious preference?
     1. Protestant   4. Islamic
     2. Catholic   5. Other   ☐
     3. Jewish   6. None

G19. Have you been in a controlled
     environment in the past 30 days?
     1. No   4. Medical Treatment   ☐
     2. Jail   5. Psychiatric Treatment
     3. Alcohol/Drug Treat 6. Other: _____
     • A place, *theoretically*, without access to drugs/alcohol

G20. How many days?
     • "NN" if Question G19 is No. Refers to total   ☐☐
       number of days detained in the past 30 days.

ADDITIONAL TEST RESULTS

_____ ☐☐☐
_____ ☐☐☐
_____ ☐☐☐
_____ ☐☐☐
_____ ☐☐☐
_____ ☐☐☐
_____ ☐☐☐
_____ ☐☐☐
_____ ☐☐☐
_____ ☐☐☐

PROBLEMS	SEVERITY PROFILE									
	0	1	2	3	4	5	6	7	8	9
MEDICAL										
EMP/SUP										
ALCOHOL										
DRUGS										
LEGAL										
FAM/SOC										
PSYCH										

GENERAL INFORMATION COMMENTS
(Include the question number with your notes)

_____
_____
_____
_____
_____
_____
_____
_____
_____
_____
_____
_____
_____
_____
_____

A. ADDICTION SEVERITY INDEX (ASI) *(Continued)*

MEDICAL STATUS

M1.* How many times in your life have you been hospitalized for medical problems?

- Include ODs and DTs. Exclude detox, alcohol/drug, psychiatric treatment, and childbirth (if no complications). Enter the number of **overnight** hospitalizations for medical problems.

M2. How long ago was your last hospitalization for a physical problem?

- If no hospitalizations in Question M1, then this is coded "NN".

Yrs.   Mos.

M3. Do you have any chronic medical problems which continue to interfere with your life?

0-No 1-Yes

- If "Yes", specify in comments.
- A chronic medical condition is a serious physical condition that requires regular care (ie, medication dietary restriction) preventing full advantage of their abilities.

M4. Are you taking any prescribed medications on a regular basis for a physical problem?

0-No 1-Yes

- If "Yes", specify in comments.
- Medication prescribed by a MD for medical conditions; **not psychiatric medicines**. Include medicines prescribed whether or not the patient is currently taking them. The intent is to verify chronic medical problems.

M5. Do you receive a pension for a physical disability?

- If "Yes", specify in comments.
- Include Worker's compensation, exclude psychiatric disability.

0-No 1-Yes

M6. How many days have you experienced medical problems in the past 30 days?

- Include flu, colds, etc. Include serious ailments related to drugs/alcohol, which would continue even if the patient were abstinent (eg, cirrhosis of liver, abscesses from needles, etc).

For Questions M7 and M8, ask the patient to use the Patient Rating scale.

M7. How troubled or bothered have you been by these medical problems in the past 30 days?

- Restrict response to problem days of Question M6.

M8. How important to you now is treatment for these medical problems?

- If client is currently receiving medical treatment, refer to the need for **additional** medical treatment by the patient.

INTERVIEWER SEVERITY RATING

M9. How would you rate the patient's need for medical treatment?

- Refers to the patient's need for **additional** medical treatment.

CONFIDENCE RATINGS

Is the above information significantly distorted by?

M10. Patient's misrepresentation?

0-No 1-Yes

M11. Patient's ability to understand?

0-No 1-Yes

MEDICAL COMMENTS

_____

_____

_____

EMPLOYMENT/SUPPORT STATUS

E1.* Education completed:
- GED = 12 years, note in comments
- Include formal education only.

Yrs.   Mos.

E2.* Training or technical education completed:
- Formal/organized training only. For military training, only include training that can be used in civilian life (eg, electronics, computers)

Mos.

E3. Do you have a profession, trade, or skill?
- Employable, transferable skill acquired through training.
- If "Yes" (specify) _____

0-No   1-Yes

E4. Do you have a valid driver's license?
- Valid license; not suspended/revoked.

0-No   1-Yes

E5. Do you have an automobile available for use?
- If answer to E4 is "No", then E5 must be "No".
Does not require ownership, only requires availability on a regular basis.

0-No   1-Yes

E6. How long was your longest full-time job?
- Full time = 35+ hours weekly; does not necessarily mean most recent job.

Yrs.   Mos.

E7.* Usual (or last) occupation? (Specify) _____
(Use Hollingshead Categories Reference Sheet)

E8. Does someone contribute to your support in any way?
- Is patient receiving any regular support (ie, cash, food, housing) from family/friend. Include spouse's contribution; exclude support by an institution.

0-No   1-Yes

E9. Does this constitute the majority of your support
- If E8 is "No", then E9 is "No"

0-No   1-Yes

E10. Usual employment pattern, past three years?

1. Full time (35+ hours)	5. Service
2. Part time (regular hours)	6. Retired/Disability
3. Part time (irregular hours)	7. Unemployed
4. Student	8. In controlled environment

- Answer should represent the majority of the last 3 years, not just the most recent selection. If there are equal times for more than one category, select that which best represents the current situation.

E11. How many days were you paid for working in the past 30?
- Include "under the table" work, paid sick days, and vacation.

EMPLOYMENT/SUPPORT COMMENTS

_____

_____

_____

A. ADDICTION SEVERITY INDEX (ASI) *(Continued)*
EMPLOYMENT/SUPPORT *(continued)*

For questions E12-17: How much money did you receive from the following sources in the past 30 days?

E12. Employment?
- Net or "take home" pay; include any "under the table" money

E13. Unemployment Compensation?

E14. Welfare?
- Include food stamps, transportation money provided by an agency to go to and from treatment.

E15. Pensions, benefits, or Social Security?
- Include disability, pensions, retirement, veteran's benefits, SSI, and workers' compensation.

E16. Mate, family, or friends?
- Money for personal expenses (ie, clothing), include unreliable sources of income. Record *cash* payments only, include windfalls (unexpected), money from loans, legal gambling, inheritance, tax returns, etc).

E17. Illegal?
- *Cash* obtained from drug dealing, stealing, fencing stolen goods, illegal gambling, prostitution, etc. *Do not* attempt to convert drugs exchanged to a dollar value.

E18. How many people depend on you for the majority of their food, shelter, etc?
- Must be regularly depending on patient, do include alimony/child support, do not include the patient or self-supporting spouse, etc

E19. How many days have you experienced employment problems in the past 30?
- Include inability to find work, if they are actively looking for work, or problems with present job in which that job is jeopardized.

For Questions E20 and E21, ask the patient to use the Patient Rating scale.

E20. How troubled or bothered have you been by these employment problems in the past 30 days?
- If the patient has been incarcerated or detained during the past 30 days, they cannot have employment problems. In that case, an "N" response is indicated.

E21. How important to you now is counseling for these employment problems?
- Stress help in finding or preparing for a job, not giving them a job.

INTERVIEWER SEVERITY RATING

E22. How would you rate the patient's need for employment counseling?

CONFIDENCE RATINGS
Is the above information significantly distorted by:

E23. Patient's misrepresentation?   0-No 1-Yes

E23. Patient's inability to understand?   0-No 1-Yes

EMPLOYMENT SUPPORT COMMENTS

ALCOHOL / DRUGS

Route of Administration Types:

| 1. Oral | 2. Nasal | 3. Smoking | 4. Non-I.V. injection | 5. I.V. |

• Note: The usual or most recent route. For more than one route, choose the most severe.
The routes are listed from least severe to most severe.

	Past 30 days	Lifetime (yrs)	Route of Admin
D1. Alcohol (any use at all, 30 days)			■
D2. Alcohol - to intoxication			■
D3. Heroin			
D4. Methadone			
D5. Other Opiates / Analgesics			
D6. Barbiturates			
D7. Sedatives / Hypnotics / Tranquilizers			
D8. Cocaine			
D9. Amphetamines			
D10. Cannabis			
D11. Hallucinogens			
D12. Inhalants			
D13. More than 1 substance per day (including alcohol)			■

D14. According to the interviewer, which substance(s) is/are the major problem?
• Interviewer should determine the major drug or drugs of abuse. Code the number next to the drug in questions 01-12, or "00" = no problem, "15" = alcohol & one or more drugs, "16" = more than one drug but no alcohol. Ask patient when not clear.

D15. How long was your last period of voluntary abstinence from this major substance? **Mos.**
• Last attempt of at least one month, not necessarily the longest. Periods of hospitalization/ incarceration **do not count.** Periods of antabuse, methadone, or naltrexone use during abstinence **do count.**
• "00" = still abstinent.

D16. How many months ago did this abstinence end? **Mos.**
• If D15 = "00", then D16 = "NN"
• "00" = still abstinent.

D17.* How many times have you had Alcohol DTs?
• **Delirium Tremens** (DTs): Occur 24-48 hours after last drink, or significant decrease in alcohol intake, shaking, severe disorientation, fever, hallucinations; they usually require medical attention.

D18.* Overdosed on Drugs?
• **Overdoses** (OD): Requires intervention by someone to recover, not simply sleeping it off, include suicide attempts by OD.

ALCOHOL/DRUGS COMMENTS

A. ADDICTION SEVERITY INDEX (ASI) *(Continued)*

ALCOHOL / DRUGS *(continued)*

D19.* How many times in your life have you been treated for:
*Alcohol abuse?
- Include detoxification, halfway houses, in/outpatient counseling, and AA (if 3+ meetings within one month period).

D21.* How many of these were detox only:
*Alcohol?

D23. How much would you say you spent during the past 30 days on:
Alcohol?

D20.* How many times in your life have you been treated for:
*Drug abuse?
- Include detoxification, halfway houses, in/outpatient counseling, and NA (if 3+ meetings within one month period).

D22.* How many of these were detox only:
*Drugs?
- If D19 = "00", then question D21 is "NN"
  If D20 = "00", then question D22 is "NN"

D24. How much would you say you spent during the past 30 days on:
Drugs?
- Only count actual *money* spent. What is the financial burden caused by drugs/alcohol?

D25. How many days have you been treated in an outpatient setting for alcohol or drugs in the past 30 days?
- Include AA/NA

D26. How many days in the past 30 have you experienced:
Alcohol problems?
- Include: Craving, withdrawal symptoms, disturbing effects of use, or wanting to stop and being unable to.

For Questions D28 + D30, ask the patient to use the Patient Rating scale. The patient is rating the need for additional substance abuse treatment.

D28. How troubled or bothered have you been in the past 30 days by these:
Alcohol problems?
- Include: Craving, withdrawal symptoms, disturbing effects of use, or wanting to stop and being unable to.

D30. How important to you now is treatment for these:
Alcohol problems?

D27. How many days in the past 30 have you experienced:
Drug problems?
- Include: Craving, withdrawal symptoms, disturbing effects of use, or wanting to stop and being unable to.

For Questions D29 + D31, ask the patient to use the Patient Rating scale. The patient is rating the need for additional substance abuse treatment.

D29. How troubled or bothered have you been in the past 30 days by these:
Drug problems?

D31. How important to you now is treatment for these:
Drug problems?

ALCOHOL / DRUGS *(continued)*

INTERVIEWER RATING

How would you rate the patient's need for treatment for:

D32. Alcohol problems? □

D33. Drug problems? □

CONFIDENCE RATINGS

Is the above information significantly distorted by:

(D34.) Patient's misrepresentation? 0-No 1-Yes □

(D35.) Patient's inability to understand? 0-No 1-Yes □

ALCOHOL/DRUGS COMMENTS

_____

_____

_____

_____

_____

_____

_____

_____

_____

_____

_____

_____

_____

A. ADDICTION SEVERITY INDEX (ASI) *(Continued)*

LEGAL STATUS

L1. Was this admission prompted or suggested by the criminal justice system?
* Judge, probation/parole officer, etc   0-No   1-Yes ☐☐

L2. Are you on parole or probation?
* Note duration and level in comments.   0-No   1-Yes ☐☐

How many times in your life have you been arrested and charged with the following:

L3.*	Shoplift/Vandal	☐☐	L10.* Assault	☐☐
L4.*	Parole/Probation Violations	☐☐	L11.* Arson	☐☐
L5.*	Drug Charges	☐☐	L12.* Rape	☐☐
L6.*	Forgery	☐☐	L13.* Homicide/Manslaughter	☐☐
L7.*	Weapons Offense	☐☐	L14.* Prostitution	☐☐
L8.*	Burglary/Larceny/B&E	☐☐	L15.* Contempt of Court	☐☐
L9.*	Robbery	☐☐	L16.* Other: _____	☐☐

* Include total number of counts, not just convictions. Do not include juvenile (pre-age 18) crimes, unless they were charged as an adult.
* Include formal charges only.

L17.* How many of these charges resulted in convictions?
* If L3-16 = "00", then question L17 = "NN."
* Do not include misdemeanor offenses from questions L18-20 below.
* Convictions include fines, probation, incarcerations, suspended sentences, guilty pleas, and plea bargaining.   ☐☐

How many times in your life have you been charged with the following:

L18.* Disorderly conduct, vagrancy, public intoxication?   ☐☐

L19.* Driving while intoxicated?   ☐☐

L20.* Major driving violations?   ☐☐
* Moving violations: Speeding, reckless driving, no license, etc.

L21.* How many months were you incarcerated in your life?
* If incarcerated 2 weeks or more, round this up to 1 month. List total number of months incarcerated.   ☐☐ Mos.

L22. How long was your last incarceration?
* Of 2 weeks or more. Enter "NN" if never incarcerated.   ☐☐ Mos.

L23. What was it for?
* Use code 03-16, 18-20. If multiple charges, choose most severe. Enter "NN" if never incarcerated.   ☐☐

L24. Are you presently awaiting charges, trial, or sentence?   0-No   1-Yes ☐

L25. What for?
* Use the number of the type of crime committed: 03-16 and 18-20
* Refers to Question L24. If more than one, choose most severe.   ☐☐

LEGAL COMMENTS

_____

_____

_____

LEGAL STATUS *(continued)*

L26. How many days in the past 30, were you detained or incarcerated?
• Include being arrested and released on the same day.

L27. How many days in the past 30, have you engaged in illegal activities for profit?
• Exclude simple drug possession. Include drug dealing, prostitution, selling stolen goods, etc. May be cross-checked with Question E17 under Employment/Family Support Section.

For Questions L28-29, ask the patient to use the Patient Rating scale.

L28. How serious do you feel your present legal problems are?
• Exclude civil problems

L29. How important to you now is counseling or referral for these legal problems?
• Patient is rating a need for referral to legal counsel for defense against criminal charges.

IINTERVIEWER SEVERITY RATING

L30. How would you rate the patient's need for legal services or counseling?

CONFIDENCE RATINGS

Is the above information significantly distorted by:

L31. Patient's misrepresentation?   0-No   1-Yes

L32. Patient's inability to understand?   0-No   1-Yes

LEGAL COMMENTS

_____

_____

_____

FAMILY HISTORY

Have any of your blood-related relatives had what you would call a significant drinking, drug use, or psychiatric problem? Specifically, was there a problem that did or should have led to treatment?

Mother's Side	Alcohol	Drug	Psych		Father's Side	Alcohol	Drug	Psych		Siblings	Alcohol	Drug	Psych
H1. Grandmother					H6. Grandmother					H11. Brother			
H2. Grandfather					H7. Grandfather								
H3. Mother					H8. Father					H12. Sister			
H4. Aunt					H9. Aunt								
H5. Uncle					H10. Uncle								

0 = Clearly No for any relatives in that category   X = Uncertain or don't know
1 = Clearly Yes for any relatives in that category   N = Never was a relative

• In cases where there is more than one person for a category, record the occurrence of problems for any in that group. Accept the patient's judgment on these questions.

FAMILY HISTORY COMMENTS

_____

_____

_____

A. ADDICTION SEVERITY INDEX (ASI) *(Continued)*

FAMILY / SOCIAL STATUS

F1. Marital Status:

1 - Married	3 - Widowed	5 - Divorced
2 - Remarried	4 - Separated	6 - Never Married

• Common-law marriage = 1. Specify in comments.

F2. How long have you been in this marital status (Q #F1)?
• If never married, then since age 18

Yrs.   Mos.

F3. Are you satisfied with this situation?
• Satisfied = generally liking the situation
• Refers to Questions F1 & F2

0-No 1-Indifferent 2-Yes

F4.* Usual living arrangements (past 3 years):

1 - With sexual partner & children	6 - With friends
2 - With sexual partner alone	7 - Alone
3 - With children alone	8 - Controlled Environment
4 - With parents	9 - No stable arrangement
5 - With family	

• Choose arrangements most representative of the past 3 years. If there is an even split in time between these arrangements, choose the most recent arrangement.

F5. How long have you lived in these arrangements?
• If with parents or family, since age 18.
• Code years and months living in arrangements from Question F4.

Yrs.   Mos.

F3. Are you satisfied with these arrangements?

0-No 1-Indifferent 2-Yes

Do you live with anyone who:

F7. Has a current alcohol problem?

0-No 1-Yes

F8. Uses nonprescribed drugs?
(or abuses prescribed drugs)

0-No 1-Yes

F9. With whom do you spend most of your free time?
• If a girlfriend/boyfriend is considered as family by patient, then they must refer to them as family throughout this section, not a friend.

1-Family 2-Friends 3-Alone

F10. Are you satisfied with spending your free time this way?
• A satisfied response must indicate that the person generally likes the situation. Referring to Question F9.

0-No 1-Indiffrerent 2-Yes

F11. How many close friends do you have?
• Stress that you mean ***close.*** Exclude family members. These are "reciprocal" relationships or mutually supportive relationships.

Would you say you have had a close reciprocal relationship with any of the following people:

F12. Mother	F15. Sexual Partner/Spouse	
F13. Father	F16. Children	
F14. Brothers/Sisters	F17. Friends	

0 = Clearly No for all in class   X = Uncertain or "I don't know"
1 = Clearly Yes for any in class   N = Never was a relative
• By reciprocal, you mean "that you would do anything you could to help them out and vice versa".

FAMILY / SOCIAL *(continued)*

Have you had significant periods in which you have experienced serious problems getting along with:

0-No 1-Yes

	Past 30 days	In Your life			Past 30 days	In Your Life
(F18.) Mother	☐	☐	(F23.) Other Significant Family		☐	☐
(F19.) Father	☐	☐	Specify _____			
(F20.) Brother/Sister	☐	☐				
(F21.) Sexual Partner/ Spouse	☐	☐	(F24.) Close Friends		☐	☐
			(F25.) Neighbors		☐	☐
(F22.) Children	☐	☐	(F26.) Co-Workers		☐	☐

- "Serious problems" mean those that endangered the relationship.
- A "problem" requires contact of some sort, either by telephone or in person. If no contact, code "N".

Has anyone ever abused you?

0-No 1-Yes

Past 30 days In Your Life

F27. Emotionally?
- Made you feel bad through harsh words.

☐ ☐

F28. Physically?
- Caused you physical harm.

☐ ☐

F29. Sexually?
- Forced sexual advances/acts.

☐ ☐

How many days in the past 30 have you had serious conflicts:

(F30.) With your family?

☐☐

For Questions F32-35, ask the patient to use the Patient Rating scale.
How troubled or bothered have you been in the past 30 days by:

(F32.) Family problems?

☐

(F34.) How important to you now is treatment or counseling for these:
Family problems
- Patient is rating his/her need for counseling for family problems, not whether they would be willing to attend.

☐

How many days in the past 30 have you had serious conflicts:

(F31.) With other people (excluding family)?

☐☐

For Questions F32-35, ask the patient to use the Patient Rating scale.
How troubled or bothered have you been in the past 30 days by:

(F33.) Social problems?

☐

(F35.) How important to you now is treatment or counseling for these:
Social problems
- Include patient's need to seek treatment for such social problems as loneliness, inability to socialize, and dissatisfaction with friends. Patient rating should refer to dissatisfaction, conflicts, or other serious problems.

☐

A. ADDICTION SEVERITY INDEX (ASI) *(Continued)*

FAMILY / SOCIAL *(continued)*

INTERVIEWER SEVERITY RATING

F36. How would you rate the patient's need for family and/or social counseling? ☐

CONFIDENCE RATING

Is the above information significantly distorted by:

(F37.) Patient's misrepresentation? 0-No 1-Yes ☐

(F38.) Patient's inability to understand? 0-No 1-Yes ☐

FAMILY / SOCIAL COMMENTS

_____

_____

_____

_____

_____

_____

_____

_____

_____

_____

_____

_____

PSYCHIATRIC STATUS

How many times have you been treated for any psychological or emotional problems:

(P1.*) In a hospital or inpatient setting?

(P2.*) Outpatient/private patient?
- Do not include substance abuse, employment, or family counseling. Treatment episode = a series or more or less continuous visits or treatment days, not the number of visits or treatment days.
- Enter diagnosis in comments, if known.

(P3.) Do you receive a pension for a psychiatric disability?　　0-No　1-Yes

---

How you had a significant period of time (that was not a direct result of alcohol/drug use) in which you have:

0-No　1-Yes

Past 30 Days　　Lifetime

(P4.) Experienced serious depression-sadness, hopelessness, loss of interest?

(P5.) Experienced serious anxiety/tension-uptight, unreasonably worried, inability to feel relaxed?

(P6.) Experienced hallucinations - saw things/heard voices that others didn't see/hear?

(P7.) Experienced trouble understanding, concentrating, or remembering?

How you had a significant period of time (despite your alcohol and drug use) in which you have:

0-No　1-Yes

Past 30 Days　　Lifetime

(P8.) Experienced trouble controlling violent behavior including episodes of rage or violence?
- Patient can be under the influence of alcohol/drugs.

(P9.) Experienced serious thoughts of suicide?
- Patient seriously considered a plan for taking his/her life. Patient can be under the influence of alcohol/drugs.

(P10.) Attempted suicide?
- Include actual suicidal gestures or attempts.
- Patient can be under the influence of alcohol/drugs.

(P11.) Been prescribed medication for any psychological or emotional problems?
- Prescribed for the patient by a physician. Record "Yes" if a medication was prescribed even if the patient is not taking it.

(P12.) How many days in the past 30 have you experienced these psychological or emotional problems?
- This refers to problems noted in Questions P4-P10.

For Questions P13-P14, ask the patient to use the Patient Rating scale.

(P13.) How much have you been troubled or bothered by these psychological or emotional problems in the past 30 days?
- Patient should be rating the problem days from Question P12.

(P13.) How important to you now is treatment for these psychological or emotion problems?

303

A. ADDICTION SEVERITY INDEX (ASI) *(Continued)*

PSYCHIATRIC STATUS *(continued)*

The following items are to be completed by the interviewer:
At the time of the interview, the patient was: 0-No 1-Yes

(P15.) Obviously depressed/withdrawn ☐

(P16.) Obviously hostile ☐

(P17.) Obviously anxious/nervous ☐

(P18.) Having trouble with reality testing, thought disorders, paranoid thinking ☐

(P19.) Having trouble comprehending, concentrating, remembering ☐

(P20.) Having suicidal thoughts ☐

INTERVIEWER SEVERITY RATING

P21. How would you rate the patient's need for psychiatric/psychological treatment? ☐

CONFIDENCE RATING

Is the above information significantly distorted by:

(P22.) Patient's misrepresentation?   0-No 1-Yes ☐

(P23.) Patient's inability to understand?   0-No 1-Yes ☐

G12. **Special Code**   ☐
   1. Patient terminated by interviewer
   2. Patient refused
   3. Patient unable to respond (language or intellectual barrier, under the influence, etc)
   N. Interview completed

PSYCHIATRIC STATUS COMMENTS

_____

_____

_____

_____

_____

_____

B. ALCOHOL USE DISORDERS IDENTIFICATION TEST (AUDIT)

OVERVIEW

The Alcohol Use Disorders Identification Test (AUDIT), developed by TF Babor and colleagues, is a screening tool to identify patterns of alcohol use that are harmful or hazardous to health. The AUDIT is not a diagnostic test for alcoholism, but rather is designed to alert clinicians to further evaluate potential for alcohol use/alcoholism-related problems. The AUDIT consists of a core assessment which may be self-rated and an optional clinical screening module which is designed to be incorporated into a medical evaluation done by a trained professional. The core assessment consists of 10 multiple choice questions that are answered using a 5-point Likert-type scale. The 10 items in the core questionnaire are scored from 0-4; total score is the sum of each individual item. The clinical screening module has 8 items, scored from 0-3; total score is the sum of each individual item. The clinical screening module includes a physical examination and laboratory testing. A score of 11 or higher on the AUDIT is usually seen in individuals with clinically-significant alcohol use. Strengths of the AUDIT include its brevity and ease of administration (no training is required). However, as the AUDIT scoring is dependent on self-report, its use may be limited in individuals with alcohol abuse who deny problem use.

GENERAL APPLICATIONS

The AUDIT is a screening tool for clinically-significant alcohol use.

SELECTED PSYCHOMETRIC PROPERTIES

The AUDIT is a well-validated and widely-used scale. Reliability is also good with Cronbach's alpha coefficient from a large undergraduate sample of 0.80.

REFERENCES

Babor TF, de la Fuente JR, Saunders J, et al, *AUDIT, The Alcohol Use Disorders Identification Test: Guidelines for Use in Primary Health Care*, Geneva: World Health Organization, 1992.

Bohn MJ, Babor TF, and Kranzler HR, "The Alcohol Use Disorders Identification Test (AUDIT): Validation of a Screening Instrument for Use in Medical Settings," *J Stud Alcohol*, 1995, 56(4):423-32.

COPYRIGHT

World Health Organization (WHO)
Program on Substance Abuse
Avenue Appia 20
1211 Geneva 27
Switzerland
Tel: (+00 41 22) 791 2111
Fax: (+00 41 22) 791 3111
e-mail: publications@who.int

The AUDIT training module is available from:
Thomas F. Babor
Alcohol Research Center
University of Connecticut Health Center
Farmington, CT 06030-0410

B. ALCOHOL USE DISORDERS IDENTIFICATION TEST (AUDIT)
(Continued)

SCALE GENERALLY DONE BY

The core questionnaire is a self-report scale; the clinical screening module is done by trained medical professionals

TIME TO COMPLETE SCALE

Less than five minutes for core questionnaire

REPRESENTATIVE STUDY UTILIZING SCALE

Isaacson JH, Nielsen C, Urbanic R, et al, "Markers for Patients With Alcohol Problems in an Outpatient General Medicine Clinic," *Subst Abus*, 1999, 20(3):141-7.

AUDIT

THE ALCOHOL USE DISORDERS IDENTIFICATION TEST

AUDIT was developed by the World Health Organization to identify persons whose alcohol consumption has become hazardous or harmful to their health. Persons at high risk include medical patients, accident victims, suicidal persons, drunk driving offenders, and armed forces personnel. Screening with AUDIT can be conducted in a variety of healthcare settings.

AUDIT is a brief structured interview that can be incorporated into a medical history. It contains questions about recent alcohol consumption, dependence symptoms, and alcohol-related problems.

The optional Clinical Screening Procedure, consists of two interview items, a brief physical examination and a laboratory test. It is designed to complement the AUDIT under conditions where additional clinical information is required.

REMEMBER:

- *Read questions as written*
- *Record answers carefully*
- *Use the ten AUDIT questions first*

*Begin the AUDIT by saying: "Now I am going to ask you some questions about your use of alcoholic beverages during the past year." Explain what is meant by "alcoholic beverages" by using local examples of beer, wine, vodka, etc. Code answers in terms of "standard drinks."

*Refer to the AUDIT guidelines for detailed instructions.

B. ALCOHOL USE DISORDERS IDENTIFICATION TEST (AUDIT)
(Continued)

CLINICAL SCREENING PROCEDURE

Record numerical score in the box at right.

TRAUMA HISTORY

Have you injured your head since your 18th birthday?

        (3) Yes   (0) No

Have you broken any bones since your 18th birthday?

        (3) Yes   (0) No

CLINICAL EXAMINATION

Code as follows:
        (0) Not present   (2) Moderate
        (1) Mild   (3) Severe

Conjunctival Infection

Abnormal Skin Vascularization

Hand Tremor

Tongue Tremor

Hepatomegaly

GGT Values
(0) Lower Normal (0-30)
(1) Upper Normal (30-50)
(3) Abnormal (50 or higher)

Record sum of individual items here.
Consult user's manual if sum is greater than 5

WARNING: AUDIT is not a diagnostic instrument.

AUDIT CORE

Place the correct answer number in the box.

1. How often do you have a drink containing alcohol?
   (0) Never   (3) 2-3 times a week
   (1) Monthly or less   (4) 4 or more times a week
   (2) 2-4 times a month

2. How many drinks containing alcohol do you have on a typical day when you are drinking?
   (0) 1 or 2   (3) 7, 8, or 9
   (1) 3 or 4   (4) 10 or more
   (2) 5 or 6

3. How often do you have six or more drinks on one occasion?
   (0) Never   (3) Weekly
   (1) < Monthly   (4) Daily or almost daily
   (2) Monthly

4. How often during the last year have you found that you were not
   able to stop drinking once you had started?
   (0) Never   (3) Weekly
   (1) < Monthly   (4) Daily or almost daily
   (2) Monthly

5. How often during the last year have you failed to do what was
   normally expected from you because of drinking?
   (0) Never   (3) Weekly
   (1) < Monthly   (4) Daily or almost daily
   (2) Monthly

6. How often during the last year have you needed a first drink in the morning
   to get yourself going after a heavy drinking session?
   (0) Never   (3) Weekly
   (1) < Monthly   (4) Daily or almost daily
   (2) Monthly

7. How often during the last year have you had a feeling of guilt or remorse after drinking?
   (0) Never   (3) Weekly
   (1) < Monthly   (4) Daily or almost daily
   (2) Monthly

8. How often during the last year have you been unable to remember what happened the
   night before because you had been drinking?
   (0) Never   (3) Weekly
   (1) < Monthly   (4) Daily or almost daily
   (2) Monthly

9. Have you or someone else been injured as a result of your drinking?
   (0) No   (4) Yes, during the last year
   (2) Yes, but not in the last year

10. Has a relative or friend or a doctor or another health worker been concerned about
    your drinking or suggested you cut down?
    (0) No   (4) Yes, during the last year
    (2) Yes, but not in the last year

Record total of specific items here.
If total is 8 or greater, consult User's Manual.

C. CAGE Questionnaire

OVERVIEW

The CAGE is, perhaps, the most widely used instrument for alcohol abuse screening. Developed by J Ewing, the CAGE consists of only four items, all self-report in format. Three of the items deal with emotional reaction to drinking, while one item focuses on morning drinking to relieve symptoms of alcohol withdrawal. If two questions or more are answered affirmatively, the scale originators found that this is a strong indicator for alcohol abuse. Strengths of the scale include its brevity and ease of administration. The CAGE is less effective at identifying individuals with alcohol abuse in outpatient populations compared to inpatient populations. The CAGE correlates more highly with a diagnosis of alcohol abuse than quantity and frequency of drinking, biological measures of alcohol abuse, or age of onset of drinking.

GENERAL APPLICATIONS

The CAGE is used as a screening tool for alcohol abuse.

SELECTED PSYCHOMETRIC PROPERTIES

The CAGE has been reported to detect 93% of excessive drinkers in survey situations. A cutoff point of "1" detects approximately 90% of individuals with alcohol abuse, with 48% false-positive diagnoses.

REFERENCES

Ewing JA, "Detecting Alcoholism: The CAGE Questionnaire," *JAMA*, 1984, 252(14):1905-7.

Ewing JA and Rouse BA, "Identifying the Hidden Alcoholic," Presented at the 29th International Congress on Alcohol and Drug Dependence, Sydney, Australia, Feb 3, 1970.

Mayfield D, McLeod G, and Hall P, "The CAGE Questionnaire: Validation of a New Alcoholism Screening Instrument," *Am J Psychiatry*, 1974, 131(10):1121-3.

COPYRIGHT

Not applicable

SCALE GENERALLY DONE BY

Self-rated scale

TIME TO COMPLETE SCALE

5 minutes or less

REPRESENTATIVE STUDY UTILIZING SCALE

Aalto M, Seppa K, Kiianmaa K, et al, "Drinking Habits and Prevalence of Drinking Among Primary Health Care Outpatients and General Population," *Addiction*, 1999, 94(9):1371-9.

THE CAGE QUESTIONNAIRE

Answer "Yes" or "No" to each of the following questions:

1. Have you ever felt you ought to **C** ut down on your drinking?

2. Have people **A** nnoyed you by criticizing your drinking?

3. Have you ever felt bad or **G** uilty about your drinking?

4. Have you ever had a drink first thing in the morning to steady your nerves or to get rid of a hangover (**E** ye opener)?

D. FAGERSTROM TEST FOR NICOTINE DEPENDENCE (FTND)

OVERVIEW

The FTND is an eight-item instrument to evaluate smoking behaviors. It is a measure of nicotine dependence. The FTND may be used as a screen for nicotine dependence and may help determine prognosis in smoking cessation treatment.

GENERAL APPLICATIONS

The FTND is used to evaluate nicotine dependence in smokers.

SELECTED PSYCHOMETRIC PROPERTIES

Test-retest reliability has been reported at 0.88. The FTND has been shown to correlate with biological measures of smoking severity, such as cotinine.

REFERENCES

Fagerstrom KO, "Measuring Degree of Physical Dependence to Tobacco Smoking With Reference to Individualization of Treatment," *Addict Behav*, 1978, 3(3-4):235-41.

Pomerleau CS, Carton SM, Lutzke ML, et al, "Reliability of the Fagerstrom Tolerance Questionnaire and the Fagerstrom Test for Nicotine Dependence," *Addict Behav*, 1994, 19(1):33-9.

Heatherton TF, Kozlowski LT, Frecker RC, et al, "The Fagerstrom Test for Nicotine Dependence: A Revision of the Fagerstrom Tolerance Questionnaire," *Br J Addict*, 1991, 86(9):1119-27.

COPYRIGHT

British Journal of Addiction
Editor: Professor Griffith Edwards, Head Office
National Addiction Centre
4 Windsor Walk
London SE5 8AF, UK
Website: www.tandf.co.uk

Publisher: World Health Organization (WHO)
Program on Substance Abuse
Avenue Appia 20
1211 Geneva 27
Switzerland
Tel: (+00 41 22) 791 2111
Fax: (+00 41 22) 791 3111
e-mail: publications@who.int

SCALE GENERALLY DONE BY

Self-rated scale

TIME TO COMPLETE SCALE

Less than 5 minutes

REPRESENTATIVE STUDY UTILIZING SCALE

Tsoh JY, Humfleet GL, Munoz RF, et al, "Development of Major Depression After Treatment for Smoking Cessation," *Am J Psychiatry*, 2000, 157(3):368-74.

FAGERSTROM TEST FOR NICOTINE DEPENDENCE

Question	Answer (Points assigned to response)*		
1. How soon after you wake up do you smoke your first cigarette?	Within 30 min (1)		After 30 min (0)
2. Do you find it hard to refrain from smoking in places where it is forbidden (eg, church, library, airplanes)?	Yes (1)		No (0)
3. Which cigarette would you hate most to give up?	The first one in the morning (1)		Any other (0)
4. How many cigarettes a day do you smoke?	15 or less (0)	16-25 (1)	26 or more (2)
5. Do you smoke more frequently during the first hours after awakening than the rest of the day?	Yes (1)		No (0)
6. Do you smoke if you are so ill that you are in bed most of the day?	Yes (1)		No (0)
7. What is the tar content of your brand?	Low (0)	Medium (1)	High (2)
8. Do you inhale?	Never (0)	Sometimes (1)	Always (2)

*Total point score of 1 to 6 indicates low to moderate nicotine dependence; score of 7 to 11 indicates high dependence.

Adapted with permission from Heatherton TF, Kozlowski LT, Frecker RC, Fagerstrom KO, "The Fagerstrom Test for Nicotine Dependence: A Revision of the Fagerstrom Tolerance Questionnaire," *Br J Addict,* 1991, 86(9):1119-27.

E. INVENTORY OF DRUG-TAKING SITUATIONS (IDTS)

OVERVIEW

The IDTS is a self-report scale developed by H Annis et al, that is designed to identify situations in which individuals drank or used drugs heavily over the past year. This information may be used to better understand relapse episodes in individuals with substance abuse. There is a version of the IDTS which focuses on drugs, and a version which focuses on alcohol. Both versions have 50 items. Each item describes a life situation (eg, "When I felt tense or uneasy in the presence of someone"), and also asks the individual to rate how frequently they used drugs/alcohol in that situation. Rating scores range from 1 = never, to 4 = almost always. A problem index score is provided which gives a general assessment of substance abuse severity, as well as several subscale scores.

GENERAL APPLICATIONS

The IDTS is used to assess situations which trigger heavy drinking/drug taking.

SELECTED PSYCHOMETRIC PROPERTIES

The scale appears to have good reliability and consistency.

REFERENCES

Annis HM, Turner NE, and Sklar SM, *Inventory of Drug-Taking Situations User's Guide*, 1997, Toronto, Canada: Addiction Research Foundation.

COPYRIGHT

HM Annis
NE Turner
SM Sklar
Addiction Research Foundation
Marketing Services
33 Russell Street
Toronto, Ontario M5S 2S1
Canada

SCALE GENERALLY DONE BY

Self-rated

TIME TO COMPLETE SCALE

15-20 minutes

REPRESENTATIVE STUDY UTILIZING SCALE

Cannon DS, Rubin A, Keefe CK, et al, "Affective Correlates of Alcohol and Cocaine Use," *Addict Behav*, 1992, 17(6):517-24.

INVENTORY OF DRUG-TAKING SITUATIONS (IDTS)

Alcohol

To be completed by the client: *(Check one)*

Is this your MAIN substance of abuse? ☐
or
your SECOND substance of abuse? ☐
or
your THIRD substance of abuse? ☐

Authors: HM Annis and G Martin, Addiction Research Foundation, © 1985

Listed below are a number of situations or events in which some people drink heav~

Read each item carefully, and answer in terms of your own drinking **over the pas~ ~ar.**

If you "NEVER" drank heavily in that situation, circle "1"
If you "RARELY" drank heavily in that situation, circle "2"
If you "FREQUENTLY" drank heavily in that situation, circle ~
If you "ALMOST ALWAYS" drank heavily in that situation ~cle ~

I DRANK HEAVILY

	~ver	Rarely	Frequently	Almost Always
1. When I was depressed about things in ge~ ~l	1	2	3	4
2. When I felt shaky, sick or nauseous		2	3	4
3. When I was happy	1	2	3	4
4. When I felt there was nowhere left to ~ ~rr	1	2	3	4
5. When I wanted to se~ whether I could ~ ~nk in moderation	1	2	3	4
6. When I was in a place where I had ~ ~ed or bought alcohol before	1	2	3	4
7. When I felt tense or uneasy in the presence of someone	1	2	3	4
8. When I was invited to someone's home and felt awkward about refusing when they offered me a drink	1	2	3	4
9. When I met some old friends and we wanted to have a good time	1	2	3	4
10. When I was unable to express my feelings to someone	1	2	3	4
11. When I felt that I had let myself down	1	2	3	4
12. When I had trouble sleeping	1	2	3	4
13. When I felt confident and relaxed	1	2	3	4

E. INVENTORY OF DRUG-TAKING SITUATIONS (IDTS) *(Continued)*

IDTS (Alcohol) continued . . .   **I DRANK HEAVILY**

	Never	Rarely	Frequently	Almost Always
14. When I was bored	1	2	3	4
15. When I wanted to prove to myself that alcohol was not a problem for me	1	2	3	4
16. When I unexpectedly found some booze or happened to see something that reminded me of drinking	1	2	3	4
17. When other people rejected me or didn't seem to like me	1	2	3	4
18. When I was out with friends and they kept suggesting we go somewhere and drink	1	2	3	4
19. When I was with an intimate friend and we wanted to feel even closer	1	2	3	4
20. When other people treated me unfairly or interfered with my plans	1	2	3	4
21. When I was lonely		2	3	4
22. When I wanted to stay awake, be more alert, or be more energetic	1	2	3	4
23. When I felt excited about something	1	2	3	4
24. When I felt anxious or tense about something	1	2	3	4
25. When I wanted to find out whether I could take a drink occasionally without getting hooked	1	2	3	4
26. When I had been using drugs and thought about drinking	1	2	3	4
27. When I felt that my family was putting a lot of pressure on me or that I couldn't measure up to their expectations	1	2	3	4
28. When others in the same room were drinking and I felt that they expected me to join in	1	2	3	4
29. When I was with friends and wanted to increase my enjoyment	1	2	3	4
30. When I was not getting along well with others at school or at work	1	2	3	4
31. When I started to feel guilty about something	1	2	3	4
32. When I wanted to lose weight	1	2	3	4
33. When I was feeling content with my life	1	2	3	4
34. When I felt overwhelmed and wanted to escape	1	2	3	4

IDTS (Alcohol) continued . . .

I DRANK HEAVILY

	Never	Rarely	Frequently	Almost Always
35. When I wanted to test out whether I could be with friends who drank without drinking	1	2	3	4
36. When I heard someone talking about their past drinking experiences	1	2	3	4
37. When there were fights at home	1	2	3	4
38. When I was pressured to drink and felt I couldn't refuse	1	2		4
39. When I wanted to celebrate with a friend	1	2	3	4
40. When someone was dissatisfied with my work or I felt pressured at school or on the job	1	2		4
41. When I was angry at the way things had turned out	1	2	3	4
42. When I had a headache or was in physical pain		2	3	4
43. When I remembered something good that had happened	1	2	3	4
44. When I felt confused about what I should	1	2	3	4
45. When I wanted to test whether ... be in place where people were drinking with ... ha... a drink	1	2	3	4
46. When I began to th... how good ha... g a few drinks or becomin... intoxica... d fe...	1	2	3	4
47. When I felt that I needed courage ... face up to someone	1	2	3	4
48. When I was with a group of people and everyone was drinking	1	2	3	4
49. When I was having a good time and wanted to increase my sexual enjoyment	1	2	3	4
50. When I felt that someone was trying to control me and I wanted to feel more independent	1	2	3	4

E. INVENTORY OF DRUG-TAKING SITUATIONS (IDTS) *(Continued)*

INVENTORY OF DRUG-TAKING SITUATIONS (IDTS)

Drugs

To be completed by the client:

    1. Type of drug: _____
(Check one)

    Is this your MAIN substance of abuse?   ☐
or
    your SECOND substance of abuse?   ☐
or
    your THIRD substance of abuse?   ☐

Authors: HM Annis and G Martin, Addiction Research Foundation, © 1985

Listed below are a number of situations or events in which some people use _____.

Read each item carefully, and answer in terms of your own use of _____ **over the past year.**

    If you "NEVER" used these drugs in that situation, circle "1"
    If you "RARELY" used these drugs in that situation, circle "2"
    If you "FREQUENTLY" used these drugs in that situation, circle "3"
    If you "ALMOST ALWAYS" used these drugs in that situation, circle "4"

I USED _____

	Never	Rarely	Frequently	Almost Always
1. When I was depressed about things in general	1	2	3	4
2. When I felt shaky, sick or nauseous	1	2	3	4
3. When I was happy	1	2	3	4
4. When I felt there was nowhere left to turn	1	2	3	4
5. When I wanted to see whether I could use these drugs in moderation	1	2	3	4
6. When I was in a place where I had used or bought these drugs before	1	2	3	4
7. When I felt tense or uneasy in the presence of someone	1	2	3	4
8. When I was invited to someone's home and felt awkward about refusing when they offered me these drugs	1	2	3	4

IDTS (Drugs) continued . . .

I USED _____

	Never	Rarely	Frequently	Almost Always
9. When I met some old friends and we wanted to have a good time	1	2	3	4
10. When I was unable to express my feelings to someone	1	2	3	4
11. When I felt that I had let myself down	1	2	3	4
12. When I had trouble sleeping	1	2	3	4
13. When I felt confident and relaxed	1	2	3	4
14. When I was bored	1	2		4
15. When I wanted to prove to myself that these drugs were not a problem for me	1	2	3	4
16. When I unexpectedly found some of these drugs or happened to see something that reminded me of these drugs	1	2	3	4
17. When other people rejected me or didn't seem to like me	1	2	3	4
18. When I was out with friends and they kept suggesting we go somewhere ___ use these drugs	1	2	3	4
19. When I was with an intimate friend ___ we wanted to feel even ___	1	2	3	4
20. When other people treated ___ ___ fair, or interfered with my ___	1	2	3	4
21. When I was lonely	1	2	3	4
22. When I wanted to stay awake, be more alert, or be more energetic	1	2	3	4
23. When I felt excited about something	1	2	3	4
24. When I felt anxious or tense about something	1	2	3	4
25. When I wanted to find out whether I could use these drugs occasionally without getting hooked	1	2	3	4
26. When I had been drinking and thought about using these drugs	1	2	3	4
27. When I felt that my family was putting a lot of pressure on me or that I couldn't measure up to their expectations	1	2	3	4
28. When others in the same room were using these drugs and I felt that they expected me to join in	1	2	3	4

E. INVENTORY OF DRUG-TAKING SITUATIONS (IDTS) *(Continued)*

IDTS (Drugs) continued . . .   **I USED** _____

	Never	Rarely	Frequently	Almost Always
29. When I was with friends and wanted to increase my enjoyment	1	2	3	4
30. When I was not getting along well with others at school or work	1	2	3	4
31. When I started to feel guilty about something	1	2	3	4
32. When I wanted to lose weight	1	2	3	4
33. When I was feeling content with my life	1	2	3	4
34. When I felt overwhelmed and wanted to escape	1	2	3	4
35. When I wanted to test out whether I could be with drug-using friends without using these drugs	1	2	3	4
36. When I heard someone talking about their past experiences with these drugs	1	2		4
37. When there were fights at home		2	3	4
38. When I was pressured to use these drugs and felt I couldn't refuse		2	3	4
39. When I wanted to celebrate with a friend		2	3	4
40. When someone was dissatisfied with my work or I felt pressured at school or on the job	1	2	3	4
41. When I was angry at the way things turned out	1	2	3	4
42. When I had a headache or was in physical pain	1	2	3	4
43. When I remembered something good that had happened	1	2	3	4
44. When I felt confused about what I should do	1	2	3	4
45. When I wanted to test whether I could be in places where these drugs were being used without using any	1	2	3	4
46. When I began to think how good a rush or a high had felt	1	2	3	4
47. When I felt that I needed courage to face up to someone	1	2	3	4
48. When I was with a group of people and everyone was using these drugs	1	2	3	4
49. When I was having a good time and wanted to increase my sexual enjoyment	1	2	3	4
50. When I felt that someone was trying to control me and I wanted to feel more independent	1	2	3	4

F. MICHIGAN ALCOHOL SCREENING TEST (MAST)

OVERVIEW

The MAST is a 24-item rating scale developed by ML Selzer to detect alcohol abuse. The MAST was developed with the premise that individuals with alcohol abuse may be reluctant to identify themselves as such. The MAST contains items that are somewhat neutral, yet help identify alcoholic symptoms. Each item is answered either "Yes" or "No". Negative answers to items 1, 4, 6, and 7 are consistent with alcoholic responses, while positive responses to the other items are consistent with alcoholic responses. The original citations assign a 1-5 weighting to each of the items, with a rating of 5 being considered diagnostic of alcoholism. The MAST may be administered by a clinician during an interview, or may be used as a self-rated questionnaire. A 13-item short form of the MAST also exists. Strengths of the MAST include its well-documented validity and ease of administration. However, the MAST reliability data has been based primarily on white males.

GENERAL APPLICATIONS

The MAST is used to screen for alcohol use and alcohol-related disabilities.

SELECTED PSYCHOMETRIC PROPERTIES

The authors report good internal consistencies of both the long and short forms of the MAST, with alphas of 0.95 and 0.93, respectively. Validity is excellent. The MAST correctly identified 92% of 99 hospitalized alcoholics.

REFERENCES

Selzer ML, "The Michigan Alcoholism Screening Test: The Quest for a New Diagnostic Instrument," *Am J Psychiatry*, 1971, 127(12):1653-8.

Selzer ML, Vinokur A, and van Rooijen L, "A Self-Administered Short Michigan Alcoholism Screening Test (SMAST)," *J Stud Alcohol*, 1975, 36(1):117-26.

COPYRIGHT

Not applicable
Additional copies of tests and scoring key are available from the author:
Melvin L Selzer
6967 Paseo Laredo
La Jolla, CA 92037

SCALE GENERALLY DONE BY

Clinician or trained rater; may also be self-rated

TIME TO COMPLETE SCALE

15-30 minutes depending on format

REPRESENTATIVE STUDY UTILIZING SCALE

Knight JR, Palacios JN, and Shannon M, "Prevalence of Alcohol Problems Among Pediatric Residents," *Arch Pediatr Adolesc Med*, 1999, 153(11):1181-3.

F. MICHIGAN ALCOHOL SCREENING TEST (MAST) *(Continued)*

MAST

Please circle either Yes or No for each item as it applies to you.

Yes	No	(2)	1.	Do you feel you are a normal drinker?
Yes	No	(2)	2.	Have you ever awakened the morning after some drinking the night before and found that you could not remember a part of the evening before?
Yes	No	(1)	3.	Does your wife, husband, parent, or other near relative ever worry or complain about your drinking?
Yes	No	(2)	4.	Can you stop drinking without a struggle after one or two drinks?
Yes	No	(1)	5.	Do you ever feel guilty about your drinking?
Yes	No	(2)	6.	Do friends or relatives think you are a normal drinker?
Yes	No	(2)	7.	Are you able to stop drinking when you want to?
Yes	No	(5)	8.	Have you ever attended a meeting of Alcoholics Anonymous (AA)?
Yes	No	(1)	9.	Have you ever gotten into physical fights when drinking?
Yes	No	(2)	10.	Has drinking ever created problems between you and your wife, husband, parent, or other near relative?
Yes	No	(2)	11.	Has your wife, husband, a parent, or other near relative ever gone to anyone for help about your drinking?
Yes	No	(2)	12.	Have you ever lost friends or girlfriends/boyfriends because of your drinking?
Yes	No	(2)	13.	Have you ever gotten into trouble at work because of drinking?
Yes	No	(2)	14.	Have you ever lost a job because of drinking?
Yes	No	(2)	15.	Have you ever neglected your obligations, your family, or your work for two or more days in a row because you were drinking?
Yes	No	(1)	16.	Do you drink before noon fairly often?
Yes	No	(2)	17.	Have you ever been told you have liver trouble? Cirrhosis?
Yes	No	(5)	18.	After heavy drinking, have you ever had delirium tremens (DTs) or severe shaking, or heard voices, or seen things that weren't really there?
Yes	No	(5)	19.	Have you ever gone to anyone for help about your drinking?
Yes	No	(5)	20.	Have you ever been in a hospital because of drinking?
Yes	No	(2)	21.	Have you ever been a patient in a psychiatric hospital or on a psychiatric ward of a general hospital where drinking was part of the problem that resulted in hospitalization?
Yes	No	(2)	22.	Have you ever been seen at a psychiatric or mental health clinic, or gone to a doctor, social worker, or clergyman for help with any emotional problem where drinking was part of the problem?
Yes	No	(2)	23.	Have you ever been arrested for drunken driving while intoxicated or driving under the influence of alcoholic beverages?
Yes	No	(2)	24.	Have you ever been arrested, even for a few hours, because of other drunken behavior?

SUICIDE RISK

ASSESSMENT SCALES

TABLE OF CONTENTS

A. BECK HOPELESSNESS SCALE (BHS)

OVERVIEW

The BHS, developed by AT Beck and RA Steer, is a 20-item self-rated scale used to evaluate hopelessness in depressed individuals. The BHS is an indirect evaluation of suicidality. The BHS was developed building upon the Beck Depression Inventory (see the BDI *on page 80*); however, it is more comprehensive in its evaluation of suicidal ideation. The authors propose that hopelessness represents negative attitudes about the future that may indicate suicide risk. The BHS consist of 20 true/false items that either endorse or deny pessimistic or optimistic statements. As with all suicide risk assessment scales, the BHS should not be considered a solitary assessment, and should be utilized in concert with a comprehensive clinical evaluation.

GENERAL APPLICATIONS

The BHS measures negative attitudes about the future and is an indirect measure of suicidality.

SELECTED PSYCHOMETRIC PROPERTIES

The BHS demonstrates high internal consistency, with KR-20 coefficients generally 0.90 or higher, retest reliability over 0.60, and concurrent validity with clinicians' rating of hopelessness ($r = 0.74$). Test-retest reliability has been reported as 0.69 at one week and 0.66 at six weeks.

REFERENCES

Beck AT, Weissman A, Lester D, et al, "The Measurement of Pessimism: The Hopelessness Scale," *J Consult Clin Psychol*, 1974, 42(6):861-5.

COPYRIGHT

Aaron T Beck
The Psychological Corporation
555 Academic Court
San Antonio, TX 78204-2498
Tel: 1-800-211-8378

SCALE GENERALLY DONE BY

Patient self-report; may also be verbally administered by a clinician or trained rater

TIME TO COMPLETE SCALE

5-10 minutes

REPRESENTATIVE STUDY UTILIZING SCALE

Rabkin JG, Goetz RR, Remien RH, et al, "Stability of Mood Despite HIV Illness Progression in a Group of Homosexual Men," *Am J Psychiatry*, 1997, 154(2):231-8.

B. BECK SCALE FOR SUICIDE IDEATION (BSS)

OVERVIEW

The BSS, developed by AT Beck and RA Steer, is a 21-item self-report scale to assess severity of suicidal ideation in adults and adolescents. Each item contains three statements that are graded in severity from 0 to 2. The first five items are screening items that limit the length and intrusiveness of the assessment for individuals who are nonsuicidal. The first part (items 1-5) evaluates an individual's attitudes toward living and dying and includes such items as wish to live, wish to die, reasons for living or dying, active suicide attempt, and passive suicide attempts. The second part (items 6-19) evaluates suicidal ideation and anticipated reactions to those thoughts. The third part (remaining items) evaluates previous suicide attempts and suicidal intent during last suicide attempt. Individuals who are nonsuicidal complete only the first and last parts of the scale, while individuals who are suicidal complete all scale items. Strengths of the BSS include its brevity and ease of administration. As with all suicide risk assessment scales, the BSS should not be considered a solitary assessment, and should be utilized in concert with a comprehensive clinical evaluation.

GENERAL APPLICATIONS

The BSS is used to assess suicide risk.

SELECTED PSYCHOMETRIC PROPERTIES

Reliability of the BSS is good, with a coefficient alpha reliability estimate of 0.90 for inpatients, and 0.87 for outpatients. Test-retest stability over one week provided a correlation of 0.54 (p <.01).

REFERENCES

Beck AT and Steer RA, *Manual for the Beck Scale for Suicide Ideation*, San Antonio, TX: The Psychological Corporation.

COPYRIGHT

Aaron T Beck
The Psychological Corporation
555 Academic Court
San Antonio, TX 78204-2498
Tel: 1-800-211-8378

SCALE GENERALLY DONE BY

Patient self-report. May also be verbally administered by a clinician or trained rater.

TIME TO COMPLETE SCALE

5-10 minutes

REPRESENTATIVE STUDY UTILIZING SCALE

Malone KM, Haas GL, Sweeny JA, et al, "Major Depression and the Risk of Attempted Suicide," *J Affect Disord*, 1995, 34(3):173-85.

C. CALIFORNIA RISK ESTIMATOR FOR SUICIDE

OVERVIEW

The California Risk Estimator for Suicide, developed by JA Motto et al, is a 15-item interviewer-rated scale to assess risk of suicide in depressed or suicidal patients. The scale items include demographic characteristics (age, occupation), psychosocial factors (stress, financial status), and clinical features (sleep time, suicidal thoughts). Items are rated based upon clinical interview. Each item is given a weighted score, with a total score used to assess relative risk of suicide. A primary strength of the Risk Estimator is its extreme brevity, although there is minimal information on validity/reliability of the scale. As with all suicide risk assessment scales, the Risk Estimator should not be considered a solitary assessment and should be utilized in concert with a comprehensive clinical evaluation.

GENERAL APPLICATIONS

The California Risk Estimator for Suicide is used to assess suicide risk.

SELECTED PSYCHOMETRIC PROPERTIES

Items from the scale by Motto, et al, were identified from a large sample of psychiatric inpatients, of whom nearly 5% committed suicide during a two-year long follow-up period. Validity/reliability have not been clearly established.

REFERENCES

Motto JA, Heilbron DC, and Juster JP, "Development of a Clinical Instrument to Estimate Suicide Risk," *Am J Psychiatry*, 1985, 142(6):680-6.

COPYRIGHT

Jerome A Motto
American Journal of Psychiatry
1400 K Street, NW
Washington, DC 20005

SCALE GENERALLY DONE BY

Clinician or trained rater

TIME TO COMPLETE SCALE

Less than 5 minutes

REPRESENTATIVE STUDY UTILIZING SCALE

Clark DC, Young MA, Scheftner WA, et al, "A Field Test of Motto's Risk Estimator for Suicide," *Am J Psychiatry*, 1987, 144(7):923-6.

THE CALIFORNIA RISK ESTIMATOR FOR SUICIDE

INSTRUCTIONS

1. The California Risk Estimator for Suicide is designed to estimate the risk of suicide in adults aged 18-70, during a 2-year period following the time of assessment.

2. The scale is primarily applicable to persons known to be at some risk, such as those in a serious depressive state, having suicidal thoughts or impulses, or having made a recent suicide attempt.

3. The scale is to be administered by a clinician, not self-administered. Responses to the items in the first column are best determined in the course of a clinical interview. The information need not be obtained in the listed order.

4. The subjective judgment of the interviewer is to be used throughout in categorizing the response, as data provided in the clinical situation may be incomplete, ambiguous, or conflicting.

5. For the one most appropriate response category in the second column, the indicated "assigned score" in the third column should be entered into the last column as the "actual score". If any data are missing or unobtainable, score that item zero.

6. Total the fifteen actual scores and determine from the Table of Risk what category of risk is scored. This is expressed in three ways:

   1) Numerically, on a scale of one to ten, representing the decile of risk,

   2) descriptively, from "Very Low" to "Very High", and

   3) an estimated percentage of risk during the two years following assessment.

The California Risk Estimator for Suicide is intended as a supplement to, not a substitute for, clinical judgment. A thorough evaluation is indicated in any serious emotional disturbance. Individual uniqueness suggests that when the scale is not consistent with clinical judgment, clinical judgment should be given precedence.

Item	Response Category	Assigned Score	Actual Score
1. Age (last birthday)	Find score in Age-Score table	See Age-Score table	
2. Occupation	Executive/Administrator	48	
	Professional	48	
	Owner of business	48	
	Semiskilled worker	48	
	Other	0	
3. Sexual orientation	Bisexual, sexually active	65	
	Homosexual, not sexually active	65	
	Other	0	
4. Financial resources	None or negative (in debt)	0	
	0 to $100	35	
	Over $100	70	
5. Threat of significant financial loss	Yes	63	
	No	0	
6. Stress unique to subject's circumstances	Severe	63	
	Other	0	
7. Hours of sleep per night (approximate)	0-2	0	
	3-5	37	
	6 or more	74	
8. Change of weight during present episode of stress (approximate)	Weight gain	60	
	Less than 10% loss	60	
	Other	0	

C. CALIFORNIA RISK ESTIMATOR FOR SUICIDE *(Continued)*

Item	Response Category	Assigned Score	Actual Score
9. Ideas of persecution or reference	Moderate or severe	45	
	Other	0	
10. Intensity of present suicidal impulses	Questionable, moderate, or severe	100	
	Other	0	
11. If current suicide attempt made, seriousness of intent to die	Unequivocal	88	
	Ambivalent, weighted toward suicide	88	
	Other or not applicable	0	
12. Number of prior psychiatric hospitalizations	None	0	
	1	21	
	2	43	
	3 or more	64	
13. Result of prior efforts to obtain help	Poor, unsatisfactory or variable	55	
	Other or not applicable	0	
14. Emotional disorder in family history	Depression	45	
	Alcoholism	45	
	Other	0	
15. Interviewer's reaction to the person	Highly positive	0	
	Moderately or slightly positive	42	
	Neutral or negative	85	
		TOTAL SCORE	

TABLE OF RISK

Total Score	Decile of Risk	Relative Risk	Approximate Suicide Rate
0-271	1	Very low	Less than 1%
272-311	2	Low	1% to 2.5%
312-344	3		
345-377	4	Moderate	2.5% to 5%
378-407	5		
408-435	6		
436-465	7		
466-502	8	High	5% to 10%
503-553	9		
Over 553	10	Very high	Over 10%

AGE-SCORE TABLE

Age	Score	Age	Score	Age	Score
18	0	36	45	54	80
19	3	37	47	55	81
20	6	38	49	56	83
21	9	39	51	57	85
22	12	40	53	58	86
23	14	41	55	59	88
24	17	42	57	60	90
25	20	43	59	61	91
26	22	44	61	62	93
27	25	45	63	63	95
28	27	46	65	64	96
29	29	47	67	65	98
30	32	48	69	66	99
31	34	49	71	67	101
32	36	50	72	68	102
33	39	51	74	69	104
34	41	52	76	70	106
35	43	53	78		

D. SUICIDE PROBABILITY SCALE (SPS)

OVERVIEW

The SPS, developed by JG Cull and WS Gill, is a 36-item, self-reported scale used to evaluate suicide risk in adolescents and adults. Each item on the SPS is a statement describing a feeling or behavior. Individuals are asked to rate how often the statement is true for them on a 4-point scale, ranging in severity from none to most or all of the time. The scale provides a total score and four subscale scores which include hopelessness, suicidal ideation, negative self-evaluation, and hostility. A fourth grade reading level is required to complete the self-reported scale. As with all suicide risk assessment scales, the SPS should not be considered a solitary assessment, and should be utilized in concert with a comprehensive clinical evaluation.

GENERAL APPLICATIONS

The SPS is used to assess suicide risk.

SELECTED PSYCHOMETRIC PROPERTIES

Internal consistency of the scale has been reported to be good, with alpha = 0.93 for the total score, and alpha coefficients ranging from .62 (negative self-evaluation) to 0.89 (suicide ideation) for the subscales. Test-retest reliability over three weeks provided a correlation of 0.92 (p <.001).

REFERENCES

Cull JG and Gill WS, "The Suicide Probability Scale," *West Psycholog Serv*, 1982.

COPYRIGHT

John G Cull, PhD
Wayne S Gill, PhD
Western Psychological Services
12031 Wilshire Blvd
Los Angeles, CA 90025-1251

SCALE GENERALLY DONE BY

Self-rated

TIME TO COMPLETE SCALE

15-20 minutes

REPRESENTATIVE STUDY UTILIZING SCALE

Cappelli M, Clulow MK, Goodman JT, et al, "Identifying Depressed and Suicidal Adolescents in a Teen Health Clinic," *J Adolesc Health*, 1995, 16(1):64-70.

SPS RATING FORM

BELOW IS A SAMPLE OF TWO STATEMENTS
USED ON THE SPS RATING SCALE

INSTRUCTIONS;

Listed below are a series of statements that some people might use to describe their feelings and behaviors. Please read each statement and determine how often the statement is true for you. Then circle the letter T in the appropriate box to indicate how often you feel the statement applies to you.

		None or a little of the time	Some of the time	Good part of the time	Most or all of the time
8.	I feel hostile toward others	T	T	T	T
32.	I think of suicide	T	T	T	T

IMPULSIVITY / AGGRESSION SCALES

TABLE OF CONTENTS

A. BARRATT IMPULSIVENESS SCALE (BIS-11)

OVERVIEW

The BIS-11, developed by E Barratt, is one of the most widely used scales in the area of impulsivity and looks at this situation in three domains: Motor impulsiveness, Nonplanning impulsiveness, and Attentional impulsiveness.

The BIS is a self-administered, 30-item questionnaire scored on a 4-point scale (1 = rarely/never to 4 = almost always/always) which usually takes between 10-15 minutes to be completed.

The scale has been tested in both clinical and nonclinical populations including psychiatric inpatients with substance abuse, and prison inmates.

The author is developing a scale which evaluates aggression. Information on this may be requested from the author.

GENERAL APPLICATIONS

The BIS-11 measures impulsivity in nonclinical and clinical populations.

SELECTED PSYCHOMETRIC PROPERTIES

The BIS has good internal consistency and the Cronbach's alpha ranges from 0.79 to 0.83 as reported by its developer who also reports good validity and moderate correlations with other measures of impulsive-related traits, especially with the Buss-Durkee Hostility Inventory *on page 336*.

REFERENCES

Barratt ES, "Impulsiveness and Aggression," *Violence and Mental Disorder: Developments in Risk Assessment,*, Monahan J and Steadman HJ, eds, Chicago, IL: University of Chicago Press, 1994, 61-79.

Patton JH, Stanford MS, and Barratt ES, "Factor Structure of the Barratt Impulsiveness Scale," *J Clin Psychol*, 1995, 51:768-74.

COPYRIGHT

Ernest S Barratt, PhD
The University of Texas Medical Branch
301 University Blvd
Galveston, TX 77555-0189

SCALE GENERALLY DONE BY

Self-rated or structured interview

TIME TO COMPLETE SCALE

10-15 minutes

REPRESENTATIVE STUDY UTILIZING SCALE

Barratt ES, Stanford MS, Kent TA, et al, "Neuropsychological and Cognitive Psychophysiological Substrates of Impulsive Aggression," *Biol Psychiatry*, 1997, 41(10):1045-61.

Personal Evaluation: BIS-11

Name: _____   *Date:* _____

Directions: People differ in the ways they act and think in different situations. This is a test to measure some of the ways in which you act and think. Read each statement carefully and **DARKEN THE APPROPRIATE CIRCLE** to the right of the statement. Answer quickly and honestly.	Rarely/Never	Occasionally	Often	Almost Always
2. I do things without thinking	○	○	○	○
8. I am self-controlled	○	○	○	○

B. BUSS-DURKEE HOSTILITY INVENTORY (BDHI)

OVERVIEW

The BDHI, developed by AH Buss and A Durkee in 1957, is perhaps the best-known hostility inventory. It is a 75-item anger and hostility questionnaire with a true-false format. The inventory has eight subscales:

> Assault
> Indirect hostility
> Irritability
> Negativity
> Resentment
> Suspicion
> Verbal hostility
> Guilt

The BDHI was developed as a tool for clinical assessments and to help in clinical research in the areas of anger and hostility. Its popularity has to do with its practicality and how easy it is to apply and score. A more recently developed version of the scale has 29 items with Likert-type ratings (Buss, 1992).

GENERAL APPLICATIONS

The BDHI measures anger and hostility in general populations.

SELECTED PSYCHOMETRIC PROPERTIES

Studies done by the developers of the scale in undergraduate populations showed Cronbach's alpha coefficients of 0.52 to 0.72. In terms of validity, the BDHI correlates well with other measures of similar domains and has the ability to distinguish between groups with different levels of hostility.

REFERENCES

Buss AH and Durkee A, "An Inventory for Assessing Different Kinds of Hostility," *J Consult Psychol*, 1957, 21:343-9.

Buss AH and Perry M, "The Aggression Questionnaire," *J Pers Soc Psychol*, 1992, 63(3):452-9.

COPYRIGHT

Journal of Consulting Psychology
A Durkee
AH Buss
Department of Psychology
University of Texas
Austin, TX 78712

SCALE GENERALLY DONE BY

Self-rated

TIME TO COMPLETE SCALE

15-20 minutes

REPRESENTATIVE STUDY UTILIZING SCALE

Lothstein LM and Jones P, "Discriminating Violent Individuals by Means of Various Psychological Tests," *J Pers Assess*, 1978, 42(3):237-43.

BUSS-DURKEE HOSTILITY INVENTORY

ASSAULT

1. I seldom strike back, even if someone hits me first.
2. Once in a while I cannot control my urge to harm others.
3. I can think of no good reason for ever hitting anyone.
4. If somebody hits me first, I let him have it.
5. Whoever insults me or my family is asking for a fight.
6. People who continually pester you are asking for a punch in the nose.
7. When I really lose my temper, I am capable of slapping someone.
8. I get into fights about as often as the next person.
9. If I have to resort to physical violence to defend my rights, I will.
10. I have known people who pushed me so far that we came to blows.

INDIRECT

1. I sometimes spread gossip about people I don't like.
2. I never get mad enough to throw things.
3. When I am angry, I sometimes sulk.
4. When I am mad, I sometimes slam doors.
5. I never play practical jokes.
6. I sometimes pout when I don't get my own way.
7. Since the age of ten, I have never had a temper tantrum.
8. I can remember being so angry that I picked up the nearest thing and broke it.
9. I sometimes show my anger by banging on the table.

IRRITABILITY

1. I lose my temper easily, but get over it quickly.
2. Sometimes people bother me just by being around.
3. I am irritated a great deal more than people are aware of.
4. I am always patient with others.
5. It makes my blood boil to have somebody make fun of me.
6. I often feel like a powder keg ready to explode.
7. I sometimes carry a chip on my shoulder.
8. I can't help being a little rude to people I don't like.
9. If someone doesn't treat me right, I don't let it annoy me.
10. I don't let a lot of unimportant things irritate me.
11. Lately, I have been kind of grouchy.

NEGATIVISM

1. Unless somebody asks me in a nice way, I won't do what they want.
2. When someone makes a rule I don't like, I am tempted to break it.
3. When someone is bossy, I do the opposite of what he asks.
4. Occasionally, when I am mad at someone, I will give him the "silent treatment."
5. When people are bossy, I take my time just to show them.

B. BUSS-DURKEE HOSTILITY INVENTORY (BDHI) *(Continued)*

RESENTMENT

1. I don't seem to get what's coming to me.
2. Other people always seem to get the breaks.
3. I don't know any people that I downright hate.
4. When I look back on what's happened to me, I can't help feeling mildly resentful.
5. Almost every week I see someone I dislike.
6. Although I don't show it, I am sometimes eaten up with jealousy.
7. If I let people see the way I feel, I'd be considered a hard person to get along with.
8. At times, I feel I get a raw deal out of life.

SUSPICION

1. I know that people tend to talk about me behind my back.
2. I tend to be on my guard with people who are somewhat more friendly than I expected.
3. There are a number of people who seem to dislike me very much.
4. There are a number of people who seem to be jealous of me.
5. I sometimes have the feeling that others are laughing at me.
6. My motto is "Never trust strangers."
7. I commonly wonder what hidden reason another person may have for doing something nice for me.
8. I used to think that most people told the truth, but now I know otherwise.
9. I have no enemies who really wish to harm me.
10. I seldom feel that people are trying to anger or insult me.

VERBAL

1. When I disapprove of my friends' behavior, I let them know it.
2. I often find myself disagreeing with people.
3. I can't help getting into arguments when people disagree with me.
4. I demand that people respect my rights.
5. Even when my anger is aroused, I don't use "strong language."
6. If somebody annoys me, I am apt to tell him what I think of him.
7. When people yell at me, I yell back.
8. When I get mad, I say nasty things.
9. I could not put someone in his place, even if he needed it.
10. I often make threats I don't really mean to carry out.
11. I generally cover up my poor opinion of others.
12. When arguing, I tend to raise my voice.
13. I would rather concede a point than get into an argument about it.

C. OVERT AGGRESSION SCALE - MODIFIED (OAS-M)

OVERVIEW

The OAS-M was developed by E Coccaro and collaborators in 1991 to assess aggressive behavior in outpatients. The scale is a 25-item, semistructured interview with nine subscales.

Aggression
> Verbal aggression
> Aggression against objects
> Aggression against others
> Auto aggression

Irritability
> Global irritability
> Subjective irritability

Suicidality
> Suicidal tendencies (ideation and behavior)
> Intent of attempt
> Lethality of attempt

Two different ways of scoring are used in this scale. Each one of the aggression subscales has seven different behaviors which are listed in order of severity, scored separately by frequency, and then multiplied by the weight assigned (1 for verbal aggression, 2 for aggression against objects, and 3 for aggression against others). The irritability and suicidality subscales use a Likert-type format with a continuous scale along seven points. The OAS-M is a short instrument, relatively easy to administer, and was developed from work with aggressive patients.

GENERAL APPLICATIONS

The OAS-M measures aggression in psychiatric patient populations.

SELECTED PSYCHOMETRIC PROPERTIES

Both data on reliability and validity are limited with high intraclass correlation (>0.91) and moderate test-retest reliability (0.46-0.54). The validity data seems to be adequate but is limited. The scales appear to be sensitive to change.

REFERENCES

Coccaro EF, Harvey PD, Kupsaw-Lawrence E, et al, "Development of Neuropharmacologically-Based Behavioral Assessments of Impulsive Aggressive Behavior," *J Neuropsych Clin Neurosci*, 1991, 3(2):S44-51.

COPYRIGHT

Emil Coccaro, MD
Department of Psychiatry
Medical College of Pennsylvania
Eastern Pennsylvania Psychiatric Institute
3200 Henry Avenue
Philadelphia, PA 19129

C. OVERT AGGRESSION SCALE - MODIFIED (OAS-M) *(Continued)*

SCALE GENERALLY DONE BY

Clinician using a semistructured interview

TIME TO COMPLETE SCALE

20-30 minutes

REPRESENTATIVE STUDY UTILIZING SCALE

Coccaro EF and Kavoussi RJ, "Fluoxetine and Impulsive Aggressive Behavior in Personality Disordered Subjects," *Arch Gen Psychiatry*, 1997, 54(12):1081-8.

OAS-M

Name:_____ Date:_____ Rater:_____

(PAST WEEK)

1. Verbal Assault:

    Assessment of verbal
    outbursts or threats made
    at spouse, boy/girl friend,
    close friends, strangers.

    0 = No events.

    1 = Snapped or yelled at someone. ____ x 1 = ____
    2 = Cursed or personally insulted
        someone. ____ x 2 = ____
    3 = Engaged in a verbal argument with
        someone. ____ x 3 = ____
    4 = Verbally threatened to hit someone
        pt knows well. ____ x 4 = ____
    5 = Verbally threatened to hit a stranger.____ x 5 = ____

    WEIGHTED "VERBAL ASSAULT" SCORE = ____ x 1 = ____

2. Assault Against Objects:

    Assessment of intentional
    physical attacks against
    one's own property, another's
    property, or animals.

    0 = No events.

    1 = Slammed door, kicked chair, threw
        clothes, in anger. ____ x 1 = ____
    2 = Broke something in anger. ____ x 2 = ____
    3 = Broke several things in anger. ____ x 3 = ____
    4 = Set a fire, vandalism, damaged
        another's property. ____ x 4 = ____
    5 = Struck, injured or tortured a pet
        or other living animal. ____ x 5 = ____

    WEIGHTED "ASSAULT AGAINST OBJECTS" SCORE = ____ x 2 = ____

3. Assault Against Others:

    Assessment of intentional
    physical attacks against
    other people.

    0 = No events.

    1 = Makes threatening gestures. ____ x 1 = ____
    2 = Assault resulting in no physical
        harm to another. ____ x 2 = ____
    3 = Assault resulting in some physical
        harm to another. ____ x 3 = ____
    4 = Assault resulting in serious
        physical injury to another. ____ x 4 = ____
    5 = Assault requiring medical attention. ____ x 5 = ____

    WEIGHTED "ASSAULT AGAINST OTHERS" SCORE = ____ x 3 = ____

C. OVERT AGGRESSION SCALE - MODIFIED (OAS-M) *(Continued)*

4. Assault Against Self:

    Assessment of intentional
    physical attacks against self,
    whether or not attacks are
    suicidal in purpose.

    0 = No events.

    1 = Hit, bit, scratched self.   ____ x 1 =   ____
    2 = Head banging, or hitting fists
        against wall.   ____ x 2 =   ____
    3 = Cut, bruised, burned self but only
        superficially.   ____ x 3 =   ____
    4 = Cut, bruised, burned self deeply or
        seriously.   ____ x 4 =   ____
    5 = Broke teeth, bone, skull.   ____ x 5 =   ____

    WEIGHTED "ASSAULT AGAINST SELF" SCORE = ____ x 3 = ____

5. Global Subjective Irritability:

    Intensity and duration of
    externally directed feelings
    of irritability/anger/resentment/
    annoyance expressed overtly
    or not.

    0 = Not at all: not clinically significance.

    1 = Slight: doubtful clinical significance.
    2 = Mild: More than called for but only occasional and
        never intense.
    3 = Moderate: often aware of feeling angry or
        occasionally, very angry.
    4 = Marked: aware of feeling angry most of the time or
        often very angry.
    5 = Extreme: almost constantly aware of feeling very angry.

6. Global Overt Irritability:

    Overt irritability or anger
    NOT associated with mania
    or psychosis.

    0 = Not at all: only subjectively felt.

    1 = Slight: Occasional snappiness of doubtful clinical
        significance.
    2 = Mild: argumentative/quick to express annoyance.
    3 = Moderate: often shouts/loses temper.
    4 = Severe: throws/breaks things, occasionally assaultive.
    5 = Extreme: repeatedly violent against things or persons.

7. Suicidal Tendencies:

    Thoughts of death or
    suicide.

    0 = None at all.

    1 = Slight: occasional thoughts of his or her death
        (w/o suicidal thoughts).
    2 = Mild: frequent thoughts of being better off dead/
        occasional thoughts of suicide (w/o plan).
    3 = Moderate: often thinks of suicide or has thought of
        specific method.
    4 = Severe: frequent suicidal thoughts, mentally rehearsed
        plan, has made a suicidal gesture.
    5 = Extreme: made preparations for a serious suicide attempt.
    6 = Very extreme: suicidal attempt with definite intent to
        die or potential for death/serious medical consequence.

If question 7 = "4, 5, or 6" (i.e., 'Severe - Very Extreme', rate questions 7a & 7b below

7a. Suicide: Intent of Attempt:

    0 = Obviously no intent, purely a manipulative gesture.

    Seriousness of suicidal
intent to kill self as judged
by overall circumstances
including likelihood of
being rescued, precautions
against discovery, action to
gain help during or after
attempt, degree of planning
and the apparent purpose
of attempt.

    1 = Not sure or only minimal intent.
2 = Definite but not very ambivalent.
3 = Serious.
4 = Very serious.
5 = Extreme (every expectation of death).

7b. Suicide: Medical Lethality:

    0 = No danger: no effects, held pills in hand.

    Actual medical threat to
life or physical condition
following the most serious
gesture or suicide attempt.

    1 = Minimal: scratch on the wrist.
2 = Mild: 10 aspirins, mild gastritis.
3 = Moderate: 10 seconds, briefly unconscious.
4 = Severe: cut throat.
5 = Extreme: respiratory arrest or prolonged coma.

OAS-M TOTAL SCORES

AGGRESSION (Q. 1-4)   ____
IRRITABILITY (Q. 5-6)   ____
SUICIDALITY (Q. 7-7b)   ____

D. STATE-TRAIT ANGER EXPRESSION INVENTORY (STAXI-2)

OVERVIEW

The STAXI was developed by C Spielberger and collaborators to assess a variety of components of anger in the evaluation of personality issues and as a contributor to an array of medical nonpsychiatric illnesses.

The STAXI-2, which is based on the original STAXI, is a 44-item, self-administered questionnaire with a 10-item scale that measures state anger and a 10-item scale that measures trait anger. Other items measure the different expressions of anger. Items are rated on a 4-point scale assessing the intensity of anger.

The STAXI-2 has a very good manual, which provides norms for a variety of populations and different age and/or special groups. In general, this inventory is a well-standardized measure with good discrimination and good clinical sense. It is easy to administer and has been tried in different populations.

GENERAL APPLICATIONS

The STAXI-2 measures anger expression in general populations.

SELECTED PSYCHOMETRIC PROPERTIES

The internal consistency for the STAXI-2 is very good with Cronbach's alphas of 0.70-0.93 for the first six scales. Test-retest reliability at two weeks was good as well with correlations of 0.62-0.81 for all scales except the anger scale.

REFERENCES

Spielberger CD, Johnson EH, Russell SF, et al, "The Experience and Expression of Anger: Construction and Validation of an Anger Expression Scale," *Anger and Hostility in Cardiovascular and Behavioral Disorders*, Chesney MA and Rosenman RH, eds, New York, NY: Hemisphere/McGraw Hill, 1985, 5-30.

COPYRIGHT

Psychological Assessment Resources, Inc
PO Box 998
Odessa, FL 33556
Tel: 1-800-331-8378

SCALE GENERALLY DONE BY

Self-rated

TIME TO COMPLETE SCALE

10-15 minutes

REPRESENTATIVE STUDY UTILIZING SCALE

Deffenbacher JL, Oetting ER, Lynch RS, et al, "The Expression of Anger and Its Consequences," *Behav Res Ther*, 1996, 34(7):575-90.

STAXI-2

The following entries are sample items from various sections of the STAXI-2 scale.

How I Feel Right Now

3. I feel angry

11. I feel like kicking somebody

How I Generally Feel

7. I have a fiery temper

21. I fly off the handle

How I Generally React or Behave When Angry or Furious

26. I control my temper

27. I express my anger

EATING DISORDERS

RATING SCALES

TABLE OF CONTENTS

A. EATING ATTITUDES TEST (EAT)

OVERVIEW

The Eating Attitudes Test (EAT), developed by DM Garner and PE Garfinkel, is a 40-item, self-rated scale for measuring the behaviors and attitudes characteristic of anorexia nervosa. The 40 items ask respondents to rate how often he or she experiences selected attitudes or behaviors related to food or eating. Responses are rated on a 1 (Always) to 6 (Never) spectrum. Items 1, 18, 19, 23, and 39 are scored: 6 = 3 points; 5 = 2 points; 4 = 1 point; 3, 2, or 1 = 0 points. The remaining items are scored: 1 = 2 points; 2 = 2 points; 3 = 1 point, and 4, 5, or 6 = 0 points. A response of "Always" for items 2-17, 20-22, 24-26, 28-38, and 40, and a response of "Never" on items 1, 18, 19, 23, and 39 are consistent with anorexia. Total score is the sum of each item. A score of 30 or higher has been identified as a rough cut off for anorectic eating concerns. Strengths of the EAT include it's brevity and ease of implementation as well as its ability to differentiate clinically recovered individuals from those with active anorexia.

GENERAL APPLICATIONS

The EAT is a self-rated scale to measure symptoms of anorexia nervosa.

SELECTED PSYCHOMETRIC PROPERTIES

The EAT has very good internal consistency, with a coefficient alpha of 0.94 for a combined sample of individuals with and without anorexia. The coefficient for anorectic individuals alone is 0.79. Average EAT scores for one sample with anorexia was 58.9 (standard deviation 13.3) compared to a clinically-recovered group with a mean score of 11.4 (standard deviation 5.1).

REFERENCES

Garner DM and Garfinkel PE, "The Eating Attitudes Test: An Index of the Symptoms of Anorexia Nervosa," *Psychol Med*, 1979, 9(2):273-9.

COPYRIGHT

Cambridge University Press
40 West 20th Street
New York, NY 10011-4211

SCALE GENERALLY DONE BY

Self-rated scale

TIME TO COMPLETE SCALE

10 minutes

REPRESENTATIVE STUDY UTILIZING SCALE

Bussolotti D, Fernandez-Aranda F, Solano R, et al, "Marital Status and Eating Disorders. An Analysis of Its Relevance," *J Psychosom Res*, 2002, 53(6):1139-45.

EAT

Please indicate on the line at the left, the answer which applies best to each of the numbered statements. All of the results will be *strictly* confidential. Most of the questions directly relate to food or eating, although other types of questions have been included. Please answer each question carefully. Thank you.

1 = Always
2 = Very often
3 = Often
4 = Sometimes
5 = Rarely
6 = Never

_____ 1. Like eating with other people.

_____ 2. Prepare foods for others but do not eat what I cook.

_____ 3. Become anxious prior to eating.

_____ 4. Am terrified about being overweight.

_____ 5. Avoid eating when I am hungry.

_____ 6. Find myself preoccupied with food.

_____ 7. Have gone on eating binges where I feel that I may not be able to stop.

_____ 8. Cut my food into small pieces.

_____ 9. Aware of the calorie content of foods that I eat.

_____ 10. Particularly avoid foods with a high carbohydrate content (eg, bread, potatoes, rice, etc).

_____ 11. Feel bloated after meals.

_____ 12. Feel that others would prefer if I ate more.

_____ 13. Vomit after I have eaten.

_____ 14. Feel extremely guilty after eating.

_____ 15. Am preoccupied with a desire to be thinner.

_____ 16. Exercise strenuously to burn off calories.

_____ 17. Weigh myself several times a day.

_____ 18. Like my clothes to fit tightly.

_____ 19. Enjoy eating meat.

_____ 20. Wake up early in the morning.

_____ 21. Eat the same foods day after day.

_____ 22. Think about burning my calories when I exercise.

_____ 23. Have regular menstrual periods.

_____ 24. Other people think that I am too thin.

_____ 25. Am preoccupied with the thought of having fat on my body.

_____ 26. Take longer than others to eat my meals.

A. EATING ATTITUDES TEST (EAT) *(Continued)*

_____ 27. Enjoy eating at restaurants.

_____ 28. Take laxatives.

_____ 29. Avoid foods with sugar in them.

_____ 30. Eat diet foods.

_____ 31. Feel that food controls my life.

_____ 32. Display self control around food.

_____ 33. Feel that others pressure me to eat.

_____ 34. Give too much time and thought to food.

_____ 35. Suffer from constipation.

_____ 36. Feel uncomfortable after eating sweets.

_____ 37. Engage in dieting behavior.

_____ 38. Like my stomach to be empty.

_____ 39. Enjoy trying new rich foods.

_____ 40. Have the impulse to vomit after meals.

B. EATING DISORDERS INVENTORY (EDI)

OVERVIEW

The Eating Disorders Inventory (EDI), developed by DM Garner, is a multidimensional self-report scale designed to assess the attitudes, behaviors, and traits present in eating disorders, particularly anorexia nervosa and bulimia nervosa. An original version of the EDI has 64 items with eight subscales. A newer version, the EDI-2 has 91 items and 11 subscales. The 11 subscales are: Drive for Thinness, Bulimia, Body Dissatisfaction, Ineffectiveness, Perfectionism, Interpersonal Distrust, Introceptive Awareness, Maturity Fears, Asceticism, Impulse Regulation, and Social Insecurity. Each item is rated on a 6-point Likert-type scale ranging from (Always true regarding oneself, Usually, Often, Sometimes, Rarely, or Never true about oneself). Responses for each item are scored from 0 to 3, with a score of 3 given to responses farthest in the symptomatic direction; scores of 2 and 1 for the next two responses; and a score of 0 for the three responses farthest in the direction of no symptoms. While a cut-off score of 14 on the Drive for Thinness subscale identifies individuals who are most likely at risk for developing an eating disorder or who have an eating disorder, the EDI is not designed to be a diagnostic scale for eating disorders. An easy reading version and a children's version of the EDI are both available.

GENERAL APPLICATIONS

The EDI is a self-report measure of attitudes, behaviors, and traits seen in eating disorders.

SELECTED PSYCHOMETRIC PROPERTIES

The EDI has good internal consistency with Cronbach's alphas ranging from 0.83-0.92 for clinical samples. The scale has good test-retest reliability at 1 week, 3 weeks, and 1 year intervals. The Drive for Thinness subscale has been shown to correlate with the Eating Attitudes Test (EAT).

REFERENCES

Garner DM, *Eating Disorder Inventory-2: Professional Manual*, Odessa, FL: Psychological Assessment Resources, 1991.

Raciti MC and Norcross JC, "The EAT and EDI: Screening, Interrelationships, and Psychometrics," *Int J Eat Disord*, 1987, 6:579-86.

COPYRIGHT

Psychological Assessment Resources, Inc
PO Box 998
Odessa, FL 33556
Tel: 1-800-331-8378

SCALE GENERALLY DONE BY

Self-rated scale

TIME TO COMPLETE SCALE

15-20 minutes

REPRESENTATIVE STUDY UTILIZING SCALE

Bussolotti D, Fernandez-Aranda F, Solano R, et al, "Marital Status and Eating Disorders. An Analysis of Its Relevance," *J Psychosom Res*, 2002, 53(6):1139-45.

B. EATING DISORDERS INVENTORY (EDI) *(Continued)*

SAMPLE ITEMS OF THE
EDI-2

David M. Garner, PhD

DIRECTIONS

Enter your name, the date, your age, sex, marital status, and occupation. Complete the questions on the rest of this page. Then turn to the inside of the booklet and carefully follow the instructions.

Name _____ Date _____

Age _____ Sex _____ Marital status _____ Occupation _____

E. What weight have you been at for the longest period of time? _____ pounds

   At what age did you first reach this weight? _____ years old

G. What is the most weight you have ever lost? _____ pounds

   Did you lose this weight on purpose? _____ Yes _____ No

   What weight did you lose to? _____ pounds

   At what age did you reach this weight? _____ years old

INSTRUCTIONS

First, write your name and the date on your EDI-2 Answer Sheet. Your ratings on the items below will be made on the EDI-2 Answer Sheet. The items ask about your attitudes, feelings, and behavior. Some of the items relate to food or eating. Other items ask about your feelings about yourself.

For each item, decide if the item is true about you ALWAYS (A), USUALLY (U), OFTEN (O), SOMETIMES (S), RARELY (R), or NEVER (N). Circle the letter that corresponds to your rating on the EDI-2 Answer Sheet. For example, if your rating for an item is OFTEN, you would circle the O for that item on the Answer Sheet.

Respond to all of the items, making sure that you circle the letter for the rating that is true about you. DO NOT ERASE! If you need to change an answer, make an "X" through the incorrect letter and then circle the correct one.

  1. I eat sweets and carbohydrates without feeling nervous.

  7. I think about dieting.

 16. I am terrified of gaining weight.

 21. I get confused about what emotion I am feeling.

 36. I hate being less than best at things.

 51. When I am upset, I don't know if I am sad, frightened, or angy.

 65. People I really like end up disappointing me.

 75. Self-denial makes me feel stronger spiritually.

 80. I feel that people give me the credit I deserve.

PREMENSTRUAL DYSPHORIC DISORDER

RATING SCALES

TABLE OF CONTENTS

A. DAILY RECORD OF SEVERITY OF PROBLEMS (DRSP)

OVERVIEW

The Daily Record of Severity of Problems (DRSP), developed by Endicott and colleagues is a 24-item rating scale to evaluate severity and change in symptoms related to premenstrual state/Premenstrual Dysphoric Disorder (PMDD). The DSRP incorporates all DSM-IV symptoms of PMDD. The first 21 items rate the psychological and physical symptoms of PMDD and the last 3 items measure 3 domains of functioning which consist of productivity at work, home, or school, interference with hobbies or social activities, and interference with relationships. Each item is self-rated on a scale of 1 (absent) to 6 (severe).

GENERAL APPLICATIONS

The DRSP evaluates symptoms of premenstrual dysphoric disorder.

SELECTED PSYCHOMETRIC PROPERTIES

The internal consistency coefficients of reliability are very high for the total scores of the DRSP, with Cronbach's alpha values ranging from 0.93-0.96 across luteal and follicular cycles (communication from Dr Endicott and colleagues). Test-retest reliability is also very high.

REFERENCES

Endicott J and Harrison W, *Daily Rating of Severity of Problems Form*, Department of Research Assessment and Training, New York, NY: New York State Psychiatric Institute, 1990.

COPYRIGHT

Jean Endicott, PhD
Chief, Department of Research, Assessment and Training
New York State Psychiatric Institute
1051 Riverside Dr, 123
New York, NY 10032

SCALE GENERALLY DONE BY

Self-rated scale

TIME TO COMPLETE SCALE

10-15 minutes

REPRESENTATIVE STUDY UTILIZING SCALE

Miner C, Brown E, McCray S, et al, "Weekly Luteal-Phase Dosing With Enteric-Coated Fluoxetine 90 mg in Premenstrual Dysphoric Disorder: A Randomized, Double-Blind, Placebo-Controlled Clinical Trial," *Clin Ther*, 2002, 24(3):417-33.

DAILY RECORD OF SEVERITY OF PROBLEMS*

Name or initials _____ ID Number _____ Date Began Rating _____

Note the degree to which you experienced each of the problems listed below. Make your ratings each evening. Circle the number which corresponds to the severity as noted here:

1 - Not at all   2 - Minimal   3 - Mild   4 - Moderate   5 - Severe   6 - Extreme

Rate under correct day of week:	MON	TUE	WED	THU	FRI	SAT	SUN **
Note date under day of wk	___	___	___	___	___	___	___ **
Note if *spotting or menses* with S or M	___	___	___	___	___	___	___
1a. Felt depressed, sad, "down," or "blue"	1 2 3 4 5 6	1 2 3 4 5 6	1 2 3 4 5 6	1 2 3 4 5 6	1 2 3 4 5 6	1 2 3 4 5 6	1 2 3 4 5 6
1b. Felt hopeless	1 2 3 4 5 6	1 2 3 4 5 6	1 2 3 4 5 6	1 2 3 4 5 6	1 2 3 4 5 6	1 2 3 4 5 6	1 2 3 4 5 6
1c. Felt worthless or guilty	1 2 3 4 5 6	1 2 3 4 5 6	1 2 3 4 5 6	1 2 3 4 5 6	1 2 3 4 5 6	1 2 3 4 5 6	1 2 3 4 5 6
2. Felt anxious, tense, "keyed up," or "on edge"	1 2 3 4 5 6	1 2 3 4 5 6	1 2 3 4 5 6	1 2 3 4 5 6	1 2 3 4 5 6	1 2 3 4 5 6	1 2 3 4 5 6
3a. Had mood swings (eg, suddenly felt sad or tearful)	1 2 3 4 5 6	1 2 3 4 5 6	1 2 3 4 5 6	1 2 3 4 5 6	1 2 3 4 5 6	1 2 3 4 5 6	1 2 3 4 5 6
3b. Was more sensitive to rejection or my feelings were easily hurt	1 2 3 4 5 6	1 2 3 4 5 6	1 2 3 4 5 6	1 2 3 4 5 6	1 2 3 4 5 6	1 2 3 4 5 6	1 2 3 4 5 6
4a. Felt angry, irritable	1 2 3 4 5 6	1 2 3 4 5 6	1 2 3 4 5 6	1 2 3 4 5 6	1 2 3 4 5 6	1 2 3 4 5 6	1 2 3 4 5 6
4b. Had conflicts or problems with people	1 2 3 4 5 6	1 2 3 4 5 6	1 2 3 4 5 6	1 2 3 4 5 6	1 2 3 4 5 6	1 2 3 4 5 6	1 2 3 4 5 6
5. Had less interest in usual activities (eg, work, school, friends, hobbies)	1 2 3 4 5 6	1 2 3 4 5 6	1 2 3 4 5 6	1 2 3 4 5 6	1 2 3 4 5 6	1 2 3 4 5 6	1 2 3 4 5 6
6. Had difficulty concentrating	1 2 3 4 5 6	1 2 3 4 5 6	1 2 3 4 5 6	1 2 3 4 5 6	1 2 3 4 5 6	1 2 3 4 5 6	1 2 3 4 5 6

A. DAILY RECORD OF SEVERITY OF PROBLEMS (DRSP) *(Continued)*

DAILY RECORD OF SEVERITY OF PROBLEMS* *(continued)*

Rate under correct day of week:	MON	TUE	WED	THU	FRI	SAT	SUN **
Note date under day of wk	___	___	___	___	___	___	___ **
Note if *spotting or menses* with S or M	___	___	___	___	___	___	___
7. Felt lethargic, tired, fatigued, or had a lack of energy	1 2 3 4 5 6	1 2 3 4 5 6	1 2 3 4 5 6	1 2 3 4 5 6	1 2 3 4 5 6	1 2 3 4 5 6	1 2 3 4 5 6
8a. Had increased appetite or overate	1 2 3 4 5 6	1 2 3 4 5 6	1 2 3 4 5 6	1 2 3 4 5 6	1 2 3 4 5 6	1 2 3 4 5 6	1 2 3 4 5 6
8b. Had cravings for specific foods	1 2 3 4 5 6	1 2 3 4 5 6	1 2 3 4 5 6	1 2 3 4 5 6	1 2 3 4 5 6	1 2 3 4 5 6	1 2 3 4 5 6
9a. Slept more, took naps, found it hard to get up when intended	1 2 3 4 5 6	1 2 3 4 5 6	1 2 3 4 5 6	1 2 3 4 5 6	1 2 3 4 5 6	1 2 3 4 5 6	1 2 3 4 5 6
9b. Had trouble getting to sleep or staying asleep	1 2 3 4 5 6	1 2 3 4 5 6	1 2 3 4 5 6	1 2 3 4 5 6	1 2 3 4 5 6	1 2 3 4 5 6	1 2 3 4 5 6
10a. Felt overwhelmed or that I could not cope	1 2 3 4 5 6	1 2 3 4 5 6	1 2 3 4 5 6	1 2 3 4 5 6	1 2 3 4 5 6	1 2 3 4 5 6	1 2 3 4 5 6
10b. Felt out of control	1 2 3 4 5 6	1 2 3 4 5 6	1 2 3 4 5 6	1 2 3 4 5 6	1 2 3 4 5 6	1 2 3 4 5 6	1 2 3 4 5 6
11a. Had breast tenderness	1 2 3 4 5 6	1 2 3 4 5 6	1 2 3 4 5 6	1 2 3 4 5 6	1 2 3 4 5 6	1 2 3 4 5 6	1 2 3 4 5 6
11b. Had breast swelling, felt "bloated," or had weight gain	1 2 3 4 5 6	1 2 3 4 5 6	1 2 3 4 5 6	1 2 3 4 5 6	1 2 3 4 5 6	1 2 3 4 5 6	1 2 3 4 5 6
11c. Had headache	1 2 3 4 5 6	1 2 3 4 5 6	1 2 3 4 5 6	1 2 3 4 5 6	1 2 3 4 5 6	1 2 3 4 5 6	1 2 3 4 5 6
11d. Had joint or muscle pain	1 2 3 4 5 6	1 2 3 4 5 6	1 2 3 4 5 6	1 2 3 4 5 6	1 2 3 4 5 6	1 2 3 4 5 6	1 2 3 4 5 6

356

DAILY RECORD OF SEVERITY OF PROBLEMS* *(continued)*

Rate under correct day of week:	MON	TUE	WED	THU	FRI	SAT	SUN **
Note date under day of wk	___	___	___	___	___	___	___ **
Note if *spotting or menses* with S or M	___	___	___	___	___	___	___
At work, at school, at home, or in daily routine, at least one of the problems noted above caused reduction of productivity or inefficiency	1 2 3 4 5 6	1 2 3 4 5 6	1 2 3 4 5 6	1 2 3 4 5 6	1 2 3 4 5 6	1 2 3 4 5 6	1 2 3 4 5 6
At least one of the problems noted above interfered with hobbies of social activities (eg, avoid or do less)	1 2 3 4 5 6	1 2 3 4 5 6	1 2 3 4 5 6	1 2 3 4 5 6	1 2 3 4 5 6	1 2 3 4 5 6	1 2 3 4 5 6
At least one of the problems noted above interfered with relationships with others	1 2 3 4 5 6	1 2 3 4 5 6	1 2 3 4 5 6	1 2 3 4 5 6	1 2 3 4 5 6	1 2 3 4 5 6	1 2 3 4 5 6

*Developed and copyrighted by Jean Endicott, PhD and Wilma Harrison, MD. Based upon suggested criteria by DSM IV work group. Used with permission.

**If ovulation is being assessed, please circle day of ovulation. Note method used: 1 = Kit; 2 = Basal temperature; 3 = Other _____

B. PREMENSTRUAL TENSION SYNDROME SCALE (PMTS)

OVERVIEW

The Premenstrual Tension Syndrome Scale (PMTS), developed by Meir Steiner and colleagues, measures premenstrual mood symptoms. The scale has an observer-derived version (PMTS-O) and a self-rated version (PMTS-SR). These scales evaluate symptoms in ten different domains including: Irritability-hostility, tension, efficiency, dysphoria, moodiness, motor coordination, mental-cognitive functioning, eating habit, sexual drive and activity, physical symptoms, and social impairment. The PMTS-SR scale contains queries on 36 individual symptoms. Each "yes" is scored as 1 point. A total maximum score is 36. The PMTS-0 scale evaluates the 10 symptom domains with a severity rating on either a 0-2 continuum or a 0-4 continuum. Maximum total score on the PMTS-0 is also 36. Visual analogue scales are sometimes paired with the PMTS to further assess symptom severity. A revised version of the PMTS, which precisely matches DSM-IV diagnostic criteria for premenstrual dysphoria, is scheduled for publication in the very near future.

GENERAL APPLICATIONS

The PMTS measures premenstrual mood symptoms.

SELECTED PSYCHOMETRIC PROPERTIES

Cronbach's alpha has been reported as 0.89 for the PMTS-0 and as 0.93 for the PMTS-SR indicating a high level of internal consistency among individual items. Correlations between PMTS-0 and PMTS-SR domain scores range from 0.67-0.80. The significant correlation between the self-administered and observer-administered PMTS demonstrates that investigators can use the version which best fits study/outcome assessment format.

REFERENCES

Steiner M, Haskett RF, and Carroll BJ, "Premenstrual Tension Syndrome: The Development of Research Diagnostic Criteria and New Rating Scales," *Acta Psychiatr Scand*, 1980, 62(2):177-90.

Steiner M, Streiner DL, Steinberg S, et al, "The Measurement of Premenstrual Mood Symptoms," *J Affect Disord*, 1999, 53(3):269-73.

COPYRIGHT

Acta Psychiatrica Scandinavia
Munksgaard
35 Norre Sogade
Postbox 173, DK-1005
Copenhagen K
Denmark
e-mail: direct@muksgaarddirect.dk

Further information on the PMTS and newly revised PMTS can be obtained from:
Meir Steiner MD, PhD, FRCPC
Women's Health Concerns Clinic
St. Joseph's Healthcare
50 Charlton Avenue East
Hamilton, Ontario L8N 4A6
Canada
Tel: 905-522-4942, ext: 3605
e-mail: mst@mcmaster.ca

SCALE GENERALLY DONE BY

PMTS-SR: Self-rated
PMRS-O: Clinician or trained rater

TIME TO COMPLETE SCALE

PMTS-SR: 10 minutes
PMTS-O: 15-20 minutes

REPRESENTATIVE STUDY UTILIZING SCALE

Critchlow DG, Bond AJ, and Wingrove J, "Mood Disorder History and Personality Assessment in Premenstrual Dysphoric Disorder," *J Clin Psychiatry*, 2001, 62(9):688-93.

B. PREMENSTRUAL TENSION SYNDROME SCALE (PMTS) *(Continued)*

PREMENSTRUAL TENSION SYNDROME SCALE (PMTS)

I am going to ask you about the premenstrual symptoms you are experiencing today.

(Based on the patient's response, circle the appropriate score.)

1. How would you rate your irritability or hostility today? This may include being irritable, hostile, having a negative attitude, being angry or short-fused, yelling and screaming at others ...

   0   **Not irritable.**

   1   **Doubtful, trivial.** Not reported without direct questioning.

   2   **Mild.** Occasional outbursts of anger.

   3   **Moderate.** Frequent outburst of irritable behavior.

   4   **Severe.** Severe interference between herself and significant others.

2. How would you rate your tension today? This may include being tense, restless, jittery, high-strung, or unable to relax ...

   0   **Not tense.**

   1   **Doubtful, trivial.** Not reported without direct questioning.

   2   **Mild.** Occasional tension.

   3   **Moderate.** Feeling tense or jittery and this behavior is evident.

   4   **Severe.** Feeling constantly tense and upset.

3 How would you rate your efficiency today? This may include experiencing decreased efficiency or being easily fatigued ...

   0   **No disturbance**

   1   **Doubtful, trivial.** Not reported without direct questioning.

   2   **Mild.** Efficiency somewhat reduced.

   3   **Moderate.** Easily fatigued, gets much less done than usual.

   4   **Severe.** Fatigue causes serious interference with functioning.

4. How would you rate your mood or depression today? (dysphoria). This may include feeling sad, depressed, blue, or moody ...

   0   **No moodiness / not depressed.**

   1   **Doubtful, trivial.** Not reported without direct questioning.

   2   **Mild.** Aware of feeling moody or emotional.

   3   **Moderate.** Marked spontaneous mood swings, occasional crying or feelings of loneliness.

   4   **Severe.** Severe, obvious and persistent moodiness / depression.

5. How would you rate your motor coordination today? This may include feeling clumsy, prone to accident, and lowered motor coordination ...

   0   **No disturbance.**

   1   **Doubtful, trivial.** Not reported without direct questioning.

   2   **Mild.** Feels clumsy or awkward.

   3   **Moderate.** Frequent accidents while doing simple housework or on the job.

   4   **Severe.** Severe impairment in motor coordination.

6. How would you rate your mental and cognitive functioning today? This may include being forgetful, having poor concentration, being confused ...

0   **No disturbance.**

1   **Doubtful, trivial.** Not reported without direct questioning.

2   **Mild.** Slight forgetfulness and distractibility.

3   **Moderate.** Performance impaired by poor concentration, disorganized thinking, forgetfulness, etc.

4   **Severe.** Marked deterioration in thinking capacity or poor judgement leading to regrettable decisions.

7. How would you rate your eating habits today? *(This scale ranges from 0 to 2)*

0   **No disturbance.**

1   **Mild.** Mild increase in food intake including eating at odd or irregular hours, mostly snacks and sweets.

2   **Severe.** An obvious, marked increase including uncontrollable cravings for sweets, chocolates, etc.

8. How would you rate your sexual drive and activity today? *(This scale ranges from 0 to 2. Circle also increase or decrease).*

0   **No disturbance.**

1   **Mild.** Mild consistent increase / decrease.

2   **Severe.** Obvious change in sexual drive and a definite change in sexual behavior increase / decrease.

9. How would you rate your physical symptoms today? These may include painful or tender breasts, swelling, water retention, weight gain, headaches, low back pain ...

0   **No physical symptoms.**

1   **Doubtful, trivial.** Not reported without direct questioning.

2   **Mild.** Some symptoms and an increased awareness of bodily changes.

3   **Moderate.** Obvious changes and complaints.

4   **Severe.** Incapacitating symptoms including pain and discomfort, marked water retention and swelling, a weight gain of more than 5 pounds, etc.

10. How would you rate your social impairment today? This may include avoidance of social activities and interactions with family at home, at work, at school, etc.

0   **No social impairment.**

1   **Doubtful, trivial.** Not reported without direct questioning.

2   **Mild.** Some avoidance of social activity.

3   **Moderate.** Obvious impairment of social activity, mainly noticeable at home with family.

4   **Severe.** Marked impairment, withdrawal or isolation from most social interactions including those at work or school.

Calculate the total score by summing all subscale scores. There should be 10 symptoms subscores for a total score ranging from 0 to 36.

___ / 4 + ___ / 4 + ___ / 4 + ___ 4 + ___ / 4 + ___ / 4 + ___ / 2 + ___ / 2 + ___ / 4 + ___ / 4 = ___ / 36

SLEEP DISORDERS

RATING SCALES

TABLE OF CONTENTS

A. PITTSBURGH SLEEP QUALITY INDEX (PSQI)

OVERVIEW

The Pittsburgh Sleep Quality Index (PSQI) was developed by Daniel J Buysse and collaborators to measure quality of sleep and to help discriminate between individuals who experience poor sleep versus individuals who sleep well. The scale has several domains which include Subjective Sleep Quality, Sleep Latency, Sleep Duration, Habitual Sleep Efficiency, Sleep Disturbances, Use of Sleep Medication, and Day Time Dysfunction. The scale has two parts: 19 self-rated questions, utilized to rate the scale, and 5 questions rated by a bed partner. Most of the items are organized in multiple choice questions and are brief and easy to understand and answer. The PSQI questions are rated from 0 = no difficulty to 3 = severe difficulty generating scores that correspond to the domains of the scale. The scores range from 0-21 and the authors suggest that a score >5 be considered as a significant sleep disturbance.

GENERAL APPLICATIONS

The PSQI was developed to provide an accurate measure of sleep quality.

SELECTED PSYCHOMETRIC PROPERTIES

The reliability of the scale is considered good with Cronbach's alpha of 0.83 for the total score. Test-retest reliability is also considered good. The validity of the scale has been described by the authors as good with a sensitivity of 89.6% and a specificity of 86.5% of patient versus control subjects.

REFERENCES

Buysse DJ, Reynolds CF 3rd, Monk TH, et al, "The Pittsburgh Sleep Quality Index: A New Instrument for Psychiatric Practice and Research," *Psychiatry Res*, 1989, 28(2):193-213.

COPYRIGHT

Daniel J Buysse, MD
Western Psychiatric Institute and Clinic
3811 O'Hara Street
Pittsburgh, PA 15213

SCALE GENERALLY DONE BY

The scale has two parts. The first part is self rated and the second is rated by a bed partner. The scale can also be given by a clinician or research assistant.

TIME TO COMPLETE SCALE

5-10 minutes

REPRESENTATIVE STUDY UTILIZING SCALE

Stein MB, Kroft CD, and Walker JR, "Sleep Impairment in Patients With Social Phobia," *Psychiatry Res*, 1993, 49(3):251-6.

PITTSBURGH SLEEP QUALITY INDEX

Instructions:
The following questions relate to your usual sleep habits during the past month only. Your answers should indicate the most accurate reply for the majority of days and nights in the past month. Please answer all questions.

1. During the past month, what time have you usually gone to bed at night?

> BED TIME _____

2. During the past month, how long (in minutes) has it usually taken you to fall asleep each night?

> NUMBER OF MINUTES _____

3. During the past month, what time have you usually gotten up in the morning?

> GETTING UP TIME _____

4. During the past month, how many hours of actual sleep did you get at night? (This may be different than the number of hours you spent in bed.)

> HOURS OF SLEEP PER NIGHT _____

For each of the remaining questions, check the one best response. Please answer all questions.

5. During the past month, how often have you had trouble sleeping because you .....

a) Cannot get to sleep within 30 minutes

| Not during the past month ____ | Less than once a week ____ | Once or twice a week ____ | Three or more times a week ____ |

b) Wake up in the middle of the night or early morning

| Not during the past month ____ | Less than once a week ____ | Once or twice a week ____ | Three or more times a week ____ |

c) Have to get up to use the bathroom

| Not during the past month ____ | Less than once a week ____ | Once or twice a week ____ | Three or more times a week ____ |

d) Cannot breath comfortably

| Not during the past month ____ | Less than once a week ____ | Once or twice a week ____ | Three or more times a week ____ |

e) Cough or snore loudly

| Not during the past month ____ | Less than once a week ____ | Once or twice a week ____ | Three or more times a week ____ |

A. PITTSBURGH SLEEP QUALITY INDEX (PSQI) *(Continued)*

f) Feel too cold

    Not during the   Less than   Once or twice   Three or more
    past month _____   once a week _____   a week _____   times a week _____

g) Feel too hot

    Not during the   Less than   Once or twice   Three or more
    past month _____   once a week _____   a week _____   times a week _____

h) Had bad dreams

    Not during the   Less than   Once or twice   Three or more
    past month _____   once a week _____   a week _____   times a week _____

i) Have pain

    Not during the   Less than   Once or twice   Three or more
    past month _____   once a week _____   a week _____   times a week _____

j) Other reason(s), please describe _____

_____

How often during the past month have you had trouble sleeping because of this?

    Not during the   Less than   Once or twice   Three or more
    past month _____   once a week _____   a week _____   times a week _____

6. During the past month, how would you rate your sleep quality overall?

    Very good _____

    Fairly good _____

    Fairly bad _____

    Very bad _____

7. During the past month, how often have you taken medicine to help you sleep (prescribed or "over-the-counter")?

    Not during the   Less than   Once or twice   Three or more
    past month _____   once a week _____   a week _____   times a week _____

8. During the past month, how often have you had trouble staying awake while driving, eating meals, or engaging in social activity?

    Not during the   Less than   Once or twice   Three or more
    past month _____   once a week _____   a week _____   times a week _____

9. During the past month, how much of a problem has it been for you to keep up enough enthusiasm to get things done?

No problem at all _____

Only a very slight problem _____

Somewhat of a problem _____

A very big problem _____

10. Do you have a bed partner or room mate?

No bed partner or room mate _____

Partner / room mate in other room _____

Partner in same room, but not same bed _____

Partner in same bed _____

If you have a room mate or bed partner, ask him / her how often in the past month you have had.....

a) Loud snoring

| Not during the past month ____ | Less than once a week ____ | Once or twice a week ____ | Three or more times a week ____ |

b) Long pauses between breaths while asleep

| Not during the past month ____ | Less than once a week ____ | Once or twice a week ____ | Three or more times a week ____ |

c) Legs twitching or jerking while asleep

| Not during the past month ____ | Less than once a week ____ | Once or twice a week ____ | Three or more times a week ____ |

d) Episodes of disorientation or confusion during sleep

| Not during the past month ____ | Less than once a week ____ | Once or twice a week ____ | Three or more times a week ____ |

e) Other restlessness while you sleep; please describe _____

_____

| Not during the past month ____ | Less than once a week ____ | Once or twice a week ____ | Three or more times a week ____ |

B. SLEEP DISORDERS QUESTIONNAIRE (SDQ)

OVERVIEW

The Sleep Disorders Questionnaire was developed by AB Douglass and collaborators to obtain reliable information for a differential diagnosis of sleep disorders. The questionnaire has several subscales which correspond to different diagnostic groups such as narcolepsy, periodic limb movement disorder, sleep apnea, psychiatric disorders, PTSD, and chronic fatigue syndrome. The SDQ scale is a self-report scale with 176 items that are rated with a 5-point scale in a session that usually lasts about 30 minutes. There is a scoring manual and computer software available from Dr Douglass. The authors have reported that the scale does not replace polysomnography as a means to obtain a diagnosis, but instead is a good initial screening instrument.

GENERAL APPLICATIONS

The SDQ is a screening scale for sleep disorders.

SELECTED PSYCHOMETRIC PROPERTIES

The reliability of the scale is good with a Cronbach's alpha range from 0.70-0.86. The test-retest reliability is good. The validity of the scale is very good. As reported by the authors, the scale was able to distinguish patients with the major cause for sleep problems including sleep apnea, narcolepsy, periodic limb movement disturbance, and psychiatric sleep disorders.

The SDQ subscales were created by canonical discriminant function analysis based on the responses of groups of patients who were diagnosed in the sleep lab as actually having the relevant disease. This makes the SDQ unique in the area, since almost all other instruments take a molar, factor-analysis approach. They end up with clusters of related sleep symptoms, rather than the specifically diagnostic approach taken by the SDQ. The SDQ was validated on patients referred by a general practitioner to a sleep disorders center, and so is not currently approved for epidemiological screening.

REFERENCES

Douglass AB, Bornstein R, Nino-Murcia G, et al, "Creation of the ASDC Sleep Disorders Questionnaire," *Sleep Research*, 1986, 15:117.

Douglass AB, *Sleep Disorders Questionnaire (SDQ) Scoring Manual — Version B*, Ann Arbor, MI: Douglass, 1993

Douglass AB, Bornstein R, Nino-Murcia G, et al, "The Sleep Disorders Questionnaire I: Creation and Multivariate Structure of SDQ," *Sleep*, 1994, 17(2):160-7.

COPYRIGHT

The SDQ is copyrighted by Alan B Douglass and colleagues, to whom only academic questions should be directed. The SDQ is licensed to SleepLab Software LTD for all sales and distribution.

SleepLab Software LTD
PO Box 131429
Ann Arbor, MI
48113-1429
e-mail: info@sleeplabsoftware.com
www.sleeplabsoftware.com

SCALE GENERALLY DONE BY

Self-rated scale

TIME TO COMPLETE SCALE

30 minutes

REPRESENTATIVE STUDY UTILIZING SCALE

Smith S and Trinder J, "Detecting Insomnia: Comparison of Four Self-Report Measures of Sleep in a Young Adult Population," *J Sleep Res*, 2001, 10(3):229-35.

B. SLEEP DISORDERS QUESTIONNAIRE (SDQ) *(Continued)*

SAMPLE ENTRIES OF THE

SDQ
SLEEP DISORDERS QUESTIONNAIRE

Instructions:

This questionnaire will give your doctor a good understanding about your problems with sleeping and waking. It is very important to answer every question, because some disorders show up as a pattern of answers to different questions.

In answering the questions, consider each question as applying to the ***past six months*** of your life, unless you have been told differently by the person who gave you this booklet.

Some people work night shift, or rotating shifts. Others have a very changeable bedtime. For these people, questions which ask about "day, daytime, morning, etc" will mean the time when they wake from their longest sleep of the day and become active. Similarly, "night, nighttime, bedtime, nocturnal" would refer to whenever they are having their longest sleep of the day.

Most of the questions are simple statements. You answer by circling a number from 1 to 5. If you strongly disagree with the statement, or if it never happens to you, answer "1". If the statement is always true in your case, or you agree strongly with it, answer "5". You may also choose "2 rarely", "3 sometimes", or "4 usually" as your answer. Notice that an "answer key" appears at the bottom of each page to remind you what is meant by the numbers. Please answer all of the questions.

Here is an example of how to fill out a question:

1. How often does it snow in Florida in July?　　　　　①2　3　4　5

IF YOU ARE CERTAIN THAT A QUESTION DOES NOT APPLY TO YOU, LEAVE IT BLANK. But...... try to answer every question if at all possible. This is important. Notice that answer "1" can mean that the things asked in the question ***never*** happen to you. If you are using the computerized answer sheet, blacken the space which corresponds to your answer, "1 to 5", instead of circling the answer in this booklet.

1.	I get too little sleep at night	1	2	3	4	5
2.	I often have a poor night's sleep	1	2	3	4	5
3.	I have trouble getting to sleep at night	1	2	3	4	5
4.	I wake up often during the night	1	2	3	4	5
5.	My bedtime varies a lot	1	2	3	4	5
6.	At bedtime, thoughts race through my mind	1	2	3	4	5
7.	At bedtime, I feel sad and depressed	1	2	3	4	5
8.	At bedtime, I worry about things	1	2	3	4	5
9.	At bedtime, I feel muscular tension	1	2	3	4	5
10.	At bedtime, I'm afraid of not being able to go to sleep	1	2	3	4	5
11.	When falling asleep, I feel paralyzed (unable to move)	1	2	3	4	5

Partial listing of SDQ; full questionnaire is 176 questions.

SEXUAL DISORDERS

RATING SCALES

TABLE OF CONTENTS

A. ARIZONA SEXUAL EXPERIENCES SCALE (ASEX)

OVERVIEW

The Arizona Sexual Experience Scale (ASEX) was developed by the Department of Psychiatry and Psychology at the University of Arizona and the Department of Psychiatry and Behavioral Sciences, Stanford University. The ASEX scale is a simple scale designed to measure 5 items identified by the authors as core elements of sexual function. These elements are sexual drive, arousal, penile erection/vaginal lubrication, ability to reach orgasm, and satisfaction from orgasm. The items are rated on a 6-point Likert scale ranging from 1 (hyperfunction) to 6 (hypofunction). The scale has two versions, one for males and one for females, with a difference in question 3 that references penile erections versus vaginal lubrication. The scales are easy to complete and the results may be used to assess current levels of sexual dysfunction or to monitor changes in sexual dysfunction over time following clinical interventions. The scale is useful in clinical trials to evaluate potential dysfunction caused by medications. A total score of more than 18 on the ASEX or a score of 5 (very difficult) or greater on any one item is associated with clinical sexual dysfunction.

GENERAL APPLICATIONS

The ASEX assesses any decrease, difficulty, and/or dissatisfaction associated with sexual function in either men or women.

SELECTED PSYCHOMETRIC PROPERTIES

The scale shows an excellent internal consistency and reliability with a Cronbach's alpha of 0.9055 and a strong test-retest reliability. The ASEX has very good validity and the items correlate relatively well with the items of other more extensive scales such as the Brief Index of Sexual Functioning (BISF). The ASEX differentiates patients from controls.

REFERENCES

McGahuey CA, Gelenberg AJ, Laukes CA, et al, "The Arizona Sexual Experience Scale (ASEX): Reliability and Validity," *J Sex Marital Ther*, 2000, 26(1):25-40.

COPYRIGHT

The Arizona Board of Regents for the University of Arizona
http://www.psychiatry.arizona.edu/

SCALE GENERALLY DONE BY

Self-rated scale but may be completed by an interviewer

TIME TO COMPLETE SCALE

5 minutes

REPRESENTATIVE STUDY UTILIZING SCALE

Gelenberg AJ, McGahuey C, Laukes C, et al, "Mirtazapine Substitution in SSRI-Induced Sexual Dysfunction," *J Clin Psychiatry*, 2000, 61(5):356-60.

ARIZONA SEXUAL EXPERIENCES (ASEX) - MALE

For each item, please indicate your OVERALL level during the PAST WEEK, including TODAY

1. How strong is your sex drive?

1	2	3	4	5	6
extremely strong	very strong	somewhat strong	somewhat weak	very weak	no sex drive

2. How easily are you sexually aroused (turned on)?

1	2	3	4	5	6
extremely easily	very easily	somewhat easily	somewhat difficult	very difficult	never aroused

3. Can you easily get and keep an erection?

1	2	3	4	5	6
extremely easily	very easily	somewhat easily	somewhat difficult	very difficult	never

4. How easily can you reach an orgasm?

1	2	3	4	5	6
extremely easily	very easily	somewhat easily	somewhat difficult	very difficult	never reach orgasm

5. Are your orgasms satisfying?

1	2	3	4	5	6
extremely satisfying	very satisfying	somewhat satisfying	somewhat unsatisfying	very unsatisfying	can't reach orgasm

Comments

_____

_____

_____

_____

A. ARIZONA SEXUAL EXPERIENCES SCALE (ASEX) *(Continued)*

ARIZONA SEXUAL EXPERIENCES (ASEX) - FEMALE

For each item, please indicate your OVERALL level during the PAST WEEK, including TODAY

1. How strong is your sex drive?

1	2	3	4	5	6
extremely strong	very strong	somewhat strong	somewhat weak	very weak	no sex drive

2. How easily are you sexually aroused (turned on)?

1	2	3	4	5	6
extremely easily	very easily	somewhat easily	somewhat difficult	very difficult	never aroused

3. How easily does your vagina become moist or wet during sex?

1	2	3	4	5	6
extremely easily	very easily	somewhat easily	somewhat difficult	very difficult	never

4. How easily can you reach an orgasm?

1	2	3	4	5	6
extremely easily	very easily	somewhat easily	somewhat difficult	very difficult	never reach orgasm

5. Are your orgasms satisfying?

1	2	3	4	5	6
extremely satisfying	very satisfying	somewhat satisfying	somewhat unsatisfying	very unsatisfying	can't reach orgasm

Comments

_____

_____

_____

_____

B. BRIEF SEXUAL FUNCTION INVENTORY (BSFI)

OVERVIEW

The Brief Sexual Function Inventory (BSFI) is a very brief self-report inventory developed by MP O'Leary and collaborators to measure the current sexual function of males. Initially it was utilized in urology studies but is now utilized to measure outcomes in other clinical research.

The scale has 11 items, scored in a 5-point Likert-type scale that covers sex drive, erectile capacity, ejaculatory function, and satisfaction with sexual performance. The inventory provides a quick, reliable way to screen the general clinical population for male sexual dysfunction. It is also helpful for utilization in clinical research.

GENERAL APPLICATIONS

The BSFI measures sexual functioning in men.

SELECTED PSYCHOMETRIC PROPERTIES

According to the authors, the internal consistency reliabilities have been in the range of 0.85-0.90 and the test-retest reliabilities, as measured by the intraclass correlation coefficient, have been in the range of 0.85-0.90.

REFERENCES

O'Leary MP, Fowler FJ, Lenderking WR, et al, "A Brief Male Sexual Function Inventory for Urology," *Urology*, 1995, 46(5):697-706.

COPYRIGHT

Michael P O'Leary, MD, MHP
Department of Surgery, Urology
Brigham and Women's Hospital
75 Francis Street
Boston, MA 02115
Tel: 781-732-6325

SCALE GENERALLY DONE BY

Self-rated

TIME TO COMPLETE SCALE

5-10 minutes

REPRESENTATIVE STUDY UTILIZING SCALE

Altwein JE and Keuler FU, "Oral Treatment of Erectile Dysfunction With Apomorphine SL," *Urol Int*, 2001, 67(4):257-63.

B. BRIEF SEXUAL FUNCTION INVENTORY (BSFI) *(Continued)*

BRIEF MALE SEXUAL FUNCTION INVENTORY

SEXUAL DRIVE					
Let's define sexual drive as a feeling that may include wanting to have a sexual experience (masturbation or intercourse), thinking about having sex, or feeling frustrated due to lack of sex.					
1. During the past 30 days, on how many days have you felt sexual drive?	No days	Only a few days	Some days	Most days	Almost every day
	0	1	2	3	4
2. During the past 30 days, how would you rate your level of sexual drive?	None at all	Low	Medium	Medium high	High
	0	1	2	3	4
ERECTIONS					
3. Over the past 30 days, how often have you had partial or full sexual erections when you were sexually stimulated in any way?	Not at all	A few times	Fairly often	Usually	Always
	0	1	2	3	4
4. Over the past 30 days, when you had erections, how often were they firm enough to have sexual intercourse?					
	0	1	2	3	4
5. How much difficulty did you have getting an erection during the past 30 days?	Did not get erections at all	A lot of difficulty	Some difficulty	Little difficulty	No difficulty
	0	1	2	3	4
EJACULATION					
6. In the past 30 days, how much difficulty have you had ejaculating when you have been sexually stimulated?	Have had no sexual stimulation in past month	A lot of difficulty	Some difficulty	Little difficulty	No difficulty
	0	1	2	3	4
7. In the past 30 days, how much did you consider the amount of semen you ejaculate to be a problem for you?	Did not climax	Big problem	Medium problem	Small problem	No problem
	0	1	2	3	4
PROBLEM ASSESSMENT					
8. In the past 30 days, to what extent have you considered a lack of sex drive to be a problem?	Big problem	Medium problem	Small problem	Very small problem	No problem
	0	1	2	3	4
9. In the past 30 days, to what extent have you considered your ability to get and keep erections to be a problem?					
	0	1	2	3	4
10. In the past 30 days, to what extent have you considered your ejaculation to be a problem?					
	0	1	2	3	4
OVERALL SATISFACTION					
11. Overall, during the past 30 days, how satisfied have you been with your sex life?	Very dissatisfied	Mostly dissatisfied	Neutral or mixed (about equally satisfied and dissatisfied)	Mostly satisfied	Very satisfied
	0	1	2	3	4

Used and reprinted with permission from O'Leary MP, Fowler FJ, Lenderking WR, et al, "A Brief Male Sexual Functioning Inventory for Urology," *Urology*, 1995, 46(5):697-706.

C. RUSH SEXUAL INVENTORY (RSI)

OVERVIEW

The Rush Sexual Inventory (RSI) is a self-rated inventory developed by John Zajecka and collaborators to be a short and comprehensive instrument designed to assess changes in sexual function over time.

The inventory consists of five visual analogs and a series of individual "yes/no" gender separated items. The inventory also includes a series of questions about premorbid and current sexual functioning. The instrument is sensitive to evaluate medication-induced changes.

GENERAL APPLICATIONS

The RSI measures changes in sexual function in both men and women.

SELECTED PSYCHOMETRIC PROPERTIES

The authors report a Cronbach's alpha of 0.77 for females and 0.75 for males. In terms of validity the RSI has significant correlation with the BISF and the BSFQ.

REFERENCES

Zajecka J, Mitchell S, and Fawcett J, "Treatment-Emergent Changes in Sexual Function With Selective Serotonin Reuptake Inhibitors as Measured With the Rush Sexual Inventory," *Psychopharmacol Bull*, 1997, 33(4):755-60.

COPYRIGHT

John M Zajecka, MD
Treatment and Research Center
Rush-Presbyterian-St Luke's Medical Center
1725 West Harrison
Chicago, IL 60612
e-mail: john_zajecka@rush.edu

SCALE GENERALLY DONE BY

Self-rated

TIME TO COMPLETE SCALE

7-10 minutes

REPRESENTATIVE STUDY UTILIZING SCALE

Zajecka J, Mitchell S, and Fawcett J, "Treatment-Emergent Changes in Sexual Function With Selective Serotonin Reuptake Inhibitors as Measured With the Rush Sexual Inventory," *Psychopharmacol Bull*, 1997, 33(4):755-60.

C. RUSH SEXUAL INVENTORY (RSI) *(Continued)*

SAMPLE ITEMS OF THE
MODIFIED RUSH SEXUAL INVENTORY

WEEK 0 VISIT

1. Have you ever experienced sexual dysfunction while taking any medications?

    1 ☐ Yes (explain): _____
    2 ☐ No

5. Have you ever been evaluated for a sexual dysfunction?

    1 ☐ Yes (explain): _____
    2 ☐ No

Rate each item as it applies in the past 8 weeks.

7. For each item below, place a mark on the line where you would place yourself.

EXAMPLE:

    |_____|_____|
    Infrequent   Very frequent

   a. How frequently do you have pleasurable sexual thoughts?

    |_____|
    Infrequent   Very frequent

   d. How often do you initiate sexual activity?

    |_____|
    Infrequent   Very frequent

---

9. Males only:
Please check Yes, No or N/A (not applicable) for each item as it applies to you over the past 8 weeks (one of the 3 choices must be checked for each item).

☐ N/A (female patient)

	Yes	No	N/A
a. Spontaneous daytime erections	☐	☐	☐
h. Requiring more stimuli than usual to maintain an erection	☐	☐	☐
r. Orgasm without erection	☐	☐	☐
t. Genital pain during sexual contact	☐	☐	☐

Females only:
Please check Yes, No or N/A (not applicable) for each item as it applies to you over the past 8 weeks (one of the 3 choices must be checked for each item).

☐ N/A (male patient)

	Yes	No	N/A
a. Increased sensitivity, other than pain, in breasts upon physical contact	☐	☐	☐
g. Inadequate swelling or vaginal lubrication during sexual arousal	☐	☐	☐
l. Experiencing orgasm without sexual provocation (spontaneously)	☐	☐	☐
p. Physical pain during sexual activity	☐	☐	☐

GERIATRIC

RATING SCALES

TABLE OF CONTENTS

A. ALZHEIMER'S DISEASE ASSESSMENT SCALE (ADAS)

OVERVIEW

The ADAS, developed by RC Mohs and WG Rosen, is a 21-item scale which measures severity of dysfunction in cognitive behaviors and noncognitive behaviors characteristic of Alzheimer's disease. Cognitive and memory task items comprise 60% of the total possible points. There is a cognitive subscale (nine items), a noncognitive subscale (ten items) and a memory task subscale (2 items). The items are rated differently depending on the domain being evaluated. This includes rating of severity of symptoms on a 1 to 5 spectrum (1 = least impaired, 5 = most impaired) and ability to complete tasks with calculation of errors/proportion of task completed. The ADAS appears sensitive to increasing dysfunction as the illness progresses, and thus may be used to track course of illness. A limitation of the scale is that its use may be less reliable in severely dysfunctional individuals with Alzheimer's disease.

GENERAL APPLICATIONS

The ADAS is used to assess cognitive and noncognitive behavioral problems in individuals with Alzheimer's disease.

SELECTED PSYCHOMETRIC PROPERTIES

Interrater reliability of the ADAS is good, with correlations ranging from 0.65 to 0.989. Test-retest reliability has been reported to range from 0.514 to 1.0 for individuals with Alzheimer's disease over 1-2 months.

REFERENCES

Rosen WG, Mohs RC, and Davis KL, "A New Rating Scale for Alzheimer's Disease," *Am J Psychiatry*, 1984, 141(11):1356-64.

COPYRIGHT

Richard Mohs, PhD
Psychiatry Service (116A)
Mt Sinai School of Medicine
VA Medical Center
130 W Kingsbridge Rd
Bronx, NY 10468

SCALE GENERALLY DONE BY

Clinician or trained rater

TIME TO COMPLETE SCALE

30-45 minutes

REPRESENTATIVE STUDY UTILIZING SCALE

Knapp MJ, Knopman DS, Solomon PR, et al, "A 30-Week Randomized Controlled Trial of High-Dose Tacrine in Patients With Alzheimer's Disease. The Tacrine Study Group," *JAMA*, 1994, 271(13):985-91.

THE ALZHEIMER'S DISEASE ASSESSMENT SCALE

Rating Scale

* = Not assessed
0 = Not present
1 = Very mild
2 = Mild
3 = Moderate
4 = Moderately severe
5 = Severe

Cognitive Behavior

_____ 1. Spoken language ability

_____ 2. Comprehension of spoken language

_____ 3. Recall of test instructions

_____ 4. Word-finding difficulty

_____ 5. Following commands

_____ 6. Naming: Objects, fingers

High: 1 2 3 4   Fingers: Thumb

Medium: 1 2 3 4   Pinky: Index

Low: 1 2 3 4   Middle: Ring

_____ 7. Constructions: Drawing

Figures correct: 1 2 3 4

Closing in: Yes ____ No ____

_____ 8. Ideational praxis

Step correct: 1 2 3 4 5

_____ 9. Orientation

Day _____ Year _____ Person _____ Time of day _____

Date _____ Month _____ Season _____ Place _____

_____ 10. Word recall: Mean error score

_____ 11. Word recognition: Mean error score

_____ **Cognition Total**

A. ALZHEIMER'S DISEASE ASSESSMENT SCALE (ADAS) *(Continued)*

Noncognitive Behavior

_____ 12. Tearful

_____ 13. Appears/reports depressed mood

_____ 14. Concentration, distractibility

_____ 15. Uncooperative to testing

_____ 16. Delusions

_____ 17. Hallucinations

_____ 18. Pacing

_____ 19. Increased motor activity

_____ 20. Tremors

_____ 21. Increase/decrease appetite

_____ **Noncognition Total**

Total Scores

_____ Cognitive behavior

_____ Noncognitive behavior

_____ Word recall

_____ Word recognition

_____ **Total**

ADMINISTRATION AND SCORING PROCEDURES

The word recall task is administered first. The next 10 minutes are spent in open-ended conversation in order to assess various aspects of expressive and receptive speech. Then the remaining cognitive tasks are administered. Noncognitive behaviors are evaluated from report of the patient or reliable informant or observed during the interview. If the patient has more than a mild memory impairment, ratings on behavioral items are based on the informant's report.

The rating scale of 0-5 reflects the degree of severity of dysfunction. A rating of 0 signifies no impairment on a task or absence of a particular behavior. A rating of 5 is reserved for the most severe degree of impairment or very high frequency of occurrence of a behavior. A rating of 1 signifies a very mild presence of a behavior or corresponds to a particular performance on a task. Ratings of 2, 3, or 4 correspond to mild, moderate, and moderately severe, respectively. Ratings on many cognitive behaviors correspond to levels of performance on task.

Cognitive Behavior

Language. Language abilities are evaluated throughout the interview and on specific tests. Questions eliciting "yes" and "no" answers assess comprehension on a very basic level. Other questions should require specific information and well-developed communication skills.

1. *Spoken language ability.* This item is a global rating of the quality of speech (ie, clarity, difficulty in making oneself understood). Quantity is **not** rated on this item.

   1 = Very mild; one instance of lack of understandability
   2 = Mild
   3 = Moderate; subject has difficulty 25% to 50% of the time
   4 = Moderately severe; subject has difficulty 50% of the time
   5 = Severe; one or two word utterances; fluent but empty speech; mute

2. *Comprehension of spoken language.* This item evaluates the patient's ability to understand speech. Do not include responses to commands.

   1 = Very mild; one instance of misunderstanding
   2 = Mild
   3 = Moderate
   4 = Moderately severe; requires several repetitions and rephrasing
   5 = Severe; patient rarely responds to questions appropriately, not due to poverty of speech

3. *Recall of test instructions.* The patient's ability to remember the requirements of the recognition task is evaluated. On each recognition trial, the patient is asked prior to presentation of the first two words, "Did you see this word before or is this a new word?" For the third word, the patient is asked, "How about this one?" If the patient responds appropriately (eg, "yes" or "no"), then recall of instructions is accurate. If the patient fails to respond, this signifies that the instructions have been forgotten. Then instruction is repeated. The procedure used for the third word is repeated for words 4-24. Each instance of recall failure is noted.

   1 = Very mild; forgets once
   2 = Mild; must be reminded 2 times
   3 = Moderate; must be reminded 3 or 4 times
   4 = Moderately severe; must be reminded 5 or 6 times
   5 = Severe; must be reminded 7 or more times

4. *Word-finding difficulty in spontaneous speech.* The patient has difficulty in finding the desired word in spontaneous speech. The problem may be overcome by circumlocution (ie, giving explanatory phrases or nearly satisfactory synonyms). Do not include finger and object naming in this rating.

   1 = Very mild; one or two instances, not clinically significant
   2 = Mild; noticeable circumlocution or synonym substitution
   3 = Moderate; loss of words without compensation on occasion
   4 = Moderately severe; frequent loss of words without compensation
   5 = Severe; nearly total loss of content words; speech sounds empty; one-two-word utterances.

5. *Following commands.* Receptive speech is assessed also on the patient's ability to carry out one- to five-step commands (26).

   1. Make a *fist.*
   2. Point to the *ceiling*, then to the *floor.*

   Line up a pencil, watch, and card, in that order, on a table in front of the patient.

   3. Put the *pencil on top of the card*, then *put it back.*
   4. Put the *watch* on the *other side of the pencil* and *turn over the card.*
   5. Tap *each shoulder twice* with *two fingers*, keeping your *eyes shut.*

   Each underlined element represents a single step. The command may be repeated once in its entirety. Each command scored is as a whole. Ratings correspond to the highest level of command correctly performed.

   0 = Five steps correct
   1 = Four steps correct
   2 = Three steps correct
   3 = Two steps correct
   4 = One step correct
   5 = Cannot do one step correctly

A. ALZHEIMER'S DISEASE ASSESSMENT SCALE (ADAS) *(Continued)*

6. *Naming objects and fingers.* The patient names the fingers of his/her dominant hand. The patient names 12 randomly presented real objects, whose frequency values (27) are high, medium, or low. Objects and their frequency are:

	Frequency	
High	*Medium*	*Low*
Flower (plastic)	Rattle	Wallet
Bed (doll house furniture)	Mask	Harmonica
Whistle	Scissors	Stethoscope
Pencil	Comb	Tongs

0 = All correct; one finger incorrect and/or one object incorrect
1 = Two-three fingers and/or two objects incorrect
2 = Two or more fingers and 3-5 objects incorrect
3 = Three or more fingers and 6-7 objects incorrect
4 = Three or more fingers and 8-9 objects incorrect

7. *Constructional praxis.* The ability to copy four geometric forms is assessed. These forms, in the order of presentation, are

1. Circle, approximately 20 cm in diameter.

2. Two overlapping rectangles.
   The vertical rectangle is 20 cm x 25 cm.
   The horizontal rectangle is 10 cm x 35 cm.

3. Rhombus.
   Each side is 20 cm.
   Acute = 50°, obtuse = 130°

4. Cube.
   Each side is 20 cm.
   Internal lines are present.

Each form is located in the upper middle of a 5-1/2" x 8-1/2" sheet of white paper. The patient is instructed, "Do you see this figure? Make one that looks like this anywhere on the paper." Two attempts are permitted.

0 = All four drawings correct
1 = One form incorrect
2 = Two forms incorrect
3 = Three forms incorrect
4 = Closing in (draws over or around model or uses parts of model); four forms incorrect
5 = No figures drawn, scribbles; parts of forms; word instead of form

Scoring criteria for each form (examples shown below*):

1. Circle. A closed curved figure.
2. Two overlapping rectangles. Forms must be 4-sided and overlap must be similar to presented form. Changes in size are not scored.
3. Rhombus (diamond). Figure must be 4-sided, obliquely oriented, and the sides approximately equal length. Four measurements are taken (see figure below*). These are ac, a'c, bc, b'c. The ratio of ac/a'c or a'c/ac ranges from .75 to 1.00. the ratio of bc/b'c or b'c/bc ranges from 0.60 to 1.00. The ratio bb'/aa' ranges from 3 to 0.75. Figure is incorrect if any ratio is outside these ranges.
4. Cube. The form is 3-dimensional, with front face in the correct orientation, internal lines drawn correctly between corners. If opposite sides of faces are not parallel by more than 20°, it is incorrect.

*2. Correct   Incorrect   3. Model   4. Incorrect

8. *Ideational praxis.* The patient is given an 8-1/2" x 11" sheet of paper and a long envelope. The patient is instructed to pretend to send the letter to himself or herself. The patient is told to put the paper into the envelope, seal it, address it to himself or herself, and stamp it. If the patient forgets part of the task, reinstruction is given. Impairment on this item should reflect dysfunction in executing an overlearned task only and not recall difficulty. The five components to the task are 1) fold letter, 2) put letter in envelope, 3) seal envelope, 4) address envelope, 5) put stamp on envelope.

      1 = Difficulty or failure to perform one component
      2 = Difficulty and/or failure to perform two components
      3 = Difficulty and/or failure to perform three components
      4 = Difficulty and/or failure to perform four components
      5 = Difficulty and/or failure to perform five components

9. *Orientation.* The components of orientation are date, month, year, day of the week, season, time of day, place, and person. One point is given for each incorrect response (maximum = 8). Acceptable answers include ±1 for the date, within 1 hour for the hour, partial name for place, naming of upcoming season within 1 week before its onset, and name of previous season for 2 weeks after its termination.

10. *Word-recall task.* The patient reads 10 high-imagery words exposed for 2 seconds each. The patient then recalls the words aloud. Three trials of reading and recall are given. The score equals the mean number of words not recalled on three trials (maximum = 10).

11. *Word-recognition task.* The patient reads aloud 12 high-imagery words. These words are then randomly mixed with 12 words the patient has not seen. The patient indicates whether or not the word was shown previously. Then two more trials of reading the original words and recognition are given. The score equals the mean number of incorrect responses for three trials (maximum = 12).

Noncognitive Behavior

The time period for evaluation includes the entire week before the interview for the following items:

    1. Appears or reports feeling sad, down, hopeless, discouraged
    2. Tearful
    3. Delusions
    4. Hallucinations
    5. Pacing
    6. Increased motor activity
    7. Increase/decrease in appetite

A. ALZHEIMER'S DISEASE ASSESSMENT SCALE (ADAS) *(Continued)*

12. *Tearful.* Patient/informant is asked about the frequency of occurrence of tearfulness.

   1 = Very mild; occurs one time during week or during test session only
   2 = Mild; occurs 2-3 times during the week
   3 = Moderate
   4 = Moderately severe; frequent crying spells nearly every day
   5 = Severe; frequent and prolonged crying spells every day

13. *Depression.* The patient or informant is asked if the patient has been sad, discouraged, down. If a positive response is given, further inquiry into the severity and pervasiveness of the mood, loss of interest or pleasure in activities, and reactivity to environmental events is made. The interviewer also assesses the patient for depressed facies and the ability to respond to encouragement and jokes.

   1 = Feels slightly dysphoric; clinically significant
   2 = Mild; appears and reports mild dysphoric mood, reactivity present, some loss of interest
   3 = Moderate; feels moderately dysphoric often
   4 = Moderately severe; feels dysphoric almost all the time with considerable loss of reactivity and interest
   5 = Severe; pervasive and severe degree of dysphoric mood; total lack of reactivity; pervasive loss of interest or pleasure

14. *Concentration/distractibility.* This item rates the frequency with which the patient is distracted by irrelevant stimuli and/or must be reoriented to the ongoing task because of loss of train of thought or the frequency with which the patient appears to be caught up in his or her own thoughts.

   1 = Very mild; one instance of poor concentration
   2 = Mild; 2-3 instances of poor concentration or distractibility
   3 = Moderate
   4 = Moderately severe; poor concentration throughout much of interview and/or frequent instances of distractibility
   5 = Severe; extreme difficulty in concentration and numerous instances of distractibility

15. *Uncooperative to testing.* This item rates the degree to which the patient objects to some aspects of the interview.

   1 = Very mild; one instance of lack of cooperation
   2 = Mild
   3 = Moderate
   4 = Moderately severe; needs frequent cajoling to complete interview
   5 = Severe; refuses to continue interview

16. *Delusions.* This item rates the extent and conviction of the patient's belief in ideas that are almost certainly not true. In rating severity, consider conviction in delusions, preoccupation, and effect they have on the patient's actions.

   1 = Very mild; one transient delusional belief
   2 = Mild; delusion definitely present but subject questions his or her belief
   3 = Moderate; patient convinced of delusion but it does not affect behavior
   4 = Moderately severe; delusion has effect on behavior
   5 = Severe; significant actions based on delusions

17. *Hallucinations.* Inquiry about visual, auditory, and tactile hallucinations is made. The frequency and degree of disruptiveness of hallucinations are rated.

   1 = Very mild; hears voice saying one word; visual hallucination once
   2 = Mild
   3 = Moderate; hallucinates numerous times during day, which interferes with normal functioning
   4 = Moderately severe
   5 = Severe; nearly constantly hallucinating, which totally disrupts normal functioning

18. *Pacing.* Rating on this item must distinguish between normal physical activity and excessive walking back and forth.

    1 = Very mild; very rare occurrence
    2 = Mild
    3 = Moderate; paces frequently each day
    4 = Moderately severe
    5 = Severe; cannot sit still and must pace excessively

19. *Increased motor activity.* This item is rated relative to the person's normal activity level or previously obtained baseline.

    1 = Very mild; very slight increase
    2 = Mild
    3 = Moderate; significant increase in amount of movement
    4 = Moderately severe
    5 = Severe; person must be moving constantly; rarely sits still

20. *Tremors.* Patient extends both hands in front of body and spreads the fingers, holding this position for approximately 10 seconds.

    1 = Very mild; very slight tremor; barely noticeable
    2 = Mild; noticeable tremor
    3 = Moderate
    4 = Moderately severe
    5 = Severe; very rapid movements with sizable displacements

21. *Increased/decreased appetite.* This item is included because appetite change may be associated with depression and because clinical observations of some Alzheimer patients reveal both increases and decreases in appetite. This item is rated relative to the person's normal appetite or previously obtained baseline.

    1 = Very mild; slight change, probably clinically significant
    2 = Mild; noticeable change, patient still eats without encouragement
    3 = Moderate; marked change; patient needs encouragement to eat; patient asks for more food
    4 = Moderately severe
    5 = Severe; patient will not eat and needs to be force-fed; patient complains of constant hunger despite consumption of sufficient quantities

B. BEHAVIORAL PATHOLOGY IN ALZHEIMER'S DISEASE (BEHAVE-AD)

OVERVIEW

The BEHAVE-AD, developed by B Reisberg et al, is a 25-item scale used to evaluate the behavioral symptoms of Alzheimer's disease. In the BEHAVE-AD all assessment measures are largely independent of the primary, cognitive symptoms of Alzheimer's disease. The separation of behavioral and cognitive symptoms, according to the authors of the scale, potentially allows researchers to evaluate the effects of psychotropic medications which may focus on psychiatric aspects of Alzheimer's disease, such as affective and psychotic symptoms. Video training material on the BEHAVE-AD is available from the author.

GENERAL APPLICATIONS

The BEHAVE-AD is used to assess behavioral symptoms of Alzheimer's disease.

SELECTED PSYCHOMETRIC PROPERTIES

Interrater reliability of the BEHAVE-AD is excellent with intraclass correlation coefficients for the BEHAVE-AD total scores of 0.95 to 0.96.

REFERENCES

Reisberg B, Borenstein J, Salob SP, et al, "Behavioral Symptoms in Alzheimer's Disease: Phenomenology and Treatment," *J Clin Psychiatry*, 1987, 48(Suppl):9-15.

COPYRIGHT

Barry Reisberg, MD
Aging and Dementia Research Program
Department of Psychiatry
New York University Medical Center
550 First Avenue
New York, NY 10016

SCALE GENERALLY DONE BY

Clinician or trained rater

TIME TO COMPLETE SCALE

10-20 minutes

REPRESENTATIVE STUDY UTILIZING SCALE

Street JS, Tollefson GD, Tohen M, et al, "Olanzapine for Psychotic Conditions in the Elderly," *Psych Ann*, 2000, 30(3):191-6.

BEHAVIORAL PATHOLOGY IN ALZHEIMER'S DISEASE (BEHAVE-AD)

(BASED UPON INFORMATION OBTAINED FROM CAREGIVER AND OTHER INFORMANTS)

Informant _____ Relationship to Patient: _____

PART 1: Symptomatology

(In preceding 2 weeks unless otherwise specified below)

Assessment Interval: _____ weeks

Circle the highest applicable severity rating (0 to 3) for each item. Each category of symptomatology (A to G) is scored independently.

A. Paranoid and Delusional Ideation
(a delusion is a false conviction, not a misidentification)

1. "People are stealing things" delusion.

   (0) Not present
   (1) Delusion that people are hiding objects.
   (2) Delusion that people are coming into the home and hiding or stealing objects.
   (3) Talking and listening to people coming into the home.

2. "One's house is not one's home" delusion.

   (0) Not present
   (1) Conviction that the place in which one is residing is not one's home (eg, packing to go home, complains while at home of "take me home").
   (2) Attempt to leave domiciliary to go home.
   (3) Violence in response to attempts to forcibly restrict exit.

3. "Spouse (or other caregiver) is an imposter" delusion.

   (0) Not present
   (1) Conviction that spouse (or other caregiver) is an imposter.
   (2) Anger towards spouse (or other caregiver) for being an imposter.
   (3) Violence towards spouse (or other caregiver) for being an imposter.

4. Delusion of abandonment (eg, to an institution).

   (0) Not present
   (1) Suspicion of caregiver plotting abandonment or institutionalization (eg, on the telephone).
   (2) Accusation of a conspiracy to abandon or institutionalize.
   (3) Accusation of impending or immediate desertion or institutionalization.

5. Delusion of infidelity (social and/or sexual unfaithfulness).

   (0) Not present
   (1) Conviction that spouse, children, and/or other caregivers are unfaithful.
   (2) Anger towards spouse, relative, or other caregiver for their infidelity.
   (3) Violence toward spouse, relative, or other caregiver for their infidelity.

B. BEHAVIORAL PATHOLOGY IN ALZHEIMER'S DISEASE (BEHAVE-AD)
(Continued)

6. Suspiciousness/Paranoia other than above

(0) Not present

(1) Suspiciousness (eg, hiding objects which they may later be unable to locate or a statement such as "I don't trust you").

(2) Paranoid (ie, fixed conviction with respect to suspicions and/or anger as a result of suspicions).

(3) Violence as a result of suspicions.

Unspecified? _____

Describe: _____

_____

_____

_____

7. Delusions (nonparanoid) other than above.

(0) Not present

(1) Delusional

(2) Verbal or emotional manifestations as a result of delusions.

(3) Physical actions or violence as a result of delusions.

Unspecified? _____

Describe: _____

_____

_____

_____

B. Hallucinations

8. Visual hallucinations

(0) Not present

(1) Vague, not clearly defined.

(2) Clearly defined hallucinations of objects and persons (eg, sees other people at the table).

(3) Verbal or physical actions or emotional responses to the hallucinations.

9. Auditory hallucinations

(0) Not present

(1) Vague, not clearly defined.

(2) Clearly defined hallucinations of words or phrases.

(3) Verbal or physical actions of emotional responses to the hallucinations.

10. Olfactory hallucinations

(0) Not present

(1) Vague, not clearly defined.

(2) Clearly defined hallucinations (eg, "smells a fire" or "something burning").

(3) Verbal or physical actions or emotional responses to the hallucinations.

11. Haptic (sense of touch) *hallucinations*

    (0) Not present
    (1) Vague, not clearly defined.
    (2) Clearly defined hallucinations (eg, "something is crawling on my body").
    (3) Verbal or physical actions or emotional responses to the hallucinations.

12. Other hallucinations

    (0) Not present
    (1) Vague, not clearly defined.
    (2) Clearly defined hallucinations.
    (3) Verbal or physical actions or emotional responses to the hallucinations.

Unspecified? _____

Describe: _____

_____

_____

_____

C. Activity Disturbances

13. Wandering (eg, away from home or caregiver).

    (0) Not present
    (1) Somewhat, but not sufficient as to require restraint.
    (2) Sufficient as to require restraint.
    (3) Verbal or physical actions or emotional responses to attempts to prevent wandering.

14. Purposeless activity (cognitive abulia).

    (0) Not present
    (1) Repetitive, purposeless activity (eg, opening and closing pocketbook, packing and unpacking clothing, repeatedly putting on and removing clothing, insistent repeating of demands or questions).
    (2) Pacing or other purposeless activity sufficient to require restraint.
    (3) Abrasions or physical harm resulting from purposeless activity.

15. Inappropriate activity.

    (0) Not present
    (1) Inappropriate activities (eg, storing and hiding objects in appropriate places, such as throwing clothing in wastebasket or putting empty plates in the oven; inappropriate sexual behavior, such as inappropriate exposure).
    (2) Present and sufficient to require restraint.
    (3) Present and sufficient to require restraint, and accompanied by anger or violence when restraint is used.

Unspecified? _____

Describe: _____

_____

_____

_____

B. BEHAVIORAL PATHOLOGY IN ALZHEIMER'S DISEASE (BEHAVE-AD)
(Continued)

D. Aggressiveness

16. Verbal outbursts.

(0) Not present
(1) Present (including unaccustomed use of foul or abusive language).
(2) Present and accompanied by anger.
(3) Present, accompanied by anger, and clearly directed at other persons.

17. Physical threats and/or violence.

(0) Not present
(1) Threatening behavior.
(2) Physical violence.
(3) Physical violence accompanied by vehemence.

18. Agitation (other than above).
(eg, nonverbal anger; negativity including refusal to bathe, dress, continue walking, take medications, etc; hyperventilation).

(0) Not present
(1) Present
(2) Present with emotional component
(3) Present with emotional component and physical component

E. Diurnal Rhythm Disturbances

19. Day/Night disturbance

(0) Not present
(1) Repetitive wakening during night (except for purpose of toileting).
(2) 50% to 75% of former sleep cycle at night.
(3) Complete disturbance of diurnal rhythm (less than 50% of former sleep cycle at night).

F. Affective Disturbance

20. Tearfulness (or whimpering or other "crying sounds").

(0) Not present
(1) Present
(2) Present accompanied by a clear affective component.
(3) Present and accompanied by affective and physical component (eg, wringing of hands or other gestures).

21. Depressed mood, other.

(0) Not present
(1) Present (eg, occasional statement "I wish I were dead," or "I'm going to kill myself," or "I feel like nothing," without clear affective concomitants).
(2) Present with clear concomitants (eg, thoughts of death).
(3) Present with emotional and physical concomitants (eg, suicidal gestures).

Unspecified? _____

Describe: _____

_____

_____

G. Anxieties and Phobias

22. Anxiety regarding upcoming events (Godot syndrome).

   (0) Not present
   (1) Present with repeated queries and/or other activities regarding upcoming appointments and/or events (eg, when are we going?).
   (2) Present and disturbing to caregivers.
   (3) Present and intolerable to caregivers.

23. Other anxieties.
   (eg, regarding money, the future, being away from home, health, memory, etc; or generalized anxiety such as thinking everything is "terribly wrong")

   (0) Not present
   (1) Present
   (2) Present and disturbing to caregivers.
   (3) Present and intolerable to caregivers.

Unspecified? _____

Describe: _____

_____

_____

24. Fear of being left alone.

   (0) Not present
   (1) Present with vocalized fear of being alone.
   (2) Vocalized and sufficient to require specific action on the part of the caregiver.
   (3) Vocalized and sufficient to require patient to be accompanied at all times (eg, patient must see the caregiver at all times).

25. Other phobias.
   (eg, fear of crowds, travel, darkness, people/strangers, bathing, etc)

   (0) Not present
   (1) Present
   (2) Present and of sufficient magnitude to require specific action by caregiver.
   (3) Present and sufficient to prevent patient activities.

Unspecified? _____

Describe: _____

_____

_____

TOTAL **SEVERITY** SCORE: _____

B. BEHAVIORAL PATHOLOGY IN ALZHEIMER'S DISEASE (BEHAVE-AD)
(Continued)

PART 2: Global Rating

Circle one choice. Are the symptoms which have been noted of sufficient magnitude as to be:

(0) Not at all troubling to the caregiver or dangerous to the patient.

(1) Mildly troubling to the caregiver or dangerous to the patient.

(2) Moderately troubling to the caregiver or dangerous to the patient.

(3) Severely troubling to the caregiver or dangerous to the patient.

Symptom most troubling to caregiver

"With respect to the symptoms which have been noted, which is the biggest problem for you and/or other caregivers?" (More than one symptom can be listed, but please give numerical order.)

_____

_____

_____

_____

_____

C. BLESSED DEMENTIA SCALE (BLS-D)

OVERVIEW

This scale, developed by G Blessed in 1968, has been utilized as a research instrument to quantify the cognitive and behavioral symptoms of patients with dementia and is part of a comprehensive package produced by Blessed. The other components are the Information Scale, the Memory Scale, and the Concentration Scale. These last three form the Blessed Information-Memory-Concentration Test (IMC). Other names for the Blessed Dementia Scale are the Blessed-Roth Dementia Scale, the Newcastle Dementia Scale, or the Dementia Rating Scale.

The BLS-D is a clinical scale that has 22 items organized in three major areas: 1. Change in performance of everyday activities (8 items), 2. Change in habits (3 items), and 3. Changes in personality, interests, and drive (11 items). The information is obtained from a caregiver and the ratings are based on a predetermined period of time, usually 6 months. The scores for each item are on a 3-point scale for the change in performance where total incompetence is 1, partial or variable incapacity is 1/2, and normal is 0. Other items in change of habits have fixed scores of 0, 1, 2, or 3. The scores go from 0 = normal to 28 = extreme incapacity.

GENERAL APPLICATIONS

The BLS-D evaluates cognitive and behavioral symptoms in individuals with dementia.

SELECTED PSYCHOMETRIC PROPERTIES

The interrater reliability for two raters is 0.59. This reliability is considered low and is probably due to the difficulty in scoring items, which call for complex judgments by the informant.

In terms of validity, the authors have reported scores correlated 0.77 with the count of plaques in the brain of several patients. The BLS-D scale correlates well with other dementia scales and has good predictive value in relation to the burden experience by caregivers.

REFERENCES

Blessed G, Tomlinson BE, and Roth M, "The Association Between Quantitative Measures of Dementia and of Senile Change in the Cerebral Gray Matter of Elderly Subjects," *Br J Psychiatry*, 1968, 114(512):797-811.

Blessed G, Tomlinson BE, and Roth M, "Blessed-Roth Dementia Scale (DS)," *Psychopharmacol Bull*, 1988, 24(4):705-8.

Cole MG, "Interrater Reliability of the Blessed Dementia Scale," *Can J Psychiatry*, 1990, 35(4):328-30.

Stern Y, Hesdorffer D, Sano M, et al, "Measurement and Prediction of Functional Capacity in Alzheimer's Disease," *Neurology*, 1990, 40(1):8-14.

COPYRIGHT

The Royal College of Psychiatrists
The British Journal of Psychiatry
17 Belgrave Square, SW1X 8PG

C. BLESSED DEMENTIA SCALE (BLS-D) *(Continued)*

SCALE GENERALLY DONE BY

Trained clinicians

TIME TO COMPLETE SCALE

15-30 minutes

REPRESENTATIVE STUDY UTILIZING SCALE

Binetti G, Locascio JJ, Corkin S, et al, "Differences Between Pick Disease and Alzheimer Disease in Clinical Appearance and Rate of Cognitive Decline," *Arch Neurol*, 2000, 57(2):225-32.

BLESSED DEMENTIA SCALE

Changes in Performance of Everyday Activities

1. Inability to perform household tasks	1	1/2	0
2. Inability to cope with small sums of money	1	1/2	0
3. Inability to remember short list of items (eg, in shopping)	1	1/2	0
4. Inability to find way about indoors	1	1/2	0
5. Inability to find way about familiar streets	1	1/2	0
6. Inability to interpret surroundings (eg, to recognize whether in hospital or at home, to discriminate between patients, doctors and nurses, relatives, and hospital staff, etc)	1	1/2	0
7. Inability to recall recent events (eg, recent outings, visits of relatives or friends, to hospital, etc)	1	1/2	0
8. Tendency to dwell in the past	1	1/2	0

Changes in Habits

9. Eating:

Cleanly with proper utensils	0
Messily with spoon only	2
Simple solids (eg, biscuits)	2
Has to be fed	3

10. Dressing:

Unaided	0
Occasionally misplaced buttons, etc	1
Wrong sequence, commonly forgetting items	2
Unable to dress	3

11. Complete sphincter control | 0

Occasional wet beds	1
Frequent wet beds	2
Doubly incontinent	3

Changes in Personality, Interests, Drive

No change	0
12. Increased rigidity	1
13. Increased egocentricity	1
14. Impairment of regard for feelings of others	1
15. Coarsening of affect	1
16. Impairment of emotional control (eg, increased petulance and irritability)	1
17. Hilarity in inappropriate situations	1
18. Diminished emotional responsiveness	1
19. Sexual misdemeanor (appearing *de novo* in old age)	1
Interests retained	0
20. Hobbies relinquished	1
21. Diminished initiative or growing apathy	1
22. Purposeless hyperactivity	1

Total ___

C. BLESSED DEMENTIA SCALE (BLS-D) *(Continued)*

Information - Memory - Concentration Test

Information Test

Name	1
Age	1
Time (hour)	1
Time of day	1
Day of week	1
Date	1
Month	1
Season	1
Year	1
Place - Name	1
Street	1
Town	1
Type of place (eg, home, hospital, etc)	1
Recognition of persons (cleaner, doctor, nurse, patient, relative; any two available)	2
Total	___

Memory:

(1) *Personal*

Date of birth	1
Place of birth	1
School attended	1
Occupation	1
Name of sibs or name of wife	1
Name of any town where patient had worked	1
Name of employers	1

(2) *Nonpersonal*

*Date of World War I	1
*Date of World War II	1
Monarch	1
Prime minister	1

(3) *Name and Address* (5-minute recall)

Mr John Brown
    42 West Street
    Gateshead
	5

Total	___

Concentration

Months of year backwards	2	1	0
Counting 1-20	2	1	0
Counting 20-1	2	1	0

* 1/2 for approximation within 3 years.

D. BURDEN INTERVIEW (BI)

OVERVIEW

The Burden Interview, developed by SH Zarit, KE Reever, and J Bach-Peterson, is a 22-item scale used to measure feelings of burden experienced by individuals caring for an elderly person with a dementing illness. The scale is focused on a primary caregiver who may be a spouse, child, or another person caring for an elderly individual with senile dementia. Each item on the Burden Interview is scored on a 5-point scale with 0 = never, and 4 = nearly always. The Burden Interview is brief to administer and potentially useful in planning of long-term care for individuals with senile dementia.

GENERAL APPLICATIONS

The Burden Interview evaluates feelings of burden experiences by caregivers of individuals with dementia.

SELECTED PSYCHOMETRIC PROPERTIES

Reliability of the BI has been reported as Cronbach's alphas ranging from 0.79 to 0.91.

REFERENCES

Zarit SH, Reever KE, and Bach-Peterson J, "Relatives of the Impaired Elderly: Correlates of Feelings of Burden," *Gerontologist*, 1980, 20(6):649-55.

Zarit SH and Zarit JM, "The Memory and Behavior Problem Checklist and the Burden Interview," (Pennsylvania State University Gerontology Center Reprint Series, No 189, Part 3), College Park, PA: Pennsylvania State University Gerontology Center, 1990.

COPYRIGHT

Steven H Zarit
Gerontology Center
105 Henderson Bldg, So
Pennsylvania State University
College Park, PA 16802-6505

SCALE GENERALLY DONE BY

Caregiver self-rated

TIME TO COMPLETE SCALE

15 minutes

REPRESENTATIVE STUDY UTILIZING SCALE

Fuh JL, Wang SJ, Liu HC, et al, "The Caregiving Burden Scale Among Chinese Caregivers of Alzheimer Patients," *Dement Geriatr Cogn Disord*, 1999, 10(3):186-91.

D. BURDEN INTERVIEW (BI) *(Continued)*

BURDEN INTERVIEW

The following is a list of statements which reflect how people sometimes feel when taking care of another person. After each statement, indicate how often you feel that way; never, rarely, sometimes, quite frequently, or nearly always. There are no right or wrong answers.

1. Do you feel that your relative asks for more help than he/she needs?

   0. Never   1. Rarely   2. Sometimes   3. Quite Frequently   4. Nearly Always

2. Do you feel that because of the time you spend with your relative that you don't have enough time for yourself?

   0. Never   1. Rarely   2. Sometimes   3. Quite Frequently   4. Nearly Always

3. Do you feel stressed between caring for your relative and trying to meet other responsibilities for your family or work?

   0. Never   1. Rarely   2. Sometimes   3. Quite Frequently   4. Nearly Always

4. Do you feel embarrassed over your relative's behavior?

   0. Never   1. Rarely   2. Sometimes   3. Quite Frequently   4. Nearly Always

5. Do you feel angry when you are around your relative?

   0. Never   1. Rarely   2. Sometimes   3. Quite Frequently   4. Nearly Always

6. Do you feel that your relative currently affects your relationship with other family members or friends in a negative way?

   0. Never   1. Rarely   2. Sometimes   3. Quite Frequently   4. Nearly Always

7. Are you afraid what the future holds for your relative?

   0. Never   1. Rarely   2. Sometimes   3. Quite Frequently   4. Nearly Always

8. Do you feel your relative is dependent upon you?

   0. Never   1. Rarely   2. Sometimes   3. Quite Frequently   4. Nearly Always

9. Do you feel strained when you are around your relative?

   0. Never   1. Rarely   2. Sometimes   3. Quite Frequently   4. Nearly Always

10. Do you feel your health has suffered because of your involvement with your relative?

    0. Never   1. Rarely   2. Sometimes   3. Quite Frequently   4. Nearly Always

11. Do you feel that you don't have as much privacy as you would like because of your relative?

    0. Never   1. Rarely   2. Sometimes   3. Quite Frequently   4. Nearly Always

12. Do you feel that your social life has suffered because you are caring for your relative?

    0. Never   1. Rarely   2. Sometimes   3. Quite Frequently   4. Nearly Always

13. Do you feel uncomfortable about having friends over because of your relative?

    0. Never   1. Rarely   2. Sometimes   3. Quite Frequently   4. Nearly Always

14. Do you feel that your relative seems to expect you to take care of him/her, as if you were the only one he/she could depend on?

    0. Never   1. Rarely   2. Sometimes   3. Quite Frequently   4. Nearly Always

15. Do you feel that you don't have enough money to care for your relative, in addition to the rest of your expenses?

    0. Never   1. Rarely   2. Sometimes   3. Quite Frequently   4. Nearly Always

16. Do you feel that you will be unable to take care of your relative much longer?

    0. Never   1. Rarely   2. Sometimes   3. Quite Frequently   4. Nearly Always

17. Do you feel you have lost control of your life since your relative's illness?

    0. Never   1. Rarely   2. Sometimes   3. Quite Frequently   4. Nearly Always

18. Do you wish you could just leave the care of your relative to someone else?

    0. Never   1. Rarely   2. Sometimes   3. Quite Frequently   4. Nearly Always

19. Do you feel uncertain about what to do about your relative?

    0. Never   1. Rarely   2. Sometimes   3. Quite Frequently   4. Nearly Always

20. Do you feel you should be doing more for your relative?

    0. Never   1. Rarely   2. Sometimes   3. Quite Frequently   4. Nearly Always

21. Do you feel you could do a better job in caring for your relative?

    0. Never   1. Rarely   2. Sometimes   3. Quite Frequently   4. Nearly Always

22. Overall, how burdened do you feel in caring for your relative?

    0. Not at all   1. A little   2. Moderately   3. Quite a bit   4. Extremely

E. DELIRIUM RATING SCALE (DRS)

OVERVIEW

The Delirium Rating Scale, developed by PT Trzepacz and colleagues, is a 10-point observer-rated scale, which evaluates a variety of symptoms seen in delirium. Each item is rated on a 0-3 or a 0-4 continuum, with higher scores indicating greater illness severity (most consistent with delirium). The DRS scoring is based upon all available information including patient interview, clinical evaluation, nursing report, family report, and laboratory testing. The total DRS score is the sum of each item; totals may range from 0-32. A cut-off score of 10 or greater has been proposed as indicating delirium. As delirium improves or resolves, an improvement in DSR score is expected. Strengths of the DSR include its brevity and ease of administration, however, the DSR may show false-positive results for individuals with dementia or other cognitive disorders.

GENERAL APPLICATIONS

The Delirium Rating Scale evaluates for presence and severity of various symptoms of delirium.

SELECTED PSYCHOMETRIC PROPERTIES

Internal consistency of the DSR is fair with significant item-total correlations of 0.37-0.53. The validity of the DSR is good with correlation with the MMSE in the order of $r = 0.43$. The DSR is sensitive to change and accurately differentiates patients with delirium from medical inpatients without delirium.

REFERENCES

Trzepacz PT, Baker RW, and Greenhouse J, "A Symptom Rating Scale for Delirium," *Psychiatry Res*, 1988, 23(1):89-97.

Trzepacz PT and Dew MA, "Further Analyses of the Delirium Rating Scale," *Gen Hosp Psychiatry*, 1995, 17(2):75-9.

COPYRIGHT

Elsevier Science
Customer Support
PO Box 945
New York, NY 10159-0945
Tel: 212-633-3730 or 1-888-YES-INFO (437-4636)
Website: www.elsevier.nl

SCALE GENERALLY DONE BY

Clinician or trained rater

TIME TO COMPLETE SCALE

5-10 minutes, may require more time with extensive clinical/observer background information

REPRESENTATIVE STUDY UTILIZING SCALE

Fann JR, Roth-Roemer S, Burington BE, et al, "Delirium in Patients Undergoing Hematopoietic Stem Cell Transplantation," *Cancer*, 2002, 95(9):1971-81.

DELIRIUM RATING SCALE

1. **Temporal onset of symptoms**

   0 — No significant change from long-standing behavior, essentially a chronic or chronic-recurrent condition.

   1 — Gradual onset of symptoms, occurring within a 6-month period.

   2 — Acute change in behavior or personality occurring over a month.

   3 — Acute change in behavior, usually occurring over a 1- to 3-day period.

2. **Perceptual disturbances**

   0 — None evident by history or observation.

   1 — Feelings of depersonalization or derealization.

   2 — Visual illusions or misperceptions including macropsia or micropsia; eg, may mistake bedclothes for something else.

   3 — Evidence that the patient is markedly confused about external reality; eg, not discriminating between dreams and reality.

3. **Hallucination type**

   0 — Hallucinations not present.

   1 — Auditory hallucinations only.

   2 — Visual hallucinations present by history or inferred by observation, with or without auditory hallucinations.

   3 — Tactile, olfactory, or gustatory hallucinations present with or without visual or auditory hallucinations.

4. **Delusions**

   0 — Not present.

   1 — Delusions are systematized, ie, well-organized and persistent.

   2 — Delusions are new and not part of a pre-existing primary psychiatric disorder.

   3 — Delusions are not well circumscribed; are transient, poorly organized, and mostly in response to misperceived environmental cues.

5. **Psychomotor behavior**

   0 — No significant retardation or agitation.

   1 — Mild restlessness, tremulousness, or anxiety evident by observation and a change from usual behavior.

   2 — Moderate agitation with pacing, removing I.V.s, etc.

   3 — Severe agitation, needs to be restrained, may be combative; or has significant withdrawal from the environment, but not due to major depression or schizophrenic catatonia.

6. **Cognitive status during formal testing**

   0 — No cognitive deficits, or deficits that can be alternatively explained by lack of education or prior mental retardation.

   1 — Very mild cognitive deficits which may be attributed to inattention, pain, etc.

   2 — Cognitive deficit largely in one major area tested, eg, memory.

   3 — Significant cognitive deficits that are diffuse; must include periods of disorientation, abnormal registration or recall, and reduced concentration.

   4 — Severe cognitive deficits, including motor or verbal perseveration, confabulations, disorientation to person, memory deficits, and inability to cooperate with formal testing.

403

E. DELIRIUM RATING SCALE (DRS) *(Continued)*

7. **Physical disorder**

   0 — None present or active.

   1 — Presence of any physical disorder that may affect mental state.

   2 — Specific drug, infection, metabolic, central nervous system lesion, or other medical problem that can be temporarily implicated in causing the altered behavior or mental status.

8. **Sleep-wake cycle disturbance**

   0 — Not present.

   1 — Occasional drowsiness during day and mild sleep continuity disturbance at night; may have nightmares but can distinguish them from reality.

   2 — Frequent napping and unable to sleep at night, constituting a significant disruption or a reversal of usual sleep-wake cycle.

   3 — Drowsiness prominent, difficulty staying alert during interview, loss of self-control over alertness and somnolence.

   4— Drifts into stuporous or comatose periods.

9. **Lability of mood**

   0— Not present.

   1— Affect/mood somewhat altered and changes over the course of the hours; patient states that mood changes are not under self-control.

   2 — Significant mood changes that are inappropriate to situation, including fear, anger, or tearfulness; rapid shifts of emotion.

   3 — Severe disinhibition of emotions, including temper outbursts, uncontrolled inappropriate laughter, or crying.

10. **Variability of symptoms**

    0 — Symptoms stable and mostly present during daytime.

    2 — Symptoms worsen at night.

    4 — Fluctuating intensity of symptoms, so that they wax and wane during a 24-hour period.

F. GERIATRIC DEPRESSION SCALE (GDS)

OVERVIEW

The GDS, developed by TL Brink et al, is a 30-item self-rated scale used to evaluate depression in the elderly. The GDS has been reported to be a useful screen for depression in elderly populations. Each item of the GDS is answered either "Yes" or "No". There are 20 items which indicate depression when answered yes, and 10 items which indicate depression when answered no (items 1, 5, 7, 9, 15, 19, 21, 27, 29, 30). A total score is provided which consists of one point from each depressive answer. Nondepressive answers are scored zero and do not add to total score. Because depression in the elderly may manifest somewhat differently than depression in younger populations, use of the GDS may be a better choice for assessment of mood disorder in later life than some of the commonly utilized scales in younger populations (see Depression Rating Scales *on page 455* in the Appendix).

GENERAL APPLICATIONS

The GDS is used to measure depression in the elderly.

SELECTED PSYCHOMETRIC PROPERTIES

The GDS has demonstrated very good internal consistency (alpha 0.94) and split-half reliability of 0.94. Stability of the GDS is also very good, with a test-retest correlation of 0.85 over one week.

REFERENCES

Yesavage JA, Brink TL, Rose TL, et al, "Development and Validation of a Geriatric Depression Screening Scale: A Preliminary Report," *J Psychiatr Res*, 1982, 17(1):37-49.

COPYRIGHT

TL Brink
Clinical Gerontologist
1103 Church St
Redlands, CA 92374

Jerome Yesavage
VA Medical Center
3801 Miranda Avenue
Palo Alto, CA 94304

SCALE GENERALLY DONE BY

Self-rated, may also be read to person being rated

TIME TO COMPLETE SCALE

15-20 minutes

REPRESENTATIVE STUDY UTILIZING SCALE

Di Iorio A, Longo AL, Mitidieri CA, et al, "Characteristics of Geriatric Patients Related to Early and Late Readmissions to Hospital," *Aging*, 1998, 10(4):339-46.

F. GERIATRIC DEPRESSION SCALE (GDS) *(Continued)*

GDS

Please circle the best answer for how you felt over the past week.

Yes	No	1.	Are you basically satisfied with your life?
Yes	No	2.	Have you dropped many of your activities and interests?
Yes	No	3.	Do you feel that you life is empty?
Yes	No	4.	Do you often get bored?
Yes	No	5.	Are you hopeful about the future?
Yes	No	6.	Are you bothered by thoughts you can't get out of your head?
Yes	No	7.	Are you in good spirits most of the time?
Yes	No	8.	Are you afraid that something bad is going to happen to you?
Yes	No	9.	Do you feel happy most of the time?
Yes	No	10.	Do you often feel helpless?
Yes	No	11.	Do you often get restless and fidgety?
Yes	No	12.	Do you prefer to stay at home rather than going out and doing new things?
Yes	No	13.	Do you frequently worry about the future?
Yes	No	14.	Do you feel you have more problems with memory than most?
Yes	No	15.	Do you think it is wonderful to be alive now?
Yes	No	16.	Do you often feel downhearted and blue?
Yes	No	17.	Do you feel pretty worthless the way you are now?
Yes	No	18.	Do you worry a lot about the past?
Yes	No	19.	Do you find life very exciting?
Yes	No	20.	Is it hard for you to get started on new projects?
Yes	No	21.	Do you feel full of energy?
Yes	No	22.	Do you feel that you situation is hopeless?
Yes	No	23.	Do you think that most people are better off than you are?
Yes	No	24.	Do you frequently get upset over little things?
Yes	No	25.	Do you frequently feel like crying?
Yes	No	26.	Do you have trouble concentrating?
Yes	No	27.	Do you enjoy getting up in the morning?
Yes	No	28.	Do you prefer to avoid social gatherings?
Yes	No	29.	Is it easy for you to make decisions?
Yes	No	30.	Is your mind as clear as it used to be?

Note: An answer of "no" is indicative of depression for questions numbered 1, 5, 7, 9, 15, 19, 21, 27, 29, and 30. For all other questions, an answer of "yes" indicates depression.

G. INSTRUMENTAL ACTIVITIES OF DAILY LIVING (IADL)

OVERVIEW

The Instrumental Activities of Daily Living (IADL), developed by MP Lawton and EM Brody is a well accepted scale to evaluate the daily living skills of older adults. One of the original functions of the IADL was to evaluate individuals residing in or applying for admission to institutions of different types. Thus, the IADL may be incorporated into the routine evaluation procedures of such facilities. The IADL focuses on concrete behavior and includes 8 domains of activities including telephoning, shopping, food preparation, housekeeping, laundering, use of transportation, use of medication, and financial behavior. A variant of the IADL also assesses household chores and driving. The IADL is scored by a trained rater, typically a mental health worker, nurse, or social worker. Scoring is based upon information from all available sources including interview of patients, staff, family members, and record review.

GENERAL APPLICATIONS

The IADL assesses functional capacity/daily living skills of older adults.

SELECTED PSYCHOMETRIC PROPERTIES

The IADL may be used as a one-time functional assessment or alternatively may be utilized within the context of a treatment plan to evaluate treatment outcome or change over time. Interrater reliability of the IADL appears good with a correlation of 0.85 between IADL total scores.

REFERENCES

Lawton MP and Brody EM, "Assessment of Older People: Self-Maintaining and Instrumental Activities of Daily Living," *Gerontologist*, 1969, 9(3):179-86.

COPYRIGHT

The Gerontological Society of America
1030 15th Street, NW
Suite 250
Washington, DC 20003-1503
Tel: 202-842-1275
Fax: 202-842-1150

SCALE GENERALLY DONE BY

Trained rater

TIME TO COMPLETE SCALE

5 minutes - not including background information collection time

REPRESENTATIVE STUDY UTILIZING SCALE

McCall WV, Dunn AG, Rosenquist P, et al, "Proxy Validation of Patient Self-Reports of ADL and IADL Function Before and After Electroconvulsive Therapy," *J ECT*, 2002, 18(2):74-9.

G. INSTRUMENTAL ACTIVITIES OF DAILY LIVING (IADL) *(Continued)*

INSTRUMENTAL ACTIVITIES OF DAILY LIVING (IADL) SCALE

A. **Ability to use the telephone**

Does not answer the telephone at all	1
Answers telephone but does not dial	2
Dials a few well-known numbers	3
Operates telephone on own initiative	4

B. **Shopping**

Completely unable to shop	1
Needs to be accompanied on any shopping trip	2
Shops independently for small purchases	3
Takes care of all shopping needs independently	4

C. **Food preparation**

Needs to have meals prepared and served	1
Heats and serves prepared meals, or prepares meals but does not maintain an adequate diet	2
Prepares adequate meals if supplied with ingredients	3
Plans, prepares, and serves adequate meals independently	4

D. **Housekeeping**

Unable to participate in any housekeeping tasks	1
Needs help with all home maintenance tasks	2
Performs light daily tasks such as dishwashing	3
Maintains house alone or with occasional assistance	4

E. **Laundry**

All laundry must be done by others	1
Launders a few small items	2
Does most small items, depends on others for large items	3
Does personal laundry completely	4

F. **Mode of Transportation**

Does not travel at all	1
Travel limited to taxi or automobile with assistance of another	2
Travels on public transportation when assisted or accompanied by another	3
Travels independently on public transportation, taxi, or drives own car	4

G. **Responsibility for own medications**

Is not capable of dispensing own medication	1
Takes responsibility if medication is prepared in advance in separate dosages	2
Takes independent responsibility but occasionally forgets a dosage	3
Is responsible for taking medication in correct dosages at correct times	4

H. **Ability to handle finances**

Incapable of handling money	1
Manages day-to-day purchases but needs help with banking, major purchases, etc	2
Manages financial matters independently but, on occasion, has forgotten to pay a bill or has been overdrawn in bank account	3
Manages financial matters independently, collects and keeps track of income	4

Note: Items can be rated as "not applicable" for persons who have never performed a particular activity (eg, driving a car) or who have no opportunity to perform a particular activity.

H. NEUROPSYCHIATRIC INVENTORY (NPI)

OVERVIEW

The Neuropsychiatric Inventory was developed in 1994 by J Cummings and collaborators at UCLA to assess behavioral problems in patients with dementia. The scale looks at 10 domains of behavioral disturbances:

Delusions
Hallucinations
Dysphoria
Anxiety
Agitation/Aggression
Euphoria
Inhibition
Irritability/lability
Apathy
Aberrant Motor Behavior

The inventory has two domains related to neurovegetative problems: Sleep and Appetite. All the items are rated on frequency and severity utilizing anchoring points provided in the manual.

There are two versions of the NPI. One version is to be used when the patient in question is in a nursing home and the Standard version is used when the patient is still at home. The only difference between the versions is the source of information. In the nursing home version, source of information is the staff member taking care of the patient, while the standard version utilizes the caregiver taking care of the patient at home. In both cases, the "caregiver" provides a rating that evaluates the burden or increased work the symptom may cause. The NPI is a structured interview done by a trained rater. It is designed to be done quickly and the questions are provided in the manual/instructions and should be asked as they are written. These questions are considered screening questions, and when the interviewee answers "no", the interviewer must proceed to the next item. If the answer is "yes", the interviewer must ask a series of follow-up questions about the presence or absence of some specific symptoms.

The NPI produces four scores: One for frequency, a second for severity, a third called total which is the multiplication of frequency by severity, and a fourth for the distress/excess work caused by the symptoms.

There is an excellent and comprehensive manual for the NPI, which may be obtained from the author. A portion of the NPI is reprinted at the end of this monograph.

GENERAL APPLICATIONS

The NPI is used to evaluate dementia.

SELECTED PSYCHOMETRIC PROPERTIES

The NPI has very good scores for reliability and agreement between raters due to the fact that the scoring is basically provided by the person being interviewed with the interviewer being a "transcriber" of the information. In terms of validity, the NPI correlates well with other measures of behavioral disturbances including the BPRS, the Behavioral Pathology in Alzheimer's Disease Rating Scale (BEHAVE-AD) *on page 388*, and the HAM-D *on page 100*.

The NPI appears to be sensitive to change and is utilized for the evaluation of treatment approaches to behavioral disturbances in these patients.

The sample scale that follows is the standard version; there is also a nursing home version available for use with professional caregivers in residential settings.

REFERENCES

Cummings JL, Mega M, Gray K, et al, "The Neuropsychiatric Inventory: Comprehensive Assessment of Psychopathology in Dementia," *Neurology*, 1994, 44(12):2308-14.

H. NEUROPSYCHIATRIC INVENTORY (NPI) *(Continued)*

COPYRIGHT

Jeffrey Cummings
Reed Neurological Research Center
University of California - Los Angeles (UCLA)
School of Medicine
710 Westwood Plaza
Los Angeles, CA 90095-1769

SCALE GENERALLY DONE BY

Clinician or trained rater

TIME TO COMPLETE SCALE

15-30 minutes

REPRESENTATIVE STUDY UTILIZING SCALE

Kaufer DI, Cummings JL, and Christine D, "Effect of Tacrine on Behavioral Symptoms in Alzheimer's Disease: An Open Label Study," *J Geriatr Psych Neurol*, 1996, 9(1):1-6.

Neuropsychiatric Inventory Worksheet

Directions: Read all items from the NPI "Instructions for Administration of the NPI." Mark Caregiver's responses on this worksheet before scoring the Frequency, Severity, and Caregiver Distress for each item.

A. DELUSIONS: Y   N   N/A

Frequency _____   Severity _____
Distress _____

____ ☐ 1. Fear of harm
____ ☐ 2. Fear of theft
____ ☐ 3. Spousal affair
____ ☐ 4. Phantom boarder
____ ☐ 5. Spouse imposter
____ ☐ 6. House not home
____ ☐ 7. Fear of abandonment
____ ☐ 8. Talks to TV, etc
____ ☐ 9. Other _____

B. HALLUCINATIONS: Y   N   N/A

Frequency _____   Severity _____
Distress _____

____ ☐ 1. Hears voices
____ ☐ 2. Talks to people not there
____ ☐ 3. Sees things not there
____ ☐ 4. Smells things not there
____ ☐ 5. Feels things not there
____ ☐ 6. Unusual taste sensations
____ ☐ 7. Other _____

C. AGITATION/AGGRESSION: Y   N   N/A

Frequency _____   Severity _____
Distress _____

____ ☐ 1. Upset with caregiver; resists ADLs
____ ☐ 2. Stubborness
____ ☐ 3. Uncooperative; resists help
____ ☐ 4. Hard to handle
____ ☐ 5. Cursing or shouting angrily
____ ☐ 6. Slams doors; kicks, throws things
____ ☐ 7. Hits, harms others
____ ☐ 8. Other _____

D. DEPRESSION/DYSPHORIA: Y   N   N/A

Frequency _____   Severity _____
Distress _____

____ ☐ 1. Tearful and sobbing
____ ☐ 2. States, acts as if sad
____ ☐ 3. Puts self down, feels like failure
____ ☐ 4. "Bad person", deserves punishment
____ ☐ 5. Discouraged, no future
____ ☐ 6. Burden to family
____ ☐ 7. Talks about dying, killing self
____ ☐ 8. Other _____

E. ANXIETY: Y   N   N/A

Frequency _____   Severity _____
Distress _____

____ ☐ 1. Worries about planned events
____ ☐ 2. Feels shaky, tense
____ ☐ 3. Sobs, sighs, gasps
____ ☐ 4. Racing heart, "butterflies"
____ ☐ 5. Phobic avoidance
____ ☐ 6. Separation anxiety
____ ☐ 7. Other _____

F. ELATION/EUPHORIA: Y   N   N/A

Frequency _____   Severity _____
Distress _____

____ ☐ 1. Feels too good, too happy
____ ☐ 2. Abnormal humor
____ ☐ 3. Childish, laughs inappropriately
____ ☐ 4. Jokes or remarks not funny to others
____ ☐ 5. Childish pranks
____ ☐ 6. Talks "big"; grandiose
____ ☐ 7. Other _____

H. NEUROPSYCHIATRIC INVENTORY (NPI) *(Continued)*

Neuropsychiatric Inventory Worksheet, *continued*

G. APATHY/INDIFFERENCE: Y   N   N/A

Frequency _____   Severity _____
Distress _____

____ ☐ 1. Less spontaneous or active
____ ☐ 2. Less likely to initiate conversation
____ ☐ 3. Less affectionate, lacking emotions
____ ☐ 4. Contributes less to household chores
____ ☐ 5. Less interested in others
____ ☐ 6. Lost interest in friends or family
____ ☐ 7. Less enthusiastic about interests
____ ☐ 8. Other _____

H. DISINHIBITION: Y   N   N/A

Frequency _____   Severity _____
Distress _____

____ ☐ 1. Acts impulsively
____ ☐ 2. Excessively familiar with strangers
____ ☐ 3. Insensitive or hurtful remarks
____ ☐ 4. Crude or sexual remarks
____ ☐ 5. Talks openly of private matters
____ ☐ 6. Inappropriate touching of others
____ ☐ 7. Other _____

I. IRRITABILITY: Y   N   N/A

Frequency _____   Severity _____
Distress _____

____ ☐ 1. Bad temper, "flies off handle" easily
____ ☐ 2. Rapid changes in mood
____ ☐ 3. Sudden flashes of anger
____ ☐ 4. Impatient, trouble coping with delays
____ ☐ 5. Cranky, irritable
____ ☐ 6. Argues, difficult to get along with
____ ☐ 7. Other _____

J. ABERRANT MOTOR BEHAVIOR: Y N N/A

Frequency _____   Severity _____
Distress _____

____ ☐ 1. Paces without purpose
____ ☐ 2. Opens or unpacks closets or drawers
____ ☐ 3. Repeatedly dresses and undresses
____ ☐ 4. Repetitive activities or "habits"
____ ☐ 5. Handling, picking, wrapping behavior
____ ☐ 6. Excessively fidgety
____ ☐ 7. Other _____

K. NIGHTTIME BEHAVIORS: Y   N   N/A

Frequency _____   Severity _____
Distress _____

____ ☐ 1. Difficulty falling asleep
____ ☐ 2. Up during the night
____ ☐ 3. Wanders, paces, inappropriate activity
____ ☐ 4. Awakens others at night
____ ☐ 5. Wakes and dresses to go out at night
____ ☐ 6. Early morning awakening
____ ☐ 7. Sleeps excessively during the day
____ ☐ 8. Other _____

L. APPETITE/EATING BEHAVIORS: Y N N/A

Frequency _____   Severity _____
Distress _____

____ ☐ 1. Loss of appetite
____ ☐ 2. Increased appetite
____ ☐ 3. Weight loss
____ ☐ 4. Weight gain
____ ☐ 5. Changes in eating habits
____ ☐ 6. Change in food preferences
____ ☐ 7. Eating rituals
____ ☐ 8. Other _____

Copies of the worksheet, scoring summary, manual, and training video are available from the author.

I. RELATIVE'S ASSESSMENT OF GLOBAL SYMPTOMATOLOGY (RAGS-E)

OVERVIEW

The RAGS, developed by A Raskin, is a 21-item scale to evaluate psychiatric and behavioral problems of elderly individuals in the community, particularly those with senile dementia. The RAGS has been tested on large numbers of elderly individuals, and has been utilized in clinical drug trials to evaluate the effects on medication in individuals with dementing illness. The RAGS is designed to be answered by relatives/caregivers of the patient, and is relatively brief and easy to administer. Each item is rated on a five point scale where 1 = not at all, and 5 = extremely. All items measure severity of a problem or symptoms except the second item, which is worded positively, and measures participation in social or recreational activities. A total pathology score may be obtained by summing the ratings for all items and dividing by 21 to get a mean score. (Item two score must be reversed before summing).

GENERAL APPLICATIONS

The RAGS is used to evaluate behavior of individuals with senile dementia in the community.

SELECTED PSYCHOMETRIC PROPERTIES

The RAGS has been demonstrated to be able to discriminate groups of individuals with senile dementia from other groups. The RAGS depression items have been reported to correlate 0.47 ($p < .01$) with the depression factor score on the Mood Scales-Elderly (Raskin et al, 1985).

REFERENCES

Raskin A and Crook T, "Relative's Assessment of Global Symptomatology (RAGS)," *Psychopharmacol Bull*, 1988, 24(4):759-63.

Raskin A, "Validation of a Battery of Tests Designed to Assess Psychopathology in the Elderly," Burrows GD, *Clinical and Pharmacological Studies in Psychiatric Disorders*, Norman TR and Dennerstein L, eds, London, England: John Libbey, 1985, 337-43.

COPYRIGHT

Not applicable

SCALE GENERALLY DONE BY

Close relative or friend of the person being rated

TIME TO COMPLETE SCALE

15-20 minutes

REPRESENTATIVE STUDY UTILIZING SCALE

Antuono PG, "Effectiveness and Safety of Velnacrine for the Treatment of Alzheimer's Disease: A Double-Blind, Placebo-Controlled Study. Mentane Study Group," *Arch Intern Med*, 1995, 155(16):1766-72.

I. RELATIVE'S ASSESSMENT OF GLOBAL SYMPTOMATOLOGY (RAGS-E) *(Continued)*

RELATIVE'S ASSESSMENT OF GLOBAL SYMPTOMATOLOGY - ELDERLY (RAGS-E)

For each of the following items, check the column which best describes the condition of your relative (friend) during the past week, including today.

To what extent does he or she:	Cues	Not at all	A little	Moderately	Quite a bit	Extremely
		1	2	3	4	5
1. Need help in caring for personal needs and appearance?	Needs help in dressing; needs assistance in eating; has to be helped in the bathroom; must be reminded to brush teeth, comb hair; appears sloppy					
2. Participate in social and recreational activities?	Makes small talk with friends; joins in social games; shows interest in hobbies, clubs, or group activities					
3. Appear depressed, blue, or despondent?	Looks sad; speaks in a sad voice; has crying spells; sighs frequently; complains of feeling blue or down in the dumps					
4. Appear tense, anxious, and inwardly distressed?	Is fidgety and nervous in movements; drums or fiddles with objects; palms feel sweaty; complains of feelings anxious; says he/she is fearful or afraid of people or objects					
5. Display irritability, annoyance, impatience, or anger?	Has temper tantrums; will not wait for things to be given to him/her; gets angry or annoyed when questioned; has an angry expression; becomes upset when things don't suit him/her					
6. Appear suspicious of people?	Feels others are against him/her or out to get him/her; feels people talk about, refer to, or watch him/her; feels he/she is being persecuted or discriminated against					
7. Report peculiar or strange thoughts or ideas?	Claims to have supernatural powers; feels he/she is being controlled by unusual forces; claims he/she has received commands from God; says he/she is dead, a zombie, or some other impossible belief					
8. Appear to be hearing or seeing things that are not there?	Hears or sees things that are not there; talks, mutters, or mumbles to himself/herself; giggles for no apparent reason					
9. Show mood swings or changes?	Mood changes frequently; seems bright and cheerful one day, down in the dumps the next					
10. Appear excited or "high" emotionally?	Talks and talks; brags or boasts of what he/she has done; has grandiose plans for the future					
11. Have difficulty in sleeping at night?	Difficulty in falling asleep (without sedatives); awakening unusually early; awakes for periods in the middle of the night					

To what extent does he or she:	Cues	Not at all	A little	Moderately	Quite a bit	Extremely
		1	2	3	4	5
12. Appear slowed-down, fatigued, and lacking in energy?	Slow in movements; speaks in a slow, drawn-out manner; acts as if everything is an effort; looks tired and worn-out; complains of physical weakness; sits or sleeps unless directed into activity					
13. Lack motor coordination?	Unsteady gait; appears clumsy, awkward; difficulty writing; difficulty eating with utensils					
14. Have difficulty speaking?	Speech is slurred; speech difficult to hear; has difficulty communicating his/her ideas through speech					
15. Express concern with own bodily health?	Complains of headache, dizziness, faintness, shortness of breath, stomach and bowel disturbances, heart racing					
16. Appear inattentive?	Fails to respond to name or questions; acts as if lost in dream world					
17. Appear confused, perplexed, or otherwise seem to be having difficulty organizing his/her thoughts?	Gives answers that have little or no bearing on topic being discussed; appears bewildered by events around him/her					
18. Seem disoriented?	Unaware of time and date; unaware of where he/she is					
19. Appear forgetful?	Forgets names; misplaces objects; forgets appointments					
20. Appear agitated?	Seems fearful and frightened; can't sit still; paces up and down; wrings hands					
21. Show variability in mental functioning?	Memory and ability to attend and concentrate good one day, poor the next. Recognizes relatives and friends one day, not the next. No difficulty maintaining a conversation one day, rambles or drifts off the topic discussed the next day.					

J. THE CAMBRIDGE MENTAL DISORDERS OF THE ELDERLY EXAMINATION (CAMDEX)

OVERVIEW

The Cambridge Mental Disorders of the Elderly Examination (CAMDEX), developed by M Roth et al, "focuses on the diagnosis of dementia, with particular reference to its mild forms and to the identification of specific types of dementia." According to the authors, the complete assessment of a patient with dementia includes scales to test cognition, severity of dementia, and changes in behavior, with the CAMDEX incorporating all these assessments in one instrument. This includes a clinical interview, cognitive tests, and an interview with a relative or caregiver to obtain reliable history about the patient's illness. The CAMDEX is a comprehensive evaluation of a patient and includes eight sections. Section A covers all the clinical information about current condition, past history, and family history. Section B incorporates the Mini-Mental State Examination. Section C includes the interviewer's observation on the patient's appearance and behavior. Section D is a physical examination. Section E includes the laboratory tests. Section F records the medication received by the patient. Section G includes miscellaneous information. Section H includes the structured interview with the relative or caregiver. A limitation of the scale is that it is lengthy, usually needs to be done with a psychiatrist as the lead person, and it may be difficult to use in research studies looking at change.

GENERAL APPLICATIONS

The CAMDEX is used to evaluate cognitive and behavioral symptoms of individuals with dementia.

SELECTED PSYCHOMETRIC PROPERTIES

According to the developers the interrater reliability has phi coefficients over 0.80 for the different sections. There is no good data on test-retest reliability. In terms of validity, Roth has reported 92% sensitivity and 96% sensitivity for the cognitive section.

The CAMDEX has shown very good correlation with other dementia scales including the MMSE *on page 418* and the Blessed Dementia Scale *on page 395*.

REFERENCES

Hendrie HC, Hall KS, Brittain HM, et al, "The CAMDEX: A Standardized Instrument for the Diagnosis of Mental Disorder in the Elderly: A Replication With a U.S. Sample," *J Am Geriatr Soc*, 1988, 36(5):402-8.

O'Connor DW, "The Contribution of CAMDEX to the Diagnosis of Mild Dementia in Community Surveys," *Psychiatr J Univ Ott*, 1990, 15(4):216-20.

Roth M, Tym E, Mountjoy CQ, et al, "CAMDEX. A Standardized Instrument for the Diagnosis of Mental Disorder in the Elderly With Special Reference to the Early Detection of Dementia," *Br J Psychiatry*, 1986, 149:698-709.

COPYRIGHT

Martin Roth
Cambridge University
Department of Psychiatry
Level 4
Addenbrooke's Hospital
Hill Road
Cambridge CB2 2QQ
England

SCALE GENERALLY DONE BY

Trained clinician

TIME TO COMPLETE SCALE

60-90 minutes

REPRESENTATIVE STUDY UTILIZING SCALE

MacKnight C, Graham J, and Rockwood K, "Factors Associated With Inconsistent Diagnosis of Dementia Between Physicians and Neuropsychologists," *J Am Geriatr Soc*, 1999, 47(11):1294-9.

K. THE MINI-MENTAL STATE EXAMINATION (MMSE)

OVERVIEW

The Mini-Mental State Examination (MMSE), developed by M Folstein in 1975, is a screening instrument that gives a brief assessment of an individual's orientation to time and place, recall ability, short memory, and arithmetic ability. The MMSE has been extensively used in clinical settings. It is important to emphasize that this instrument should not be used to diagnose dementia but, rather, is utilized as a bedside instrument to assess the cognitive function of a patient.

The 11-item MMSE is divided in two sections. The first section requires verbal responses to orientation, memory, and attention questions. The second section requires reading, writing, and the ability to copy a geometric figure (a polygon).

All the questions must be asked and usually are done in sequence. The test can be scored immediately with a maximum of 30 (no impairment). The cut-off point to indicate cognitive impairment is generally between 23-25.

Questions that are not answered should be treated as errors. The problem of questions not answered because of lack of education or blindness has not been addressed properly, and has been handled according to previously agreed upon conventions such as treating them as errors or prorating the responses. The MMSE is brief, easy to use, and can be administered by a nonprofessional. It has been reported to potentially miss mild impairments and individuals with limited education tend to give false-positive responses.

GENERAL APPLICATIONS

The MMSE is used to measure cognitive functioning in adults.

SELECTED PSYCHOMETRIC PROPERTIES

The internal consistency of the scales has reported an alpha of 0.68 to 0.96. Test-retest reliability has been examined in many studies with values over 0.80. The interrater reliability has been widely studied with Pearson correlations of 0.90 and Kendall coefficients of 0.70 or more.

In terms of content validity, the MMSE measures most of the different aspects used to evaluate cognitive status.

In terms of concurrent validity, the MMSE correlates well with the WAIS and with other dementia rating scales such as the Reisberg's Global Deterioration Scale and the Blessed Dementia Scale.

REFERENCES

Folstein MF, Folstein SE, and McHugh PR, "Mini-Mental State. A Practical Method for Grading the Cognitive State of Patients for the Clinician," *J Psychiatr Res*, 1975, 12(3):189-98.

Mitrushina M and Satz P, "Reliability and Validity of the Mini-Mental State Exam in Neurologically Intact Elderly," *J Clin Psychol*, 1991, 47(4):537-43.

Salmon DP, Thal LJ, Butters N, et al, "Longitudinal Evaluation of Dementia of the Alzheimer Type: A Comparison of 3 Standardized Mental Status Examinations," *Neurology*, 1990, 40(8):1225-30.

Tombaugh TN and McIntyre NJ, "The Mini-Mental State Examination: A Comprehensive Review," *J Am Geriatr Soc*, 1992, 40(9):922-35.

COPYRIGHT

MiniMental, LLC
John Gonsalves, Jr
31 St James Avenue, Suite 1
Boston, MA 02116
Tel: 617-587-4215

SCALE GENERALLY DONE BY

Trained rater or clinician

TIME TO COMPLETE SCALE

5-10 minutes

REPRESENTATIVE STUDY UTILIZING SCALE

Mori E, Shimomura T, Fujimori M, et al, "Visuoperceptual Impairment in Dementia With Lewy Bodies," *Arch Neurol*, 2000, 57(4):489-93.

K. THE MINI-MENTAL STATE EXAMINATION (MMSE) *(Continued)*

SAMPLE ITEMS OF THE
MINI MENTAL SCALE (MMSE)

ORIENTATION TO TIME

Ask:

What is the date?_____

REGISTRATION OF THREE WORDS

Say: "Listen carefully, I am going to say three words. You say them back after I stop.
Ready? Here they are.... HOUSE (pause), CAR (pause), LAKE (pause).
Now, repeat those words back to me."

_____

_____

_____

(Repeat up to 5 times, but score only the first trial.)

NAMING

Ask:
"What is this?" (Point to a pencil or pen) _____

READING

Say:
"Please read this and do what it says." (Show examinee the words on the stimulus form.)

Close your eyes

RATING SCALES
FOR CHILDREN*

TABLE OF CONTENTS

* Clinicians/researchers often utilize scales for children which have been modified from adult psychopathology rating scales. Examples include the PANSS, the Young Mania Rating Scale, and the YBOCS. Commonly utilized diagnostic scales for children include the National Institute of Mental Health Diagnostic Interview Schedule for Children (NIMH-DISC) and the Schedule for Affective Disorders for School Age Children (Kiddie-SADS).

A. ADAPTIVE BEHAVIOR SCALE (AAMR ABS)

OVERVIEW

The ABS, developed by N Lambert et al, is a tool to evaluate functioning and behavior disorder in children and adolescents with mental retardation, autism, or other developmental disabilities. The ABS consists of two parts. The first part covers nine behavioral domains and assesses the adaptive coping skills and personal independence in these areas. The second part covers seven behavior domains and evaluates social maladaptive behavior. Five factors are measured in the ABS, including personal self-sufficiency, community self-sufficiency, personal-social responsibility, social adjustment, and personal adjustment. The ABS may be particularly useful in determining which children may require special educational settings.

GENERAL APPLICATIONS

The ABS evaluates functioning and behavioral problems in children and adolescents with developmental disorders.

SELECTED PSYCHOMETRIC PROPERTIES

Interrater reliability of the ABS has been reported to range from 0.83 to 0.99. Internal consistency coefficients range from 0.80 to 0.98 for scale domains and 0.92 to 0.99 for factors.

REFERENCES

Lambert N, Nihira K, and Leland H, *Adaptive Behavior Scale - School*, 2nd ed, Austin, TX: Pro-Ed, Inc, 1993.

COPYRIGHT

Nadine Lambert
Henry Leland
Kazuo Nihira
Pro-Ed
8700 Shoal Creek Blvd
Austin, TX 78757
Tel: 1-800-897-3202

SCALE GENERALLY DONE BY

Clinician or trained rater

TIME TO COMPLETE SCALE

15-30 minutes

REPRESENTATIVE STUDY UTILIZING SCALE

Rousey A, Best S, and Blacher J, "Mothers and Fathers Perceptions of Stress and Coping With Children Who Have Severe Disabilities," *Am J Ment Retard*, 1992, 97:99-109.

SAMPLE ITEMS OF THE
AAMR ABS SCALE

PART TWO: DOMAIN X

Social Behavior

INSTRUCTIONS:
Circle the "0" if the behavior never occurs (signified by N), the "1" if the behavior occurs occasionally (signified by O), or the "2" if it occurs frequently (signified by F).

Use the space for "Other" when:
1. The person has related behavior problems in addition to those circled.
2. The person has behavior problems that are not covered by any of the examples listed.

ITEM 1	**Threatens or Does Physical Violence**	N	O	F
	Uses threatening gestures	0	1	2
	Indirectly causes injury to others	0	1	2
	Spits on others	0	1	2
	Pushes, scratches, or pinches others	0	1	2
	Pulls others' hair, ears, etc	0	1	2
	Bites others	0	1	2
	Kicks, strikes, or slaps others	0	1	2
	Throws objects at others	0	1	2
	Chokes others	0	1	2
	Uses objects as weapons against others	0	1	2
	Hurts animals	0	1	2
Other (specify) _____		0	1	2

ITEM 2	**Has Violent Temper or Temper Tantrums**			
	Cries and screams	0	1	2
	Stamps feet while banging objects or slamming doors, etc	0	1	2
	Stamps feet, screaming and yelling	0	1	2
	Throws self on floor, screaming and yelling	0	1	2
Other (specify) _____		0	1	2

ITEM 3	**Teases or Gossips About Others**			
	Gossips about others	0	1	2
	Tells untrue or exaggerated stories about others	0	1	2
	Teases others	0	1	2
	Picks on others	0	1	2
	Makes fun of others	0	1	2
Other (specify) _____		0	1	2

ITEM 4	**Bosses and Manipulates Others**			
	Tries to tell others what to do	0	1	2
	Demands services from others	0	1	2
	Pushes others around	0	1	2
	Causes fights among other people	0	1	2
	Manipulates others to get them in trouble	0	1	2
Other (specify) _____		0	1	2

ITEM 5	**Uses Angry Language**			
	Uses hostile language, eg, "stupid jerk," "dirty pig," etc	0	1	2
	Swears, curses, or uses obscene language	0	1	2
	Yells or screams threats of violence	0	1	2
	Verbally threatens others, suggesting physical violence	0	1	2
Other (specify) _____		0	1	2

ITEM 6	**Reacts Poorly to Frustration**			
	Blames own mistakes on others	0	1	2
	Withdraws or pouts when thwarted	0	1	2
	Becomes upset when thwarted	0	1	2
	Throws temper tantrums when does not get own way	0	1	2
Other (specify) _____		0	1	2

ITEM 7	**Disrupts Others' Activities**			
	Is always in the way	0	1	2
	Interferes with others' activities, eg, blocking passage, upsetting wheelchairs, etc	0	1	2
	Upsets others' work	0	1	2
	Knocks around articles that others are working with, eg, puzzles, card games, etc	0	1	2
	Snatches things out of others' hands	0	1	2
Other (specify) _____		0	1	2

B. CHILD BEHAVIOR CHECKLIST (CBCL)

OVERVIEW

The CBCL, developed by TM Achenbach, is an assessment tool that is intended to be one part of a comprehensive, multi-informant evaluation of a child's behavior. The CBCL is intended to evaluate pathological behaviors and social competence in children ages $1\frac{1}{2}$ to 18 years of age. The CBCL/4-18 is a 113-item behavioral problems checklist with a seven-part social competency checklist. There is also a version for younger, preschool children, the CBCL/$1\frac{1}{2}$-5 which contains only a 100-item behavioral checklist. In addition to the behavioral and social competency checklists, there are a youth self-report version, a teacher's report form, a direct observation form, and a semistructured clinical interview for children and adolescents which includes a videotape and computer scoring programs. The CBCL has been tested in large populations and is fairly easy and brief to administer. It is used both in clinical settings and in research. A limitation of the CBCL is that syndromes from the scale do not necessarily correspond with DSM-IV diagnostic categories. Forthcoming versions have DSM-oriented scales based on ratings of CBCL items by highly experienced mental health researchers from 8 countries. A computerized version of the CBCL is available from the author as well as manuals/detailed instructions for scale administration.

GENERAL APPLICATIONS

The CBCL is used to assess pathological behaviors and social competence in children.

SELECTED PSYCHOMETRIC PROPERTIES

Reliability of the CBCL, as with all scales, depends on the raters. Interparent agreement coefficients on the CBCL average 0.66. The reliability of the composite behavioral problems scores is excellent, with internal consistency and one-week test-retest coefficients above 0.89. The CBCL is the standard in the child psychopathology field against which other instruments are often measured.

REFERENCES

Achenbach TM and Rescorla LA, *Manual for the ASEBA Preschool Forms and Profiles*, Burlington, VT: Department of Psychiatry, 2000.

Achenbach TM, *Integrative Guide for the 1991 CBCL/4-18, YSR, and TRF Profiles*, Burlington, VT: University of Vermont, Department of Psychiatry, 1991.

Achenbach TM, *Manual for the Child Behavior Checklist/4-18 and 1991 Profile*, Burlington, VT: University of Vermont, Department of Psychiatry, 1991.

COPYRIGHT

Thomas M Achenbach
1 South Prospect Street, Room 6436
Burlington, VT 05401-3456
Tel: 802-656-8313
e-mail: checklist@uvm.edu
Website: http://checklist.uvm.edu

SCALE GENERALLY DONE BY

Varies depending on format: Includes ratings by parents, self-report, teachers, clinicians/ trained observers, daycare providers

TIME TO COMPLETE SCALE

Approximately 15 minutes; may vary by format.

REPRESENTATIVE STUDY UTILIZING SCALE

Guralnick MJ, "Peer Social Networks of Young Boys With Developmental Delays," *Am J Ment Retard*, 1997, 101(6):595-612.

B. CHILD BEHAVIOR CHECKLIST (CBCL) *(Continued)*

CBCL SCALE

Below is a list of items that describe children and youth. For each item that describes your child **now or within the past 6 months**, please circle the **2** if the item is **very true or often true** of your child. Circle the **1** if the item is **somewhat or sometimes true** of your child. If the item is **not true** of your child, circle the **0**. Please answer all items as well as you can, even if some do not seem to apply to your child.

> **0 = Not True (as far as you know)   1 = Somewhat or Sometimes True**
> **2 = Very True or Often True**

0	1	2	1. Acts too young for his/her age
0	1	2	2. Allergy (describe): _____
0	1	2	3. Argues a lot
0	1	2	4. Asthma
0	1	2	5. Behaves like opposite sex
0	1	2	6. Bowel movements outside toilet
0	1	2	7. Bragging, boasting
0	1	2	8. Can't concentrate, can't pay attention for long
0	1	2	9. Can't get his/her mind off certain thoughts; obsessions (describe):
			_____
0	1	2	10. Can't sit still, restless, or hyperactive
0	1	2	11. Clings to adults or too dependent
0	1	2	12. Complains of loneliness
0	1	2	13. Confused or seems to be in a fog
0	1	2	14. Cries a lot
0	1	2	15. Cruel to animals
0	1	2	16. Cruelty, bullying, or meanness to others
0	1	2	17. Daydreams or gets lost in his/her thoughts
0	1	2	18. Deliberately harms self or attempts suicide
0	1	2	19. Demands a lot of attention
0	1	2	20. Destroys his/her own things
0	1	2	21. Destroys things belonging to his/her family or others
0	1	2	22. Disobedient at home
0	1	2	23. Disobedient at school
0	1	2	24. Doesn't eat well
0	1	2	25. Doesn't get along with other kids
0	1	2	26. Doesn't seem to feel guilty after misbehaving
0	1	2	27. Easily jealous
0	1	2	28. Eats or drinks things that are not food - **don't** include sweets (describe):
			_____
0	1	2	29. Fears certain animals, situations, or places, other than school (describe):
			_____
0	1	2	30. Fears going to school
0	1	2	31. Fears he/she might think or do something bad
0	1	2	32. Feels he/she has to be perfect
0	1	2	33. Feels or complains that no one loves him/her
0	1	2	34. Feels others are out to get him/her
0	1	2	35. Feels worthless or inferior
0	1	2	36. Gets hurt a lot, accident-prone
0	1	2	37. Gets in many fights
0	1	2	38. Gets teased a lot

0	1	2	39. Hangs around with others who get in trouble
0	1	2	40. Hears sounds or voices that aren't there (describe): _____
0	1	2	41. Impulsive or acts without thinking
0	1	2	42. Would rather be alone than with others
0	1	2	43. Lying or cheating
0	1	2	44. Bites fingernails
0	1	2	45. Nervous, highstrung, or tense
0	1	2	46. Nervous movements or twitching (describe): _____
0	1	2	47. Nightmares
0	1	2	48. Not liked by other kids
0	1	2	49. Constipated, doesn't move bowels
0	1	2	50. Too fearful or anxious
0	1	2	51. Feels dizzy
0	1	2	52. Feels too guilty
0	1	2	53. Overeating
0	1	2	54. Overtired
0	1	2	55. Overweight
			56. Physical problems **without known medical cause:**
0	1	2	a. Aches or pains (**not** stomach or headaches)
0	1	2	b. Headaches
0	1	2	c. Nausea, feels sick
0	1	2	d. Problems with eyes (**not** if corrected by glasses) (describe:) _____
0	1	2	e. Rashes or other skin problems
0	1	2	f. Stomach aches or cramps
0	1	2	g. Vomiting, throwing up
0	1	2	h. Other (describe): _____
0	1	2	57. Physically attacks people
0	1	2	58. Picks nose, skin, or other parts of body (describe): _____
0	1	2	59. Plays with own sex parts in public
0	1	2	60. Plays with own sex parts too much
0	1	2	61. Poor school work
0	1	2	62. Poorly coordinated or clumsy
0	1	2	63. Prefers being with older kids
0	1	2	64. Prefers being with younger kids
0	1	2	65. Refuses to talk
0	1	2	66. Repeats certain acts over and over; compulsions (describe): _____
0	1	2	67. Runs away from home
0	1	2	68. Screams a lot
0	1	2	69. Secretive, keeps things to self
0	1	2	70. Sees things that aren't there (describe): _____
0	1	2	71. Self-conscious or easily embarrassed
0	1	2	72. Sets fires
0	1	2	73. Sexual problems (describe): _____
0	1	2	74. Showing off or clowning
0	1	2	75. Shy or timid
0	1	2	76. Sleeps less than most kids
0	1	2	77. Sleeps more than most kids during day and/or night (describe): _____
0	1	2	78. Smears or plays with bowel movements

427

B. CHILD BEHAVIOR CHECKLIST (CBCL) *(Continued)*

0	1	2	79.	Speech problem (describe): _____
0	1	2	80.	Stares blankly
0	1	2	81.	Steals at home
0	1	2	82.	Steals outside the home
0	1	2	83.	Stores up things he/she doesn't need (describe): _____
0	1	2	84.	Strange behavior (describe): _____
0	1	2	85.	Strange ideas (describe): _____
0	1	2	86.	Stubborn, sullen, or irritable
0	1	2	87.	Sudden changes in mood or feelings
0	1	2	88.	Sulks a lot
0	1	2	89.	Suspicious
0	1	2	90.	Swearing or obscene language
0	1	2	91.	Talks about killing self
0	1	2	92.	Talks or walks in sleep (describe): _____
0	1	2	93.	Talks too much
0	1	2	94.	Teases a lot
0	1	2	95.	Temper tantrums or hot temper
0	1	2	96.	Thinks about sex too much
0	1	2	97.	Threatens people
0	1	2	98.	Thumb-sucking
0	1	2	99.	Too concerned with neatness or cleanliness
0	1	2	100.	Trouble sleeping (describe): _____
0	1	2	101.	Truancy, skips school
0	1	2	102.	Underactive, slow moving, or lacks energy
0	1	2	103.	Unhappy, sad, or depressed
0	1	2	104.	Unusually loud
0	1	2	105.	Uses alcohol or drugs for nonmedical purposes (describe): _____
				_____
0	1	2	106.	Vandalism
0	1	2	107.	Wets self during the day
0	1	2	108.	Wets the bed
0	1	2	109.	Whining
0	1	2	110.	Wishes to be of opposite sex
0	1	2	111.	Withdrawn, doesn't get involved with others
0	1	2	112.	Worries
0	1	2	113.	Please write in any problems your child has that were not listed above:
0	1	2		_____
0	1	2		_____
0	1	2		_____

C. CHILDREN'S DEPRESSION INVENTORY (CDI)

OVERVIEW

The CDI, developed by M Kovacs, is a widely utilized 27-item rating scale to evaluate depressive symptoms in children 7-17 years of age. The scale is a self-report scale. First-grade reading level skills are required to complete the scale. Each item has three response choices which correspond to increasing levels of illness severity. A total score is provided as well as five subfactors which include negative mood, ineffectiveness, negative self-esteem, interpersonal problems, and anhedonia. There is also a 10-item short form of the scale available which may be used for a quick depression screening.

GENERAL APPLICATIONS

The CDI is used to evaluate depression in children and adolescents.

SELECTED PSYCHOMETRIC PROPERTIES

The CDI has been reported to have internal consistency alpha coefficients ranging from 0.71 to 0.89. The validity of the scale has been well established in clinical and research settings over the past two decades.

REFERENCES

Kovacs M, "Rating Scales to Assess Depression in School Age Children," *Acta Paedopsychiatrica*, 1981, 46:305-15.

COPYRIGHT

Maria Kovacs, PhD
Multi-Health Systems, Inc
P.O. Box 950
North Tonawanda, NY 14120-0950
Tel: 1-800-456-3003

SCALE GENERALLY DONE BY

Self-rated scale

TIME TO COMPLETE SCALE

Longer form: 15 minutes; short form: 10 minutes or less

REPRESENTATIVE STUDY UTILIZING SCALE

Linna SL, Moilanen I, Ebeling H, et al, "Psychiatric Symptoms in Children With Intellectual Disability," *Eur Child Adolesc Psychiatry*, 1999, 8(Suppl 4):77-82.

C. CHILDREN'S DEPRESSION INVENTORY (CDI) *(Continued)*

SAMPLE ENTRIES OF THE
CDI

Kids sometimes have different feelings and ideas.

This form lists the feelings and ideas in groups. From each group of three sentences, pick one sentence that describes you **best** for the past two weeks. After you pick a sentence from the first group, go on to the next group.

There is no right answer or wrong answer. Just pick the sentence that best describes the way you have been recently. Put a mark like this ☒ next to your answer. Put the mark in the box next to the sentence that you pick.

*Remember, pick out the sentences that describe you best in the **PAST TWO WEEKS.***

Item 1	Item 7
☐ I am sad once in a while.	☐ I hate myself.
☐ I am sad many times.	☐ I do not like myself.
☐ I am sad all the time.	☐ I like myself.

Item 14	Item 22
☐ I look OK.	☐ I have plenty of friends.
☐ There are some bad things about my looks.	☐ I have some friends but I wish I had more.
☐ I look ugly.	☐ I do not have any friends.

Item 24	Item 22
☐ I can never be as good as other kids.	☐ Nobody really loves me.
☐ I can be as good as other kids if I want to.	☐ I am not sure if anybody loves me.
☐ I am just as good as other kids.	☐ I am sure that somebody loves me.

D. CHILDREN'S DEPRESSION RATING SCALE (CDRS)

OVERVIEW

The CDRS, developed by EO Poznanski and SC Cook, is a 16-item scale used to evaluate the severity of depression in children. The scale is designed to be administered to children between the ages of 6 and 12 years. Each item is scored on either a 0 to 3 scale (0 = no information, 3 = most severe) or a 0 to 5 scale (0 = no information, 5 = most severe) except for the last item, reversal of affect, which is answered by a yes or no. The scale was derived from the Hamilton Rating Scale for Depression *on page 100*, and may be used for repeated measures. A score of 15 on the CDRS is equivalent to a score of 0 on the HAM-D. The scale is based upon utilization of all available information including child/parent interview and school information. It has been reported that the CDRS may be easily used by relatively inexperienced raters, as well as experienced clinician/raters.

GENERAL APPLICATIONS

The CDRS evaluates severity of depression in children.

SELECTED PSYCHOMETRIC PROPERTIES

Correlation of individual items from the CDRS with Total CDRS Score and Global Ratings have been reported to range from 0.036 (self-esteem) to 0.94 (depressed mood).

REFERENCES

Freeman LN, Mokros H, and Poznanski EO, "Violent Events Reported by Normal Urban School-Aged Children: Characteristics and Depression Correlate," *J Am Acad Child Adolesc Psychiatry*, 1993, 32(2):419-23.

Poznanski EO, Cook SC, and Carroll BJ, "A Depression Rating Scale for Children," *Pediatrics*, 1979, 64(4):442-50.

Poznanski EO, Cook SC, Carroll BJ, et al, "Use of the Children's Depression Rating Scale in an Inpatient Psychiatric Population," *J Clin Psychiatry*, 1983, 44(6):200-3.

COPYRIGHT

American Academy of Pediatrics
141 Northwest Point Blvd
Elk Grove Village, IL 60007-1098
Tel: 847-228-5005

SCALE GENERALLY DONE BY

Clinician or trained rater

TIME TO COMPLETE SCALE

20 minutes

REPRESENTATIVE STUDY UTILIZING SCALE

Emslie GJ, Rush AJ, Weinberg WA, et al, "A Double-Blind, Randomized, Placebo-Controlled Trial of Fluoxetine in Children and Adolescents With Depression," *Arch Gen Psychiatry*, 1997, 54(11):1031-7.

D. CHILDREN'S DEPRESSION RATING SCALE (CDRS) *(Continued)*

CHILDREN'S DEPRESSION RATING SCALE
(Age 6-12)

1. *Depressed Mood (0-5)*. Affect may be aroused (eg, sad, forlorn, gloomy, anguished) or suppressed. Note nonverbal behavior (eg, facial expression, eye contact, body posture). Child may or may not verbalize feelings of sadness.

   0   No information
   1   Definitely not depressed - facial expression and voice animated during interview.
   2   Doubtful - mild suppression of affect during interview and/or some loss of spontaneity.
   3   Mild - overall some loss of spontaneity. Child looks unhappy during parts of interview. May still be able to smile when discussing nonthreatening areas.
   4   Moderate - may have a moderate restriction of affect throughout most of interview and have brief periods where looks unhappy.
   5   Severe - child looks sad, withdrawn with little verbal interaction throughout interview. May look like crying.

2. *Weeping (0-3)*. Information usually from parents, teachers, but occasionally from child.

   0   No information
   1   Normal for age
   2   Suggestive statements that child cries more frequently than peers.
   3   Cries frequently - more than reasonable for age or provocation.

3. *Self-Esteem (0-5)*. The child's ability to describe self is very concrete at 6 and 7, becoming more sophisticated at 9 and 10. Note affective tones around the child's responses. Inappropriate guilt rates 3 or 4.

   0   No information
   1   Child describes self in mostly positive terms.
   2   Doubtful evidence of lowered self-esteem.
   3   Child describes self using a mixture of attributes, with both affectively positive and negative tones.
   4   Child uses both affectively positive and negative terms, but preponderance of negative attributes, or if concept understood, gives minimal bland answers.
   5   Child either refers to self in derogatory terms (eg, unpleasant nicknames) or completely avoids any question dealing with self-concepts, self-image, or self-esteem.

4. *Morbid Ideation (0-4)*.

   0   No information
   1   None expressed
   2   Some morbid thoughts - all related to a recent reality event.
   3   Admits to morbid thoughts on questioning, but does not dwell on them, or parents report morbid thoughts of child.
   4   Death themes spontaneously discussed or elaborate and extensive morbid ideation.

5. *Suicide and Suicide Ideation (0-5)*.

   0   No information
   1   None
   2   Has thoughts about suicide - usually when angry.
   3   Recurrent thoughts of suicide.
   4   Thinks about suicide and names methods or if depressed, strongly denies thinking about suicide.
   5.   Suicide attempt within the last month or actively suicidal.

6. *Irritability (0-5)*. Information usually from parents, nurses, etc, and direct observation. This can range from whining, "chip on the shoulder" attitudes to temper outbursts and other direct displays of hostility and anger. Rate on frequency of irritable behavior. Some children may directly display whining, irritable behavior during the interview.

0   No information
1   Normal
2   Occasional - slightly more than normal
3   Episodic
4   Frequent
5. Constant

7. *Schoolwork (0-5)*. Consider current function as opposed to usual or expected function. Expected function should take into consideration the intelligence of the child and specific learning disabilities, cultural and family expectations.

0   No information
1   Performing at or above the expected level.
3   "Not working to capacity" or recent disinterest in schoolwork with minimal interference with performance.
4   Doing poorly in most subjects or evidence of a recent major interference with performance.
5   Incapable of doing productive schoolwork at time of rating.

8. *Capacity to Have Fun (0-5)*. Often reflected in hobbies and interests outside of school.

0   No information
1   Child's interests and hobbies appropriate for age, personality, and environment. No appreciable change during present illness.
2   Child has interests - hobbies outside of school, but activities mainly passive. Shows some interest but not enthusiasm.
3   Child easily bored. May frequently complain of nothing to do, or child expresses interest and hobbies which are realistically unavailable to the child.
4   In structured activities, may "go through the motions" without real interest or enthusiasm.
5. Child doesn't take initiative to involve self in any activities. Tends to passively watch others or watch TV. Takes pushing and coaxing to involve in any activities.

9. *Social Withdrawal (0-5)*.

0   No information
1   Enjoys good friendships with peers at school and home or never has had adequate peer relationships.
2   Child names several friends, but relationships sound meager or has one or two friends, but not able to integrate into larger peer group.
3   Child *changes* from actively seeking out friendships to a passive role (ie, waits for others to initiate a relationship). Observes rather than participates in groups unless pushed.
4   Child frequently rejects opportunities for seemingly desirable interaction with other children.
5. Child does not relate to other children. Either states he has "no friends" or actively rejects former friends and any new children.

D. CHILDREN'S DEPRESSION RATING SCALE (CDRS) *(Continued)*

10. *Expressive Communication (0-3)*. Refers primarily to possible psychomotor retardation of language. Rate on the quantity and quality of verbal material. Consider the cultural background and intelligence of child in the interview situation.

   0   No information
   1   Normal
   2   Doubtful - mild. Monotonous voice. Mild delay in answering questions. Gives monosyllabic or short answers in all areas of interview.
   3   Moderate - severe. Same as (1) except delay in answering questions prolongs the interview. Even greater reduction in verbal content, may also have poverty of facial expression.

11. *Sleep (0-3)*. This information usually most reliable from child interview.

   0   No information
   1   No difficulty or occasional difficulty sleeping.
   2   Mild - frequent difficulty sleeping. Child and/or parent may report this.
   3   Moderate - difficulty with sleeping nearly every night. May be evidence of sleep deprivation (eg, child looks tired).

Circle if difficulty with sleep is:

   0   No information/does not apply
   1   Initial
   2   Middle
   3   Early morning wakening

12. *Disturbance of Eating Pattern (0-3)*.

   0   No information
   1   No problem
   2   Mild. Mother complains of change in eating pattern or chronic problem with food, either some variety of "poor eater" or overeats.
   3   Moderate. More severe disturbance of eating pattern. If undereats, accompanied by weight loss. If overeats, has moderate obesity. May steal and hoard food or show more bizarre pattern such as eating out of garbage cans. Unable to follow a medically necessary diet prescribed by a physician.

13. *Frequent Physical Complaints (0-4)*. Child may complain of stomach pains, headaches, or other bodily aches and pains. Rate frequency. Parents and nurses generally more reliable.

   0   No information
   1   No complaints
   2   Occasional complaints. Child is easily reassured.
   3   Frequent complaints, but can be distracted or reassured (eg, school phobic who feels fine if allowed to stay home from school).
   4   Preoccupied with aches and pains - may keep child from other activities.

14. *General Somatic (0-3).*

 0 No information
 1 Normal
 2 Occasional complaints of fatigue.
 3 Frequent - complains of being tired, doesn't feel like doing things used to enjoy.

15. *Hypoactivity (0-3).* Consider current activity level as opposed to usual activity level. Check with parents, school teachers, nurses.

 0 No information
 1 Activity at usual level.
 2 Minimal retardation activity.
 3 Talks slowly, walks slowly, slow to move during play.

16. *Reversal of Affect.*

 0 No information
 1 No
 2 Yes

E. COMPREHENSIVE BEHAVIOR RATING SCALE FOR CHILDREN (CBRSC)

OVERVIEW

The CBRSC, developed by R Neeper et al, is a 70-item scale intended to measure child school functioning. The scale is intended for use with children/adolescents ages 6 through 14 years of age. The CBRSC is generally rated by a teacher or other adult who has direct contact with the child being evaluated. The CBRSC assesses cognitive, social, emotional, and behavioral dimensions of functioning. Each item is rated on a five-point scale from 1 to 5 (1 = not at all, 5 = very much). There are nine subscales in the CBRSC including inattention-disorganization, reading problems, cognitive deficits, oppositional-conduct disorders, motor hyperactivity, anxiety, sluggish tempo, daydreaming, and social competence.

GENERAL APPLICATIONS

The CBRSC is used to assess child school functioning.

SELECTED PSYCHOMETRIC PROPERTIES

Much of the available psychometric data is cited on previous slightly different versions of the CBRSC. The authors have reported that test-retest reliability over a 2-week period ranges from 0.84 to 0.97.

REFERENCES

Frick PJ, O'Brien BS, Wootton JM, et al, "Psychopathy and Conduct Problems in Children," *J Abnorm Psychol*, 1994, 103(4):700-7.

COPYRIGHT

Ronald Neeper
Benjamin B. Lahey
Paul J. Frick
The Psychological Corporation
555 Academic Court
San Antonio, Texas 78204-2498
Tel: 1-800-211-8378

SCALE GENERALLY DONE BY

Teacher

TIME TO COMPLETE SCALE

10-15 minutes

REPRESENTATIVE STUDY UTILIZING SCALE

Schaughency EA, Vannatta K, Langhinrichsen J, et al, "Correlates in Sociometric Status in School Children in Buenos Aires," *J Abnorm Child Psychol*, 1992, 20(3):317-26.

F. CONNERS' RATING SCALE
(CRS, CRS-R, and CASS)

OVERVIEW

The CRS, developed by CK Conners, is a scale that evaluates a broad range of psychopathology and behavioral problems in children. There are multiple formats of the scale, which was revised in 1997 (CRS-R). The CRS-R is intended for use in children 3 to 17 years of age. There is a self-report instrument for children/adolescents 12-17 years of age (CASS), and also parent ratings and teacher ratings. The CRS-R includes an Attention-Deficit Hyperactivity Disorder (ADHD) scale and a global index which is particularly useful for monitoring of change during treatment. The CRS-R has DSM-IV scales which are directly linked to DSM-IV diagnostic criteria. The CRS exists in a long form and short form version.

GENERAL APPLICATIONS

The CRS is used to assess psychopathology and behavioral problems in children and adolescents.

SELECTED PSYCHOMETRIC PROPERTIES

Internal consistency coefficients for all the CRS-R versions have been calculated. Cronbach's alphas range from 0.77 to 0.95. Internal consistency coefficients for the subscales are also high.

REFERENCES

Conners CK, Sitarenios G, Parker JD, et al, "The Revised Conners' Parent Rating Scale (CPRS-R): Factor Structure, Reliability and Criterion Validity," *J Abnorm Child Psychol*, 1998, 26(4):257-68.

COPYRIGHT

C Keith Conners
Multi-Health Systems, Inc
P.O. Box 950
North Tonawanda, NY 14120-0950
Tel: 1-800-456-3003

SCALE GENERALLY DONE BY

Rater varies by format; includes parent, self-rating, teacher, clinician, or trained rater.

TIME TO COMPLETE SCALE

Varies by format; long versions generally 15-20 minutes, short versions generally 5-10 minutes.

REPRESENTATIVE STUDY UTILIZING SCALE

McCormick LH, "Improving Social Adjustment in Children With Attention-Deficit/Hyperactivity Disorder," *Arch Fam Med*, 2000, 9(2):191-4.

F. CONNERS' RATING SCALE
(CRS, CRS-R, and CASS) *(Continued)*

SAMPLE ENTRIES OF THE
CONNERS-WELLS ADOLESCENT SELF-REPORT SCALE (L)

By C. Keith Conners, PhD and Karen Wells, PhD

Name: _____   Gender: M   F
(Circle one)

Birthdate: _____ / _____ / _____   Age: _____   School Grade: _____   Today's Date: _____ / _____ / _____
　　　　　Month　Day　Year　　　　　　　　　　　　　　　　　　　　　　　　Month　Day　Year

Instructions: For the items below, circle the number that indicates whether the item is Not At ___, Just A Little, Pretty Much, or Very Much True for you. "Not at all" means that the item is seldom or nev___ problem. "Very Much" means that the item is very often a problem or occurs very frequently. "Just a Litt___ d "Pre___ Much" are in between. Please respond to all the items.

	NOT TRUE AT ALL (Never, seldom)	JUST A LITTLE TRUE (Occasionally)	MUCH TRUE (Often, Quite a Bit)	VERY MUCH TRUE (Very Often, Very Frequent)
2. I feel like crying		1	2	3
6. I cannot sit still for very long		1	2	3
10. I am discouraged	0	1	2	3
19. I feel sad and gl___	0	1	2	3
23. I have a hot temper	0	1	2	3
32. I feel restless inside even if I am sitting still	0	1	2	3

SAMPLE ENTRIES OF THE
Conners' Parent Rating Scale - Revised (S)

by C. Keith Conners, PhD

Child's Name: _____ _____ Gender: M   F

Birthdate: ____/____/____ Age: _____ School Grade: __
Month Day Year

Parent's Name: _____ _____ Today's Date: ____/____/____
Month Day Year

Instructions: Below are a number of common problems that children have. Please rate each item according to your child's behavior in the last month. For each item, ask yourself, "How much of a problem has this been in the last month?", and circle the best answer for each one. If none, not at all, seldom, or very infrequently, you would circle 0. If very much true, or it occurs very often or frequently, you would circle 3. You would circle 1 or 2 for ratings in between. Please respond to each item.

	NOT TRUE AT ALL (Never, seldom)	JUST A LITTLE TRUE (Occasionally)	PRETTY MUCH TRUE (Often, Quite a Bit)	VERY MUCH TRUE (Very Often, Very Frequent)
1. Inattentive, easily distracted	0	1	2	3
2. Angry and resentful	0	1	2	3
3. Difficulty doing or completing homework	0	1	2	3

G. DIAGNOSTIC INTERVIEW SCHEDULE FOR CHILDREN (DISC)

OVERVIEW

The National Institute of Mental Health Diagnostic Interview Schedule for Children Version IV (NIMH DISC-IV) is a highly structured diagnostic interview designed to assess more than 30 common mental disorders occurring in children and adolescents. The DISC-IV has grown out of the original NIMH DISC, developed in 1979, to provide a highly structured diagnostic instrument designed for use by nonclinicians. A rater may administer the interview after minimal training. The DISC begins with an introductory module that includes demographic information and an information component that teaches respondents about the scope of the interview, the format in which their answers are to be given, and what they should do if they have more to say than just "yes" or "no". The remainder of the interview is organized into 6 modules, each containing related diagnoses (anxiety, mood, disruptive, substance use, schizophrenia, and miscellaneous disorders). The DISC-IV assesses the presence of diagnoses occurring within both the past 12 months and the past 4 weeks. The NIMH DISC-IV compares favorably with earlier versions of the DISC, although its more lengthy. The DISC-IV is available in English and Spanish versions, scales in development include a teacher version and a quick version. There are parallel parent and youth versions, and the instrument is computer-assisted for ease of administration and scoring.

GENERAL APPLICATIONS

The DISC is used to diagnose mental disorders in children and adolescents.

SELECTED PSYCHOMETRIC PROPERTIES

In general, the DISC shows moderate to good diagnostic reliability for the parent interview and using information from both parent and youth interviews in combined algorithms.

REFERENCES

Shaffer D, Fisher P, Lucas CP, et al, "NIMH Diagnostic Interview Schedule for Children Version IV (NIMH DISC-IV): Description, Differences From Previous Versions, and Reliability of Some Common Diagnoses," *J Am Acad Child Adolesc Psychiatry*, 2000, 39(1):28-38.

COPYRIGHT

Not applicable

The computerized version of the NIMH DISC-IV is owned and distributed by the Division of Child and Adolescent Psychiatry at Columbia University. To obtain further information about the NIMH DISC-IV or its derivatives contact:

Columbia DISC Development Group
1051 Riverside Dr
New York, NY 10032
Tel: 1-888-814-DISC
Fax: 212-543-5966
e-mail: disc@worldnet.att.net

SCALE GENERALLY DONE BY

Trained rater

TIME TO COMPLETE SCALE

70-120 minutes

REPRESENTATIVE STUDY UTILIZING SCALE

Luis CA and Mittenberg W, "Mood and Anxiety Disorders Following Pediatric Traumatic Brain Injury: A Prospective Study," *J Clin Exp Neuropsychol*, 2002, 24(3):270-9.

H. REVISED CHILDREN'S MANIFEST ANXIETY SCALE (RCMAS)

OVERVIEW

The RCMAS, developed by C Reynolds and B Richmond, is a 37-item scale used to evaluate anxiety in children. The scale is designed to be utilized for school children grades 1 to 12. The revised version of the scale is a modified version of an original scale consisting of 73 items. Each item on the RCMAS may either be read and answered by the child, or may be read to the child to answer for children in the younger grades. Most children grades 3 and higher are able to read and complete the scale themselves. Each question is answered either "Yes" or "No". There are 28 items which make up an "Anxiety" subscale, an example is "I worry a lot of the time." There are nine items which make up a "Lie" scale, an example is "I like everyone I know". The revised version of the scale is relatively easy to administer and widely used in clinical trial settings. A limitation of the scale is that high Lie scores make the scale less useful for children in grades one and two.

GENERAL APPLICATIONS

The RCMAS is used to evaluate anxiety in children.

SELECTED PSYCHOMETRIC PROPERTIES

The RCMAS has reliability estimates of 0.83 with item selection sample, and 0.85 with a cross-validation group. There is an overall trend for anxiety scores to increase somewhat with age.

REFERENCES

Reynolds CR and Richmond BO, "What I Think and Feel: A Revised Measure of Children's Manifest Anxiety," *J Abnorm Child Psychol*, 1978, 6(2):271-80.

Reynolds CR and Richmond BO, "What I Think and Feel: A Revised Measure of Children's Manifest Anxiety," *J Abnorm Child Psychol*, 1997, 25(1):15-20.

COPYRIGHT

Western Psychological Service
12031 Wilshire Blvd
Los Angeles, CA 90025-1251
Tel: 800-648-8851; 310-478-2061
e-mail: custsvc@wpspublish.com

SCALE GENERALLY DONE BY

Self-rated, clinician, or trained rater

TIME TO COMPLETE SCALE

15-20 minutes

REPRESENTATIVE STUDY UTILIZING SCALE

Hagborg WJ, "Adolescent Clients and Perceived Counselor Characteristics: A Study of Background Characteristics, Therapeutic Progress, Psychological Distress and Social Desirability," *J Clin Psychol*, 1991, 47(1):107-13.

SAMPLE ITEMS OF THE

CMAS REVISION (RCMAS)

Items and item statistics, p and r_{bis}, for all anxiety and lie items retained on the revision of the CMAS.

Item Number	Item Type[a]	Item	p[b]	r_{bis}[b]
2	A	I get nervous when things do not go the right way for me.	61	47
6	A	I worry a lot of the time.	45	50

[a]A = Anxiety Scale; L = Lie Scale; [b]Decimals omitted, all signs are positive; [c]New test item.

I. REYNOLDS ADOLESCENT DEPRESSION SCALE (RADS)

OVERVIEW

The Reynolds Adolescent Depression Scale (RADS), developed by WM Reynolds, is a self-report scale to measure depressive symptoms in adolescents (13-18 years of age). The RADS is a widely recognized instrument which consists of 30 items, each item rated on a 4-point continuum. Scoring for each item ranges from 1 (Never) to 4 (Most of the time). Teens are asked to rate how they feel in a variety of domains consistent with depression. The RADS evaluates multiple dimensions of teen depression including cognitive symptoms, motoric-vegetative, somatic, and interpersonal symptoms. Total possible scores for the RADS range from 30-120 with higher scores indicating more depressive symptoms. A cut-off of 77 or higher on the RADS has been identified as a marker of clinically-significant adolescent depression.

GENERAL APPLICATIONS

The RADS is used to screen for and measure depression in adolescents.

SELECTED PSYCHOMETRIC PROPERTIES

The author reports excellent internal consistency for the RADS (Cronbach's alpha) ranging from 0.90-0.95. Reliability for both Caucasian and African American populations is very good as well, with alpha coefficients between 0.90 and 0.93. Test-retest reliabilities have been reported at 0.80 at 6 weeks and 0.79 at 3 months. The RADS correlates very well with the HAM-D.

REFERENCES

Reynolds WM, "A Model for the Screening and Identification of Depressed Children and Adolescents in School Settings," *Professional School Psychology*, 1986, 1:117-29.

Reynolds WM, *Reynolds Adolescent Depression Scale: Professional Manual*, Odessa, FL: Psychological Assessment Resources, 1987.

Reynolds WM and Mazza JJ, "Reliability and Validity of the Reynolds Adolescent Depression Scale With Young Adolescents," *Journal of School Psychology*, 1998, 36:353-76.

COPYRIGHT

Psychological Assessment Resources, Inc
PO Box 998
Odessa, FL 33556
Tel: 1-800-331-8378

SCALE GENERALLY DONE BY

Self-rated scale

TIME TO COMPLETE SCALE

15 minutes

REPRESENTATIVE STUDY UTILIZING SCALE

King CA, Hovey JD, Brand E, et al, "Prediction of Positive Outcomes for Adolescent Psychiatric Inpatients," *J Am Acad Child Adolesc Psychiatry*, 1997, 36(10):1434-42.

SAMPLE ITEMS OF THE
RADS-2

by William M. Reynolds, PhD

Name: _____ Age: _____ Sex: ☐ M ☐ F Today's Date: ___/___/___
                                                                        mo day yr

Grade in School: _____ Ethnicity/Race: _____ School/Agency: _____

Directions: Listed below are some sentences about how you feel. Read each sentence and decide how often you feel this way. Decide if you feel this way almost never, hardly ever, sometimes, or most of the time. To answer each item, circle the number under the answer that best describes how you really feel. Remember, there are no right or wrong answers. Just choose the answer that tells how you usually feel.

	Almost never	Hardly ever	Some-times	Most of the time
2. I worry about school	1	2	3	4
13. I feel like running away	1	2	3	4
14. I feel like hurting myself	1	2	3	4
27. I get stomachaches	1	2	3	4

Adapted and reproduced by special permission of the Publisher, Psychological Assessment Resources, Inc. 16204 North Florida Avenue, Lutz, Florida 33549, from the Reynolds Adolescent Depression Scale, by William M. Reynolds, PhD. Copyright © 1981, 1986 by Psychological Assessment Resources, Inc. Further reproduction is prohibited without permission from PAR, Inc.

APPENDIX TABLE OF CONTENTS

SELECTED PSYCHOMETRIC TERMS USED TO DESCRIBE RATING SCALES

Term	Definition
Reliability	Ability of the scale to convey consistent and reproducible information
Validity	Degree to which the scale measures what it is supposed to measure
Interrater Reliability	The consistency between different individuals doing the ratings
Test-Retest Reliability	The consistency of the ratings being done on multiple occasions
Content Validity	How adequately the sampling of questions, drawn from the proper domain of content, reflect the aim of the scale
Criterion Validity	The degree of agreement between the scores obtained with the scale and a selected set of external criteria
Face Validity	Degree to which the scale seems to measure what it is supposed to measure
Predictive Validity	The capacity that the scale has to provide information about a particular outcome

COMMON STATISTICAL TECHNIQUES USED IN RATING SCALE ANALYSIS

Statistical Technique	Common Application
t-test	This tool provides a simple means of testing differences between two independent groups, such as a treatment and a control group.
Analysis of Variance	This tool tests differences between two or more independent groups. It can also test differences on more than one characteristic simultaneously (ie, diagnostic groups and treatment groups).
Logistic Regression	This tool is used to predict group membership or group differences. An example is recovered patients vs those who remain ill.
Survival Analysis	This tool can be used to predict the eventual occurrence of an event or to predict the time to an event. An example is relapse of illness.
Ordinary Least Squares Regression	This tool can be used to predict the level of an outcome variable. For example, it could be used to identify clinical variables that predict more severe symptoms.

SELF-RATED SCALES

Name of Scale	Condition Assessed
Brief Fear of Negative Evaluation Scale	Social phobia
Fear Questionnaire	Phobias
Sheehan Patient-Rated Anxiety Scale	Panic disorder
Post-Traumatic Stress Diagnostic Scale	Post-traumatic stress
Mississippi Scale	Post-traumatic stress in Vietnam Veterans
Children's Depression Inventory	Childhood depression
Child Behavior Checklist*	Childhood behavior
Conner's Rating Scale*	Childhood behavior
Revised Children's Manifest Anxiety Scale*	Anxiety
Reynolds Adolescent Depression Scale	Adolescent depression
Beck Depression Inventory	Depression
Zung Depression Scale	Depression
Carroll Depression Scale	Depression
The Duke Health Profile	General health status
The Short Form 36 Health Survey	General health status
The COOP Charts for Adult Primary Care Practice	General health status
Symptom Checklist-90-Revised	General health status
Burden Interview	Caregiver burden
Geriatric Depression Scale	Geriatric depression
The Client Satisfaction Questionnaire	Satisfaction with healthcare services
The Service Satisfaction Scale	Satisfaction with healthcare services
Patient Satisfaction Questionnaire	Satisfaction with medical care
Drug Attitude Inventory	Subjective response to neuroleptic medication
Psychological General Well Being Schedule	Quality of life/inner personal state
The Sickness Impact Profile	Quality of life
The Nottingham Health Profile	Quality of life
The Quality of Well Being Scale*	Quality of life
CAGE Questionnaire	Alcohol abuse
Michigan Alcohol Screening Test	Alcohol abuse
Inventory of Drug-Taking Situations	Alcohol/drug abuse

(continued)

Fagerstrom Test for Nicotine Dependence	Nicotine dependence
Beck Scale for Suicide Ideation	Suicide risk
Beck Hopelessness Scale	Suicidality
Suicide Probability Scale	Suicide risk
Barratt Impulsiveness Scale	Impulsivity
Buss-Durkee Hostility Inventory	Anger/hostility
State-Trait Anger Expression Inventory	Anger expression
Arizona Sexual Experiences	Sexual disorders
Brief Sexual Function Inventory	Sexual functioning in men
Rush Sexual Inventory	Sexual function
Sleep Disorders Questionnaire	Differential diagnosis of sleep disorders
Eating Disorders Inventory	Eating disorders
Eating Attitudes Test	Anorexia nervosa
Daily Record of Severity of Problems	Premenstrual dysphoric disorder
Premenstrual Tension Syndrome Scale*	Premenstrual mood symptoms
Social Adjustment Scale*	Social functioning
Multidimensional Scale of Perceived Social Support	Perceived social support
Family Assessment Device	Family functioning
Mood Disorders Questionnaire	Bipolar spectrum disorder

*Multiple versions exist, including a self-rated version.

"TIPS" TO INCREASE RELIABILITY OF RATING SCALES

- Be familiar with the scale, it's manual, and the definition of items as well as their anchoring points.

- Use all available information when doing the ratings unless specifically requested NOT to do so in the rating manual instructions.

- A clinical interview yields the most comprehensive information.

- Score all items.

- In case of indecision, use consultation.

- Two raters are better than one.

- When unable to decide between two scores (example "3" or example "4") always "rate up" and use the higher score.

- Do not look for "explanations" for symptoms. For example, if a patient reports inability to sleep due to concern about a future job interview, rate the symptom as reported, and do not "rate down" because you feel that some anxiety-related insomnia might be expected given the circumstances.

ANXIETY RATING SCALES

Scale Name	Acronym	Type of Administration	Time to Complete
Acute Panic Inventory	API	Rater-administered	10-15 minutes
Brief Fear of Negative Evaluation Scale	Brief-FNE	Self-rated	5-10 minutes
Clinician-Administered PTSD Scale	CAPS	Rater-administered	50-60 minutes
Covi Anxiety Scale	—	Rater-administered	10 minutes
Davidson Trauma Scale	DTS	Rater-administered	10 minutes
Fear Questionnaire	FG	Self-rated	10 minutes
Hamilton Rating Scale for Anxiety	HAM-A, HARS	Rater-administered	20 minutes
Leyton Obsessional Inventory	LOI	Rater-administered	15-20 minutes
Liebowitz Social Anxiety Scale	LSAS	Rater-administered	15 minutes
Mississippi Scale	MSS	Self-rated	10-20 minutes
Post-Traumatic Stress Diagnostic Scale	PDS®	Self-rated	10-15 minutes
Sheehan Disability Scale	—	Rater-administered	5 minutes or less
Sheehan Patient-Rated Anxiety Scale	SPRAS	Self-rated	15 minutes
Social Phobia and Anxiety Inventory	SPAI	Rater-administered	20-30 minutes
State-Trait Anxiety Inventory	STAI	Rater-administered	10 minutes
Yale-Brown Obsessive-Compulsive Scale	Y-BOCS	Rater-administered	20 minutes

RATING SCALES FOR CHILDREN

Scale Name	Acronym	Type of Administration	Time to Complete
Adaptive Behavior Scale	AAMR, ABS	Rater-administered	15-30 minutes
Child Behavior Checklist	CBCL	Multiple formats	15 minutes
Children's Depression Inventory	CDI	Self-rated	10-15 minutes
Children's Depression Rating Scale	CDRS	Rater-administered	20 minutes
Comprehensive Behavior Rating Scale for Children	CBRSC	Rater-administered	10-15 minutes
Conner's Rating Scale	CRS, CRS-R	Multiple formats	5-10 minutes - short form 15-20 minutes - long form
Revised Children's Manifest Anxiety Scale	RCMAS	Rater-administered	15-20 minutes
Reynolds Adolescent Depression Scale	RADS	Self-rated	15 minutes

DEPRESSION RATING SCALES

Scale Name	Acronym	Type of Administration	Time to Complete
Beck Depression Inventory	BDI	Self-rated	5-10 minutes
Carroll Depression Scale	CDS, CRS	Self-rated	20 minutes
Cornell Dysthymia Rating Scale	CDRS	Rater-administered	20 minutes
Depression Outcomes Module	DOM	Variable formats	Patient: 25 minutes Clinician: 5-10 minutes Medical Records: 5-10 minutes
Hamilton Rating Scale for Depression	HAM-D, HRSD	Rater-administered	30 minutes
Montgomery-Asberg Depression Rating Scale	MADRS	Rater-administered	20 minutes
Raskin Depression Rating Scale	—	Rater-administered	10-15 minutes
Zung Depression Scale A. Self-rated B. Clinician-rated	SDS DSI	Self-rated Rater-administered	10 minutes 10 minutes

DIAGNOSTIC SCALES IN PSYCHIATRY

Scale Name	Acronym	Time to Complete*
Composite International Diagnostic Interview	CIDI	60-90 minutes
Diagnostic Interview Schedule	DIS	90-120 minutes
Diagnostic Interview Schedule for Children	DISC	70-120 minutes
Mini International Neuropsychiatric Inventory	MINI	15-20 minutes
Present State Examination	PSE	90 minutes
Primary Care Evaluation of Mental Disorders	PRIME-MD	10-20 minutes
Schedule for Affective Disorders and Schizophrenia	SADS	60 minutes
Schedule for Clinical Assessment in Neuropsychiatry	SCAN	90-120 minutes
Structured Clinical Interview for Axis I DSM-IV Disorders	SCID	60-90 minutes

*All scales may require longer to administer with some psychiatric populations.

GERIATRIC RATING SCALES

Scale Name	Acronym	Type of Administration	Time to Complete
Alzheimer's Disease Assessment Scale	ADAS	Rater-administered	30-45 minutes
Behavioral Pathology in Alzheimer's Disease	BEHAVE-AD	Rater-administered	10-20 minutes
Blessed Dementia Scale	BLS-D	Rater-administered	15-30 minutes
Burden Interview	BI	Self-rated	15 minutes
Delirium Rating Scale	DRS	Rater-administered	5-10 minutes
Geriatric Depression Scale	GDS	Self-rated	15-20 minutes
Instrumental Activities of Daily Living	IADL	Rater-administered	5 minutes
Neuropsychiatric Inventory	NPI	Rater-administered	15-20 minutes
Relatives Assessment of Global Symptomatology	RAGS-E	Rater-administered	15-20 minutes
The Cambridge Mental Disorders of the Elderly Examination	CAMDEX	Rater-administered	60-90 minutes
The Mini-Mental State Examination	MMSE	Rater-administered	5-10 minutes

PSYCHOSIS RATING SCALES

Scale Name	Acronym	Type of Administration	Time to Complete
Brief Psychiatric Rating Scale	BPRS	Rater-administered	30 minutes
Comprehensive Psychopathological Rating Scale	CPRS	Rater-administered	45-60 minutes
Manchester Scale	—	Rater-administered	10-15 minutes
Nurses' Observation Scale for Inpatient Evaluation	NOSIE	Rater-administered	5-10 minutes
Positive and Negative Symptom Scale for Schizophrenia	PANSS	Rater-administered	30-40 minutes
Scale for Assessment of Negative Symptoms	SANS	Rater-administered	15-20 minutes
Scale for Assessment of Positive Symptoms	SAPS	Rater-administered	15-20 minutes

QUALITY OF LIFE SCALES

Scale Name	Acronym	Type of Administration	Time to Complete
Lehman Quality of Life Interview	QOLI	Rater-administered	45 minutes
Psychological General Well Being Schedule	PGWB	Self-rated	10-15 minutes
Quality of Life Scale	—	Rater-administered	30-45 minutes
The Nottingham Health Profile	NHP	Self-rated	10-15 minutes
The Quality of Well Being Scale	QWB	Self-rated	Under 10 minutes
The Sickness Impact Profile	SIP	Self-rated	20 minutes

SUBSTANCE ABUSE RATING SCALES

Scale Name	Acronym	Type of Administration	Time to Complete
Addiction Severity Index	ASI	Rater-administered	60 minutes
Alcohol Use Disorders Identification Test	AUDIT	Questionnaire: Self-rated Screening module: Rater-administered	Less than 5 minutes for Questionnaire
CAGE Questionnaire	CAGE	Self-rated	5 minutes or less
Fagerstrom Test for Nicotine Dependence	FTQ	Self-rated	5 minutes or less
Inventory of Drug-Taking Situations	IDS	Self-rated	20 minutes
Michigan Alcohol Screening Test	MAST	Rater-administered	15-30 minutes

ACRONYMS INDEX OF RATING SCALES

ALPHABETICAL INDEX OF RATING SCALES

AUTHORS INDEX

AUTHORS INDEX

NOTES

NOTES

NOTES

NOTES

NOTES

NOTES

NOTES

Other books offered by
LEXI-COMP, INC.

PHARMACOGENOMICS HANDBOOK
by Humma, Ellingrod, Kolesar

This exciting new title by Lexi-Comp, introduces Pharmacogenomics to the forward-thinking healthcare professional and student! It presents information concerning key genetic variations that may influence drug disposition and/or sensitivity. Brief introductions to fundamental concepts in genetics and genomics are provided in order to bring the reader up-to-date on these rapidly emerging sciences. This book provides a foundation for all clinicians who will be called on to integrate rapidly expanding genomic knowledge into the management of drug therapy. A great introduction to pharmacogenetic principles as well as a concise reference on key polymorphisms known to influence drug response!

NATURAL THERAPEUTICS POCKET GUIDE
by Daniel L. Krinsky, RPh, MS; James B. LaValle, RPh, DHM, NMD, CCN; Ernest B. Hawkins, RPh, MS; Ross Pelton, RPh, PhD, CCN; Nancy Ashbrook Willis, BA, JD

Provides condition-specific information on common uses of natural therapies. Each condition discussed includes the following: review of condition, decision tree, list of commonly recommended herbals, nutritional supplements, homeopathic remedies, lifestyle modifications, and special considerations.

Provides herbal/nutritional/nutraceutical monographs with over 10 fields including references, reported uses, dosage, pharmacology, toxicity, warnings & interactions, and cautions & contraindications.

The Appendix includes: drug-nutrient depletion, herb-drug interactions, drug-nutrient interaction, herbal medicine use in pediatrics, unsafe herbs, and reference of top herbals.

INFECTIOUS DISEASES HANDBOOK
by Carlos M. Isada, MD; Bernard L. Kasten Jr., MD; Morton P. Goldman, PharmD; Larry D. Gray, PhD; and Judith A. Aberg, MD

A four-in-one quick reference concerned with the identification and treatment of infectious diseases. Each of the four sections of the book contains related information and cross-referencing to one or more of the other three sections. The Disease Syndrome section provides the clinical presentation, differential diagnosis, diagnostic tests, and drug therapy recommended for treatment of more common infectious diseases. The Organism section presents the microbiology, epidemiology, diagnosis, and treatment of each organism. The Laboratory Diagnosis section describes performance of specific tests and procedures. The Antimicrobial Therapy section presents important facts and considerations regarding each drug recommended for specific diseases of organisms. Also contains an International Brand Name Index with names from 58 different countries.

DRUG-INDUCED NUTRIENT DEPLETION HANDBOOK
by Ross Pelton, RPh, PhD, CCN; James B. LaValle, RPh, DHM, NMD, CCN; Ernest B. Hawkins, RPh, MS; Daniel L. Krinsky, RPh, MS

A complete and up-to-date listing of all drugs known to deplete the body of nutritional compounds.

This book is alphabetically organized and provides extensive cross-referencing to related information in the various sections of the book. Drug monographs identify the nutrients depleted and provide cross-references to the nutrient monographs for more detailed information on effects of depletion, biological function & effect, side effects & toxicity, RDA, dosage range, and dietary sources. this book also contains a studies & abstracts section, a valuable appendix, and alphabetical & pharmacological indexes.

Other books offered by
LEXI-COMP, INC.

DRUG INFORMATION HANDBOOK FOR DENTISTRY
by Richard L. Wynn, BSPharm, PhD; Timothy F. Meiller, DDS, PhD; Harold L. Crossley, DDS, PhD

For all dental professionals requiring quick access to concisely-stated drug information pertaining to medications commonly prescribed by dentists and physicians. Designed and written by dentists for all dental professionals as a portable, chairside resource. Includes drugs commonly prescribed by dentists or being taken by dental patients and written in an easy-to-understand format. There are 24 key points of information for each drug including **Local Anesthetic/Vasoconstrictor, Precautions, Effects on Dental Treatment,** and **Drug Interactions**. Includes information on dental treatment for medically-compromised patients and dental management of specific oral conditions.

Also contains Canadian & Mexican brand names.

MANUAL OF DENTAL IMPLANTS
by David P. Sarment, DDS, MS and Beth Peshman, RDH

Contains over 220 quality color photos, plus diagrams and decision trees. The diagnosis and treatment plans are explained in detail. Restorative step-by-step illustrations are included for each case type. Hygiene techniques and protocols are also included as well as assistant and staff training guidelines.

MANUAL OF CLINICAL PERIODONTICS
by Francis G. Serio, DMD, MS and Charles E. Hawley, DDS, PhD

A reference manual for diagnosis and treatment including sample treatment plans. It is organized by basic principles and is visually-cued with over 220 high quality color photos. The presentation is in a "question & answer" format. There are 12 chapters tabbed for easy access: 1) Problem-based Periodontal Diagnosis; 2) Anatomy, Histology, and Physiology; 3) Etiology and Disease Classification; 4) Assessment, Diagnosis, and Treatment Planning; 5) Prevention and Maintenance; 6) Nonsurgical Treatment; 7) Surgical Treatment: Principles; 8) Repair, Resection, and Regeneration; 9) Periodontal Plastic Surgery; 10) Periodontal Emergencies; 11) Implant Considerations; 12) Appendix

YOUR ROADMAP TO FINANCIAL INTEGRITY IN THE DENTAL OFFICE
by Donald P. Lewis, Jr., DDS, CFE

A Teamwork Approach to Fraud Protection & Security. Ideal practice management reference, designed and written by a dentist in private practice. Covers four basic areas of financial security. Utilizes tabbed paging system with 8 major tabs for quick reference. **Part I: Financial Transactions Incoming:** Financial Arrangements, Billing, Accounts Receivable, Banking, Cash, Checks, and Credit Cards; **Part II: Financial Transactions Outgoing:** Accounts Payable, Supplies, Cash-on-hand, Payroll; **Part III: Internal Controls:** Banking, General Office Management, Human Resource (H/R) issues; **Part IV: Employees:** Employee Related Issues and Employees Manual Topics **Part V: Report Checklist:** Daily, Weekly, Monthly, Quarterly, Semi-annually, Annually; **Additional Features:** Glossary terms for clarification, alphabetical index for quick reference, 1600 bulleted points of interest, over 180 checklist options, 12 real-life stories (names changed to protect the innocent!), 80-boxed topics of special interest for quick review.

To order call toll free anywhere in the U.S.: 1-800-837-LEXI (5394)
Outside of the U.S. call: 330-650-6506 or online at www.lexi.com

Other books offered by
LEXI-COMP, INC.

Patient Education Desk Charts

A Patient Guide to Mental Health Issues

8 Titles

Designed specifically for healthcare professionals dealing with mental health patients. Combines EIGHT of our popular Patient Chart titles into one, convenient, desktop presentation. This will assist in explaining the most common mental health issues to your patients on a level that they will understand!

Contains:

❶ **Alzheimer's Disease**
❷ **Anxiety**
❸ **Bipolar Disorder**
❹ **Depression**
❺ **Insomnia**
❻ **Obsessive-Compulsive Disorder**
❼ **Panic Attacks**
❽ **Schizophrenia**

An excellent reference to have on display in your office!

Diseases Explained ™

See the following pages for wall posters and patient booklets covering these same mental health diseases.

A PATIENT GUIDE TO ROOT THERAPY
Contributor Thom C. Dumsha, M.S., D.D.S., M.S.

Dentistry Explained
Patient Guide to Root Canal Therapy

Contributor
Thom C. Dumsha, M.S., D.D.S., M.S.

- An ideal tool used to educate and explain to your patients about root canals

- 8 1/2" x 11" colorful tabbed flip chart explaining each of the steps involved in a root canal

- Actual clinical photographs, radiographs, and diagrams

PATIENT GUIDE TO DENTAL IMPLANTS
Contributor Marvin L. Baer, D.D.S., M.Sc.

Dentistry Explained
Patient Guide to Dental Implants

Contributor
Marvin L. Baer, D.D.S., M.Sc.

- An ideal tool used to educate and explain to your patients about dental implants

- 8 1/2" x 11" colorful tabbed flip chart explaining each of the steps involved in:
  1.) Single tooth restoration
  2.) Replacement of several teeth
  3.) Implants supported overdenture
  4.) Screw-retained denture

To order call toll free anywhere in the U.S.: 1-800-837-LEXI (5394)
Outside of the U.S. call: 330-650-6506 or online at www.lexi.com

LEXI-COMP ON-HAND™
SOFTWARE LIBRARY

Lexi-Comp's handheld software solutions provide quick, portable access to clinical information needed at the point-of-care. Whether you need laboratory test or diagnostic procedure information, to validate a dose, or to check multiple medications and natural products for drug interactions, Lexi-Comp has the information you need in the palm of your hand. Lexi-Comp also provides advanced linking technology to allow you to hyperlink to related information topics within a title or to the same topic in another title for more extensive information. No longer will you have to exit one database (such as Griffith's 5-Minute Clinical Consult) to look up a drug dose in Lexi-Drugs® or lab test information in Lexi-Lab & Diagnostic Procedures™. Seamless linking between all databases to **saves valuable time and helps to improve patient care.**

Palm OS® Device

New Navigational Tools:

❶ **"Jump"** provides a drop down list of available fields to easily navigate through information.

❷ **Back arrow** returns to the index from a monograph or to the "Installed Books" menu from the Index.

❸ **"H"** provides a linkable History to return to any of the last 12 Topics viewed during your session.

❹ **Title bar:** Tap the monograph or topic title bar to activate a menu to "Edit a Note" or return to the "Installed Books" menu.

❺ **Linking:** Link to another companion database by clicking the topic or monograph title link or within a database noted by various hyperlinked (colorized and underlined) text.

Databases Available
for Palm OS® and Windows™ Powered Pocket PC devices

Lexi-COMPLETE™ $225.00
Lexi-Comp's Clinical Suite™ $175.00
Lexi-Drugs®
Lexi-Interact™
Pediatric Lexi-Drugs™
Nursing Lexi-Drugs™ $50.00
Dental Lexi-Drugs™
Lexi-Natural Products™
Griffith's 5-Minute Clinical Consult

Lexi-Diagnostic Medicine™
Lexi-Infectious Diseases™
Lexi-Poisoning & Toxicology™
Lexi-Pharmacogenomics™
Medical Abbreviations $35.00
Stedman's Medical Dictionary $35.00
Lexi-PALS™ (Patient Advisory Leaflets)
Lexi-Comp's NBC Agent Exposures
Lexi-Calc™ (Medical Calculations)

PRICING: Single database - $75.00 (unless otherwise noted) Add any other database of equal or lesser value - $40.00 each